Other books by
Glade B. Curtis, MD, MPH, OB/GYN, and Judith Schuler, MS

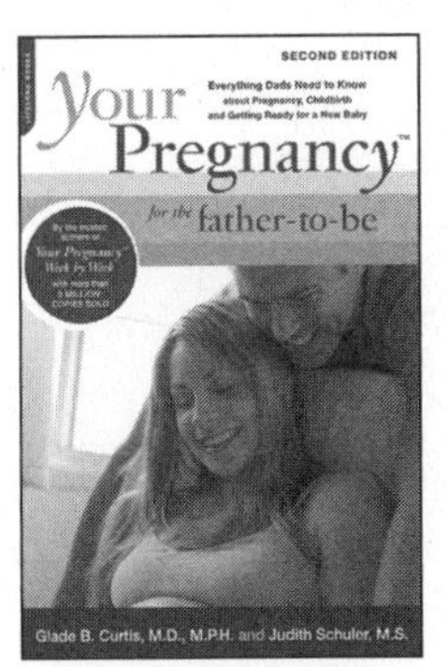

Your Pregnancy for the Father-To-Be
978-0-7382-1275-3

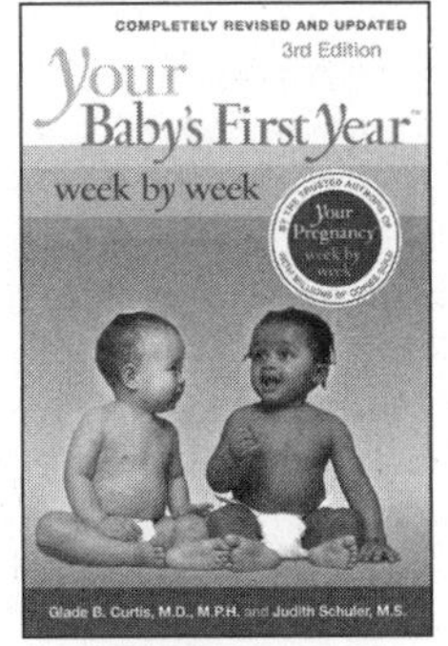

Your Baby's First Year, Week by Week
978-0-7382-1371-2

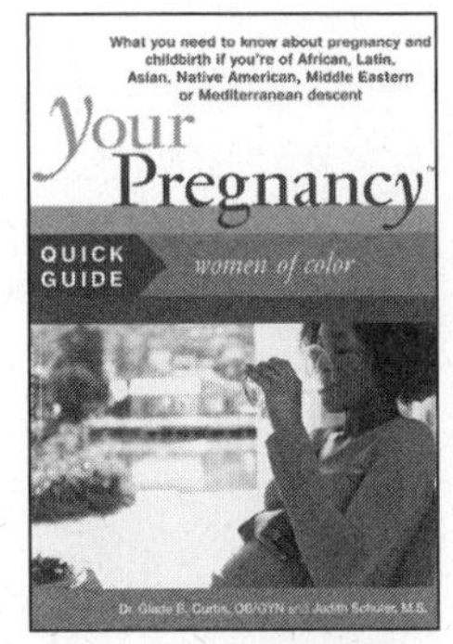

Your Pregnancy Quick Guide: Women of Color
978-0-7382-1060-5

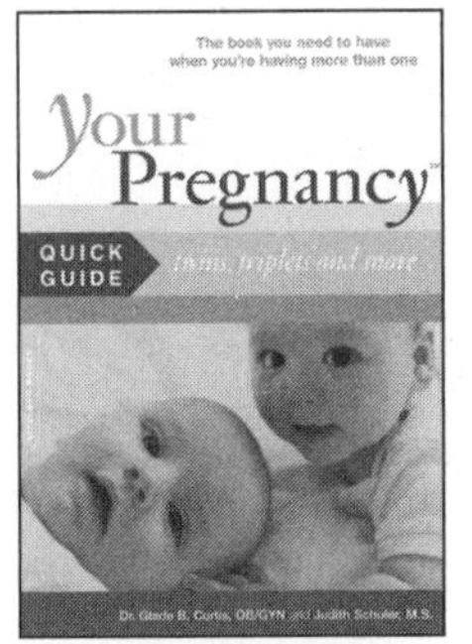

Your Pregnancy Quick Guide: Twins, Triplets, and More
978-0-7382-1008-7

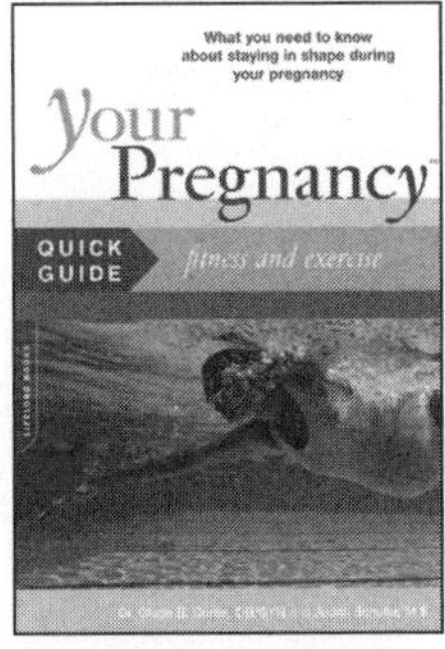

Your Pregnancy Quick Guide: Fitness and Exercise
978-0-7382-0952-4

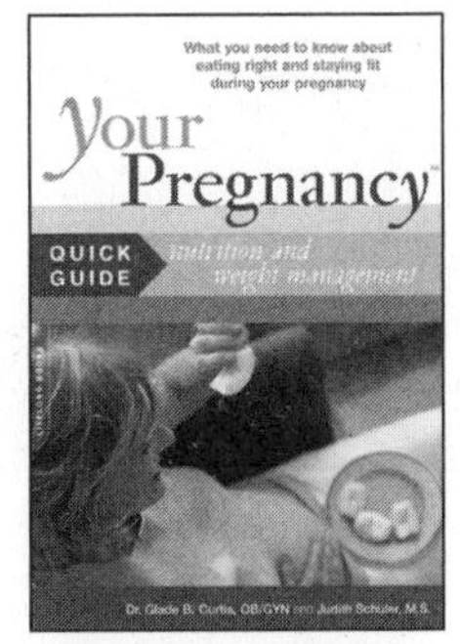

Your Pregnancy Quick Guide: Nutrition and Weight Management
978-0-7382-0954-8

What Doctors Are Saying About *Your Pregnancy Week by Week*

"*Your Pregnancy Week by Week* is the primary book I recommend to patients during pregnancy. I know I can trust it. It's organized, up to date and provides women with terrific information."

—Elizabeth D. Warner, M.D., OB/GYN,
Rochester Gynecologic and Obstetric Associates

"*Your Pregnancy Week by Week* is an extraordinarily well-written and accessible book. Dr. Glade Curtis's years of practice make him familiar with what really concerns patients and with what they most want to know. *Your Pregnancy* covers not only the specific issues every pregnant woman experiences, but deals with the whole wide array of potential concerns that can arise in pregnancy. All this, together with the elegant side-bars and skillful drawings, make *Your Pregnancy* not only the most comprehensive of the pregnancy books available for the lay public but also the most readable."

—Henry M. Lerner, M.D., OB/GYN, Newton-Wellesley Hospital,
Clinical Instructor in Obstetrics and Gynecology
at Harvard Medical School

"Regular contact with an obstetrician is an important part of a healthy pregnancy. And that's why I can so strongly recommend *Your Pregnancy Week by Week* to patients who want to have a doctor's advice in addition to my own. It's written by a doctor, it's full of trustworthy and up-to-date information, and its 'bedside manner' is excellent."

—Henry Hess, M.D., Associate Clinical Professor of Obstetrics and
Gynecology, University of Rochester School of Medicine

What Other Women Are Saying
About Your Pregnancy Week by Week

"Most books only give you a month-by-month breakdown of what's going on with baby and mom. I like how this one gives you week-by-week information. I look forward to reading it each week." —RACHEL M., OHIO

"*Your Pregnancy Week by Week* has been a good friend. Reading each week and knowing what changes my baby was going through was important to me."
—ANITA A., CALIFORNIA

"I have other pregnancy books but when I started reading *Your Pregnancy Week by Week*, I put the others down. This book is excellent. I highly recommend it to all mothers-to-be." —CRYSTAL L., VIRGINIA

"The week-by-week style is wonderful. It lets you know what is happening as it happens." —HEATHER H., LOUISIANA

"I liked how it went week by week because that is how my doctor thinks, too."
—REBECCA C., VIRGINIA

"The detailed week-by-week information about changes in me and my baby's changing body was excellent. It gave me something to read weekly, not just monthly."
—DEANA S., MASSACHUSETTS

"*Your Pregnancy Week by Week* was my second Bible. I used it so much I have almost memorized it! I recommend it to everyone!"
—CHRISSY M., ILLINOIS

"*Your Pregnancy Week by Week* was very comforting. It put my mind at ease."
—JENNIFER W., KENTUCKY

"This book is full of helpful ideas that both new and experienced mothers-to-be can put to immediate use."
—ZENAIDA M., FLORIDA

"This book is the 'A, B, C book to pregnancy.'"
—DORIS H., INDIANA

"Reading this book is like talking to your mom about how it was being pregnant."
—AMANDA S., KENTUCKY

"All the information on a weekly basis is wonderful. I highly recommend this book to every woman expecting."
—THERESA C., CALIFORNIA

"This book should be read by every mother-to-be. It gives you information week by week instead of month by month, and it helped me so much."
—KRISTI C., GEORGIA

your pregnancy™ week by week

Also by Glade B. Curtis, M.D., M.P.H, OB/GYN, and Judith Schuler, M.S.

Bouncing Back after Your Pregnancy

Su Embarazo Semana a Semana

Your Baby's First Year Week by Week

Your Pregnancy after 35

Your Pregnancy—Every Woman's Guide

Your Pregnancy for the Father-to-Be

Your Pregnancy Journal Week by Week

Your Pregnancy Questions & Answers

Your Pregnancy Quick Guide: Feeding Your Baby

Your Pregnancy Quick Guide: Fitness and Exercise

Your Pregnancy Quick Guide: Labor and Delivery

Your Pregnancy Quick Guide: Nutrition and Weight Management

Your Pregnancy Quick Guide: Postpartum Wellness

Your Pregnancy Quick Guide: Tests and Procedures

Your Pregnancy Quick Guide: Twins, Triplets and More

Your Pregnancy Quick Guide: Understanding and Enhancing Your Baby's Development

Your Pregnancy Quick Guide: Women of Color

7TH EDITION

your pregnancy™ week by week

Glade B. Curtis, M.D., M.P.H., OB/GYN

Judith Schuler, M.S.

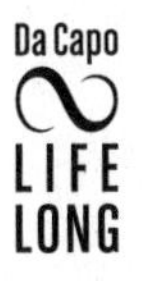

A Member of the Perseus Books Group

Medical illustrations by David Fischer
Exercise Illustrations by Neal Rohrer
Designed by Lisa Kreinbrink
Set in 11.5 point Minion Pro by The Perseus Books Group

Cataloging-in-Publication Data for this book is available from the Library of Congress

Hardcover ISBN: 978-0-7382-1463-4
Paperback ISBN: 978-0-7382-1464-1

First Da Capo Press printing 2011

Published by Da Capo Press
A Member of the Perseus Books Group
http://www.dacapopress.com

Note: The information in this book is true and complete to the best of our knowledge. This book is intended only as an informative guide for those wishing to know more about pregnancy. In no way is this book intended to replace, countermand or conflict with the advice given to you by your own physician. The ultimate decision concerning your care should be made between you and your doctor. We strongly recommend you follow his or her advice. The information in this book is general and is offered with no guarantees on the part of the authors or Da Capo Press. The authors and publisher disclaim all liability in connection with the use of this book. The names and identifying details of people associated with events described in this book have been changed. Any similarity to actual persons is coincidental.

Da Capo Press books are available at special discounts for bulk purchases in the U.S. by corporations, institutions, and other organizations. For more information, please contact the Special Markets Department at the Perseus Books Group, 2300 Chestnut Street, Suite 200, Philadelphia, PA, 19103, call (800) 255-1514, or e-mail special.markets@perseusbooks.com.

10 9 8 7 6 5 4 3 2 1

About the Authors

Glade B. Curtis, *M.D., M.P.H., F.A.C.O.G.,* is board-certified by the American Board of Obstetrics and Gynecology and a Fellow of the American College of Obstetricians and Gynecologists. He has over 25 years of experience and has participated in more than 5,000 deliveries.

Dr. Curtis is a graduate of the University of Utah with a Bachelor of Science and a Master's Degree in Public Health (M.P.H.). He attended the University of Rochester School of Medicine and Dentistry in New York. He interned and was a resident and chief resident in Obstetrics and Gynecology at the University of Rochester Strong Memorial Hospital, Rochester, New York.

Judith Schuler, *M.S.,* has worked with Dr. Curtis for over 25 years, as his co-author and editor. They have collaborated together on 18 books dealing with pregnancy, women's health and children's health.

Ms. Schuler earned a Master of Science degree in Family Studies from the University of Arizona in Tucson. Before becoming an editor for HPBooks, where she and Dr. Curtis first began working together, Ms. Schuler taught at the university level in California and Arizona.

Their Goal as Authors

One of Dr. Curtis's goals as a doctor has been to provide patients with information about gynecological and obstetrical conditions they may have, problems they may encounter and procedures they may undergo. In pursuit of that goal, he and Ms. Schuler have co-authored several additional books for pregnant women and their partners, including *Your Pregnancy for the Father-to-Be, Your Pregnancy Questions & Answers, Your Pregnancy after 35, Your Pregnancy—Every Woman's Guide, Your Pregnancy Journal Week by Week, Bouncing Back after*

Your Pregnancy, Your Baby's First Year Week by Week and the *Your Pregnancy Quick Guide Series*, including *Understanding and Enhancing Your Baby's Development, Exercise and Fitness, Feeding Your Baby, Labor and Delivery, Twins, Triplets and More, Nutrition and Weight Management, Postpartum Wellness, Tests and Procedures,* and *Women of Color.*

Acknowledgments

Special thanks to Courtney Gordon, M.S., PA-C, and Melinda Mossman, FNP-C, for their valuable assistance in reading and suggesting changes to our information on Certified Nurse Midwives, Physician Assistants and Nurse Practitioners.

Glade B. Curtis. In this, the 7th edition of *Your Pregnancy Week by Week*, I continue to draw upon the many questions from discussions with my patients and their partners, and my professional colleagues. I have gained new insights and a greater understanding of the joy and anticipation of impending parenthood. I have rejoiced in my patients' happiness and thank all of them for allowing me to be part of this miraculous process.

Credit must also be given to my understanding and generous wife, Debbie, and our family, who support me in a profession that requires much of them. Beyond that commitment, they have supported and encouraged me to pursue the challenge of this project. Thanks to David Stevens, D.D.S., for his dental expertise. And my parents have always offered their unconditional love and support.

Judith Schuler. I wish to thank my friends, family members and people I have met all over the world who have shared with me their questions and concerns about their journey through pregnancy. They have helped me immensely in our efforts to provide for all our readers the pregnancy information they seek.

To my mother, Kay Gordon, I appreciate your love and continued support. To my son, Ian, thank you for your interest, friendship and love. And thanks to Bob Rucinski for helping me in so many ways—for your professionalism, your expertise and your encouragement.

Contents

Preparing for Pregnancy

Nothing compares with the miracle and magic of pregnancy. It's your chance to be involved in life's creative process. Planning ahead for this experience can improve your chances of doing well yourself and giving birth to a healthy baby. Getting in shape for pregnancy means physical and mental preparation.

Your lifestyle affects you and your baby. If you live healthfully, you can control many things you and baby are exposed to. The first 3 to 8 weeks of pregnancy are the most critical; many women don't even know they're pregnant during this important time. By the time most women realize it, they may be 4 to 8 weeks pregnant. By the time they see their healthcare provider, they're 8 to 12 weeks along. Many important things can happen in the first few weeks of pregnancy.

Pregnancy is a condition, not an illness; you're not sick. However, you will experience major changes. Being in good health before pregnancy can help you deal with physical and emotional stresses during pregnancy, and labor and delivery.

Your General Health

In the past, the emphasis was to be healthy during pregnancy. Today, most experts suggest looking at pregnancy as lasting 12 months or more instead of just 9 months; this includes a 3-month preparation period.

Some medical experts now suggest *all* women of childbearing age should live their lives as if they were trying to get pregnant. Why? Because 50% of all pregnancies are unplanned. That means half of all mothers-to-be may not have been taking the best care of themselves, which could impact the baby. Live every day as if this is the day you get pregnant, and you'll help make certain any child you give birth to has a good start in life.

> You will find many boxes in each weekly discussion, which will provide you with information you will *not* find in the text. Our boxes do not repeat information contained in a discussion. Each box is unique, so read them for specific information.

Prepare for Pregnancy

There are a lot of things you can do to get ready for pregnancy. Reach your ideal weight. Overweight women often have more pregnancy complications. Underweight women may have a harder time getting pregnant.

Eat lots of fruits and vegetables. Choose foods low in saturated fat to help keep your metabolism healthy.

Begin exercising regularly, and stick with it. Exercise 30 minutes a day, at least 5 days a week. Exercising before and during pregnancy can help you feel good for the entire 9 months.

See your healthcare provider to talk about any medicine you take regularly. If you have medical problems, get them under control. Schedule medical tests before you stop contraception. Be sure you're up to date on vaccinations. Have your immunity to rubella and chicken pox checked. If you need vaccinations, find out how long you have to wait after you have them before you try to get pregnant.

Find out your HIV status. Know your blood type and the blood type of your baby's father. Together with your partner, write down your family medical histories.

Ask your healthcare provider to check your iron level. Iron deficiency before pregnancy could make you feel more tired. Get a thyroid test.

Check your cholesterol level; reduce high levels by eating foods high in fiber and low in saturated fat. High cholesterol may contribute to high blood pressure during pregnancy.

Take time off the pill—at least 3 months. Keep a record of your fertility cycle by using charts. Or check your fertility cycle with ovulation-predictor devices. See the discussion that begins on page 589 in Appendix A.

Start taking prenatal vitamins, and *stop* taking your daily multivitamin. *More is not better* in this situation. Take folic acid—400mcg/day is recommended—to help prevent some types of birth defects. Taking folic acid *before* pregnancy gives you protection during the first 28 days of pregnancy, which is very important.

Stop taking aspirin and ibuprofen. Instead, use acetaminophen (Tylenol)—this may help reduce chances of miscarriage. Be careful about taking some herbs, such as St. John's wort, saw palmetto and echinacea; they may interfere with conception.

Have a dental checkup, and have any treatments you need. Get gum disease under control; if you have it during pregnancy, it may increase your risk of problems.

Stop smoking. Avoid second-hand and third-hand smoke. Stop drinking alcohol. Stay away from hazardous chemicals at work and at home. Reduce stress in your life.

Some of the above actions may be hard to begin *during* pregnancy. If you know you're healthy, you won't have to worry about the risks they may pose while you're pregnant.

> *Tip for Prepregnancy*
>
> **Even though you aren't pregnant, treat your body as if you were. When you do get pregnant, you'll be on the right track for eating, exercising and avoiding harmful substances.**

See Your Healthcare Provider *before* Pregnancy

See your healthcare provider before you get pregnant. Have a checkup and discuss pregnancy plans. You'll know when you do get pregnant, you're in good health.

Your general medical history will be covered. You may be asked many things about your health and lifestyle. Your answers provide clues as to what needs to be done once you do get pregnant to keep you healthy.

Your healthcare provider will ask you about your gynecologic history. Answer all questions as clearly and honestly as you can. Answers help him or her understand how pregnancy may affect you. Areas often covered include date of your last menstrual period, how long your cycle lasts, the age at which menstruation began, questions about Pap smears and any STDs you may have had. A pregnancy history will also be taken.

If you have had any type of surgery in the past, you'll be asked about it. Previous Cesarean delivery or other surgeries may affect your pregnancy, so be sure to share this information.

The Father-to-Be

A father-to-be can have an impact on his partner's ability to get pregnant and to have a healthy pregnancy. To learn more, read the information in the fertility discussion, Appendix A, page 589.

Your healthcare provider will also want to know about your family's medical history, especially on your side of the family. Talk to your mother, aunts and sisters about pregnancy complications they may have had. It's good to know if anyone in the family had twins, triplets or more. If birth defects occurred, get as much information as possible about them. If there is a history of any inherited problems in your family or your partner's family, let your healthcare provider know.

Be prepared to talk about any medicine you take and any tests you may be having. Cover all medical problems you're being treated for. Include all over-the-counter medicines, herbs, supplements and vitamins you may use. It's easier to answer questions about these things before you get pregnant rather than after you are pregnant.

Don't be surprised if you're asked about your lifestyle and any substances you take or use. These include cigarettes, alcohol, illicit drugs, legal drugs you may be using, your exercise program, your job and chemical substances you may be exposed to at work or at home. Domestic violence may also be addressed because it can often appear for the first time, or it can escalate, during pregnancy.

Be honest in your answers; your healthcare provider is trying to evaluate your situation. Concealing facts because you're embarrassed or scared doesn't help you or the baby you hope to conceive.

You may have heard a couple shouldn't have sex too often when they're trying to conceive. A new study states having sex several times in one week may actually *increase* a man's sperm production by as much as 30%.

If You Have Problems

The odds of getting pregnant in any menstrual cycle are about 20 to 25%; nearly 60% of all couples conceive within 6 months. But if you have trouble getting pregnant, talk to your healthcare provider. If you're over 35 and have had trouble getting pregnant, your healthcare provider may be able to advise you about lifestyle changes and other factors that could increase your chances.

If your menstrual cycle is longer than 36 days or shorter than 23 days, ovulation may be an issue. Your healthcare provider can advise you of various ways to determine whether you are ovulating and when you ovulate. Also see the discussion that begins on page 589 in Appendix A.

Tests for You

Have a physical exam before you get pregnant. A Pap smear and a breast exam should be included in this physical. Lab tests may include tests for rubella, blood type and Rh-factor. If you're 40 or older, a mammogram is also a good idea.

If you think you may have been exposed to HIV or hepatitis, ask about testing. If you have a family history of other medical problems, such as diabetes, ask about tests to rule them out. If you have a chronic medical problem, such as anemia, your healthcare provider may suggest other tests.

Ask for a pregnancy test *before* having any test involving radiation, including dental work. Tests involving radiation include *X-rays, CT scans* and *MRIs*. Use reliable contraception before these tests to make sure you're not pregnant. Schedule a test right after the end of your period. If you need a series of tests, continue birth control.

Possible Prepregnancy Tests

Your healthcare provider may do a lot of tests to identify any problems that could affect your pregnancy. You can deal with them now instead of later. The following tests may be done at a prepregnancy visit. You may have had some of them in the past, and they may not need to be repeated:

- a physical exam
- pelvic exam and a Pap smear
- breast exam (mammogram if you are at least 40)
- rubella (German measles) and varicella (chicken pox)
- blood type and Rh-factor
- HIV/AIDS (if you have risk factors)
- hepatitis screen (if you have risk factors)
- vaccination and immunization screens
- screening for sexually transmitted diseases (if you have risk factors)
- screening for genetic disorders based on racial and ethnic background, including cystic fibrosis, sickle-cell disease, thalassemia, Tay-Sachs disease, Gaucher disease, Canavan disease, Niemann-Pick disease
- screening for other genetic disorders, based on family history, including fragile-X syndrome, hemophilia, Duchenne muscular dystrophy

Tests for Women of Color and Jewish Women

If you are a woman of color (Black/African American, Latina/Hispanic, Native American/Alaska Native, Asian/Pacific Islander or Mediterranean) or of Jewish descent, you may be advised to have some tests to help determine if you could pass a particular disease or condition to your baby. For example, if you are of Mediterranean descent, you may be told a screening test for beta-thalassemia is a good idea. Asian/Pacific Islanders might be screened for alpha-thalassemia. If you're Black/African American, your healthcare provider may suggest screening for sickle-cell disease.

Although a woman of Jewish descent may not be a woman of color, there are diseases that might affect her. These conditions usually affect women who are Ashkenazi or Sephardi Jews.

The American College of Obstetricians and Gynecologists recommends Tay-Sachs carrier screening be offered before pregnancy to women who are at high risk. This includes those of Ashkenazi Jewish, French-Canadian or Cajun descent, and those with a family history of Tay-Sachs disease.

If you have any questions about these conditions, discuss them with your healthcare provider. He or she can give you information and guidance.

Discontinuing Contraception

It's important to continue some form of contraception until you're ready to get pregnant. If you're in the middle of treatment for a medical problem or if you're having tests, finish the treatment or tests before trying to conceive. (If you're not using some form of birth control, you're basically trying to get pregnant.)

After stopping your regular contraceptive, use some other birth-control method until your periods become normal. You can choose from condoms, spermicides, the sponge or a diaphragm.

If you use birth-control pills, patches or rings, most healthcare providers recommend you have two or three normal periods after you stop using them before trying to get pregnant. If you get pregnant immediately, it may be hard to determine when you conceived. This can make it harder to figure out your due date. It may not seem important now, but it'll be very important during pregnancy and before you deliver.

If you have an IUD (intrauterine device), have it taken out before you try to conceive. However, pregnancy can occur while an IUD is in place. The best time to remove an IUD is during a menstrual period.

If you use Implanon or other implantable contraception, have at least two or three normal menstrual cycles after it's removed before trying to get pregnant. It may take a few months for your periods to return to normal. If you get pregnant immediately, it may be difficult to determine when you got pregnant and what your due date is.

Depoprovera should be discontinued for at least 3 to 6 months before trying to conceive. Wait until you have had at least two or three normal periods.

Your Health before Pregnancy

Discuss any chronic medical problems you have with your healthcare provider. You may need extra care before and during pregnancy. Some common chronic medical problems are discussed below.

Anemia

Anemia means you do not have enough hemoglobin in your blood to carry oxygen to your body's cells. Symptoms include weakness, fatigue, shortness of breath and pale skin.

Iron plays an important part in anemia. It's possible to develop anemia during pregnancy because the baby makes great demands on your body for iron. If you have low iron levels, pregnancy can tip the balance and make you anemic.

If you have a family history of anemia (such as sickle-cell disease or thalassemia), discuss it with your healthcare provider *before* you get pregnant. If you take hydroxyurea, discuss whether you should continue using it. We don't know whether this medication is safe during pregnancy.

Asthma

Most asthma medications are safe to take during pregnancy, but talk to your healthcare provider about your medication. Try to get asthma under good control before trying to get pregnant.

Bladder or Kidney Problems

Bladder infections, such as urinary-tract infections or UTIs, may occur more often during pregnancy. If a urinary-tract infection is not treated, it can cause an infection of the kidneys, called *pyelonephritis*. Kidney stones may also cause problems during pregnancy.

If you've had kidney or bladder surgery, major kidney problems or if your kidney function is less than normal, tell your healthcare provider. It may be necessary to evaluate your kidney function with tests before you become pregnant.

If you have an occasional bladder infection, don't be alarmed. Your healthcare provider will decide whether further testing is necessary before you become pregnant.

Celiac Disease

Celiac disease affects the small intestine and interferes with nutrient absorption. It occurs when you eat gluten, which is found in foods made from white flour, wheat, barley, rye and oats. If you have celiac disease, discuss any intestinal problems you have.

It's best to have the disease under control for 1 to 2 years before pregnancy to help heal your digestive tract. Better nutrient absorption helps ensure the good health of you and your baby. If you can manage your celiac disease and take in enough of the nutrients your body needs before pregnancy, you decrease your risks of problems.

Diabetes

It may be harder for you to become pregnant if you have diabetes. If your diabetes is *not* under control when you get pregnant, the risk increases of having a child with a birth defect.

Most healthcare providers recommend having diabetes under control for at least 2 to 3 months before pregnancy begins. Get your blood sugar under control, manage blood pressure, reach a healthy weight and take care of any other problems you may have. When it isn't under control, you increase the chance of problems. Many problems occur during the first trimester (the first 13 weeks of pregnancy).

Pregnancy may increase your need for insulin. Being pregnant increases your body's resistance to insulin; some oral antidiabetes medications can cause problems for your baby. You may have to check your blood sugar several times a day.

If you're diabetic, you may have more prenatal visits and more testing during pregnancy. Your healthcare provider may have to work very closely with the healthcare provider who treats your diabetes.

Epilepsy and Seizures

Before you become pregnant, talk to your healthcare provider about therapies for treating epilepsy. Some anticonvulsant medicine shouldn't be used during pregnancy. If you take several medications in combination, you may be advised to take only one.

Seizures can be dangerous to a mother and baby. It's important for you to take your medication regularly and as prescribed by your healthcare provider. Do not decrease or discontinue any medication on your own!

Heart Disease

Consult your physician about any heart condition before you become pregnant. Some heart problems may be serious during pregnancy and may require antibiotics at the time of delivery. Other heart problems may seriously affect your health. Your healthcare provider will advise you.

High Blood Pressure (Hypertension)

High blood pressure, or hypertension, can cause problems for a pregnant woman and her growing baby. If you have high blood pressure before pregnancy, you'll need to work with your healthcare provider(s) to lower your blood pressure. If necessary, start exercising now and lose any extra weight. Take blood-pressure medication as prescribed.

Some high-blood-pressure medications are safe to take during pregnancy; others are not. *Do not stop or decrease any medication on your own!* If you're planning pregnancy, ask your healthcare provider about your medication.

Lupus

Lupus treatment is individual and may involve taking steroids. There is an increased risk of problems in women with lupus, which requires extra care during pregnancy.

If you take methotrexate, discontinue it before you try to get pregnant. But don't just stop taking it. Talk to your healthcare provider so you can plan alternative treatment.

Migraine Headaches

About 15 to 20% of all pregnant women suffer from migraine headaches. Many women notice fewer or less-intense headaches while they're pregnant. If you take medication for headaches, check with your healthcare provider now so you'll know whether the one you take is safe to use during pregnancy.

Rheumatoid Arthritis (RA)

If you have rheumatoid arthritis, talk to your healthcare provider about the medicine you take to treat your disease. Some medication can be dangerous to a pregnant woman. Methotrexate should *not* be used during pregnancy because it may cause miscarriage and birth defects.

Thyroid Problems

Thyroid problems can appear as either too much or too little thyroid hormone. Pregnancy can change medication requirements, so you should be tested before pregnancy to determine the correct amount of medication for you. You will also need to be checked during pregnancy.

Back Surgery

If you've had back surgery, discuss pregnancy plans with your surgeon. If you had surgery on your lower back, you may be advised to wait 3 to 6 months before trying to become pregnant. If you had fusion surgery, the wait is often 6 months to a year.

Why wait? Waiting lets your back heal before taking on the stress of pregnancy. You may have fewer problems or complications. Be sure to check with your surgeon before you plan to become pregnant.

Current Medications

It's important for you and your healthcare providers to consider the possibility of pregnancy each time you are given a prescription or advised to take a medicine. When you're pregnant, many things change with regard to medication usage.

> ### *Be Careful with Medications*
>
> Before pregnancy, play it safe with medicines. Keep in mind the following.
>
> - If you use birth control, don't stop unless you want to get pregnant.
> - Take prescriptions exactly as they are prescribed.
> - Tell your healthcare provider if you think you might be pregnant or if you are not using birth control when a medication is prescribed.
> - Don't self-treat or use medicine you were given for other problems.
> - Never use someone else's medication.
> - If you're unsure about taking something, call your healthcare provider *before* you use it!

Medicine that is safe when you aren't pregnant may have harmful effects during pregnancy. Most organ development in the baby occurs in the first 13 weeks of pregnancy. This is an important time to avoid exposing baby to unnecessary or harmful substances. You'll feel better and do better during pregnancy if you have medication use under control before you try to get pregnant.

Some medicine is intended for short-term use, such as antibiotics for infections. Others are for chronic or long-lasting problems, such as high blood pressure or diabetes. Some medications are OK to take while you're pregnant and may help make your pregnancy successful. Other medications may not be safe to take during pregnancy.

Vaccinations

When you have a vaccination, use reliable contraception. Research shows it's better to receive vaccinations for various diseases *before* you get pregnant than during pregnancy. Some vaccinations cannot be given to pregnant women; others can.

At your prepregnancy visit, ask your healthcare provider if you're up to date on your vaccinations. A good rule of thumb is to complete vaccinations at least 3 months before trying to get pregnant.

Vaccinations are usually most harmful in the first trimester. If you need a vaccination for rubella, MMR (measles, mumps, rubella) or chicken pox before you get pregnant, experts recommend you wait at least 4 weeks after receiving it before you try to get pregnant.

An exception to this rule is the flu vaccine; you can get it at any time during pregnancy. However, don't get the nasal mist type of flu vaccine—it's not advised for pregnant women. If you're advised to take the flu vaccine because of your job or for some other reason, go ahead. It will help protect you and baby.

Genetic Counseling

If you're planning your first pregnancy, you are probably not considering genetic counseling. However, there may be circumstances in which genetic counseling could help you and your partner make informed decisions about having children.

Genetics is the study of how traits and characteristics are passed from parent to child through chromosomes and genes. *Genetic counseling* is an information session between you and your partner and a genetic counselor or group of counselors.

In actuality, the occurrence of birth defects is *very* low—they occur in about 0.04% of all births. The primary goal in genetic counseling is prevention and/or early diagnosis of these problems. Certain groups have a higher incidence of problems, and certain medications, chemicals and pesticides can put a couple at risk.

Genetic disorders may be caused in various ways. If you have an *inherited disorder,* it comes from your parents. A *chromosomal disorder* can happen even when parents don't have any risk factors. *Multifactorial disorders* can occur from more than one source; the cause is generally unknown.

Genetic counseling aims to help you and your partner understand what might happen in your particular situation. A counselor won't make decisions for you. He or she will give you information on tests you might take and what test results may mean. So don't hide information you feel is embarrassing or hard to talk about. It's important to tell a counselor what he or she needs to know.

Most couples who need genetic counseling do not find out they needed it until after they have a child born with a birth defect. You might consider genetic counseling if any of the following apply to you.

- You will be at least 35 years old at the time of delivery.
- You have delivered a child with a birth defect.
- You or your partner have a birth defect.
- You or your partner have a family history of Down syndrome, mental retardation, cystic fibrosis, spina bifida, muscular dystrophy, bleeding disorders, skeletal or bone problems, dwarfism, epilepsy, congenital heart defects or blindness.
- You or your partner have a family history of inherited deafness.
- You and your partner are related (consanguinity).
- You have had recurrent miscarriages (usually three or more).
- You *and* your partner are descended from Ashkenazi Jews. There is an increased risk of Tay-Sachs disease, Canavan disease and other problems. See the discussion of Jewish Disorders in Week 7.
- You or your partner are Black/African American (risk of sickle-cell disease).
- Your partner is at least 40 years old.

Some information may be difficult to gather, especially if you or your partner are adopted. You may know little about your family's medical history. Discuss this with your healthcare provider before you get pregnant. If you learn about the chances of problems before pregnancy, you won't have to make difficult decisions after you get pregnant.

Genetic Testing

Your genetic counselor may talk about various tests with you. More than 1000 disorders can be detected using genetic tests, but most are rare. The conditions regularly tested for include cystic fibrosis, Down syndrome, neural-tube defects, thalassemia, Tay-Sachs and sickle-cell disease.

There are three types of tests that may be done—carrier testing, screening tests and diagnostic tests. *Carrier testing* involves testing both partners to determine if either or both is a carrier of a particular genetic defect. *Screening tests* may be done during pregnancy to determine whether there is an increased risk of a problem; it does not positively identify the problem. *Diagnostic tests* often determine whether a problem is present.

Pregnancy after 35

More women are choosing to marry after they have established a career, and more couples are choosing to start their families at a later age. Today, healthcare providers are seeing more older first-time mothers; many have safe, healthy pregnancies. You may also want to read our book, *Your Pregnancy after 35*, which focuses primarily on pregnancy in older women.

An older woman considering pregnancy often has two major concerns. She wants to know how the pregnancy will affect her and how her age will affect her pregnancy. A pregnant woman older than 35 may face increased risks of:

- a baby born with Down syndrome
- high blood pressure
- pelvic pressure or pelvic pain
- pre-eclampsia
- Cesarean delivery
- multiple births
- placental abruption
- bleeding and other complications
- premature labor

You may find it easier to be pregnant when you're 20 than it is when you're 40. You may have a job or other children making demands on your time. You may find it harder to rest, exercise and eat right. But these concerns shouldn't dissuade you from having children when you're older.

Through medical research, we know older women are at higher risk of giving birth to a child with Down syndrome. Various tests may be offered to an older woman during pregnancy to determine whether a baby will have Down syndrome. It's the most common chromosomal defect detected by amniocentesis.

The risk of delivering a baby with Down syndrome increases as you get older. But there's a positive way to look at these statistics. If you're 45, you have a 97% chance of *not* having a baby with Down syndrome. If you're 49, you have a 92% chance of delivering a child without Down syndrome. If you're concerned about the risk of Down syndrome because of your age or family history, discuss it with your healthcare provider.

Research shows a father's age may be important. Chromosomal abnormalities that cause birth defects occur more often in older women and in men over 40. Some researchers recommend men father children before age 40, but there's still some controversy about this.

If you're older, you can maximize your chances of having a successful pregnancy by being as healthy as possible *before* you become pregnant. Most experts recommend a baseline mammogram be done at age 40. Have this test before you become pregnant. Paying attention to general recommendations for your diet and your health care is also important in preparing for pregnancy.

Weight Management before Pregnancy

Most people feel better and work better when they eat a well-balanced diet. Planning and following a healthy eating plan before pregnancy helps provide your growing baby good nutrition during the first few weeks or months of pregnancy.

Usually a woman takes good care of herself once she knows she's pregnant. By planning ahead, you can be sure baby has a healthy environment for the entire 9 months of pregnancy, not for just the 6 or 7 months after you find out you're pregnant.

Weight Management

Some researchers believe your weight may affect your chances of getting pregnant. Being underweight or overweight can alter sex hormones, your menstrual cycle, ovulation and may even affect the lining of your uterus. Any of these can make it harder for you to get pregnant.

If you're *underweight,* your body may not produce enough hormones for you to ovulate every month. You may also have problems getting the best nutrition for your baby.

If you're *overweight,* don't diet while you're trying to conceive, and don't take diet pills. You may have a harder time getting pregnant if you're overweight or obese. *Overweight* is defined as having a body-mass index (BMI) between 26 and 30. *Obesity* is defined as having a BMI over 30. See the discussion in Week 14.

Examine your eating habits. Determine what you need to work on to make your food intake healthy for you and baby. It may be very helpful to lose weight before trying to get pregnant, which may help reduce pregnancy complications and birth defects.

Consult your healthcare provider if you're thinking about starting a special diet to lose or gain weight before you try to get pregnant. Dieting may cause a drop in vitamins and minerals that both you and your developing baby need.

If You've Had Weight-Loss Surgery

Some women have weight-loss surgery to help them lose weight. *Bariatric surgery* is defined as surgery related to the prevention and control of obesity and related diseases. Women who have had bariatric surgery have been shown to have less-complicated pregnancies than obese women who don't have surgery, and their children are also less likely to be obese.

If you had gastric-bypass surgery to lose weight, you may be at increased risk of getting pregnant after the procedure. This happens because you lose weight, which may lead to more-regular ovulation. This could result in pregnancy.

If you plan to become pregnant soon, having lap-band surgery may be your best choice. Unlike gastric-bypass surgery, lap banding is fully reversible. It's possible to have your stomach outlet size opened so you can meet the increased nutritional needs of pregnancy.

You should probably delay getting pregnant for 12 to 18 months following surgery because this is the time you will be losing weight very rapidly. You may not have sufficient nutrients available for you and your growing baby.

Be Careful with Vitamins, Minerals and Herbs

Don't self-medicate with large amounts or unusual combinations of vitamins, minerals or herbs. You *can* overdo it! Certain vitamins, such as vitamin A, can cause birth defects if used in excessive amounts. Some experts believe various herbs can temporarily reduce fertility in men *and* women, so you and your partner should not take St. John's wort, echinacea and gingko biloba.

Stop all extra supplements at least 3 months before pregnancy. Eat a well-balanced diet and take a multivitamin or prenatal vitamin. Most healthcare providers are happy to prescribe prenatal vitamins if you're planning a pregnancy.

Green Tea Warning

Don't drink green tea while you're trying to get pregnant—not even a glass or two! It may increase your chances of having a baby with a neural-tube defect. The problem is the antioxidant in green tea decreases the effectiveness of folic acid. Enough folic acid during the first few weeks of pregnancy may help lower the risk. Wait until after baby comes to drink green tea again.

Folic Acid

Folic acid is a B vitamin (B_9) that can contribute to a healthy pregnancy. Taking folic-acid for at least 1 year before pregnancy may help reduce your risk of certain birth defects and pregnancy problems. If you take 0.4mg (400 micrograms) of folic acid each day before pregnancy, it may help protect your baby against birth defects of the spine and brain, called *neural-tube defects*. Once pregnancy is confirmed, it may be too late to prevent these problems.

In 1998, the U.S. government ordered that some grain products, such as flour, breakfast cereals and pasta, be fortified with folic acid. It is now also found in many other foods. Eat a well-balanced, varied diet to help you reach your goal. Many foods that contain folate (the natural form of folic acid found in food) include asparagus, avocados, bananas, black beans, broccoli, citrus fruits and juices, egg yolks, green beans, leafy green vegetables, lentils, liver, peas, plantains, spinach, strawberries, tuna, wheat germ, yogurt and fortified breads and cereals.

Begin Good Eating Habits

A woman often carries her prepregnancy eating habits into pregnancy. Many women eat on the run and pay little attention to what they eat most of the day. Before pregnancy, you may be able to get away with this. However, because of the increased demands on you and the needs of your baby, it won't work when you do become pregnant.

Eat a balanced diet. Going to extremes with vitamins or fad diets may be harmful.

If you have various problems, such as polycycstic ovarian syndrome, some

Can You Help Avoid Morning Sickness in Pregnancy?

If you eat high amounts of saturated fat—the kind found in cheese and red meat—in the year *before* you get pregnant, you may have severe morning sickness during pregnancy. If you're planning to get pregnant, cut down on these foods. Taking a multivitamin regularly before you get pregnant may also lower your risk.

foods may improve your chances of conceiving. Foods to consider adding to your diet include broccoli, spinach, cabbage, nuts, fruit, kelp, nori, beans and fish.

Before getting pregnant, talk to your healthcare provider if you have special dietary needs. This includes whether you are a vegetarian, how much exercise you do, whether you skip meals, your diet plan (are you trying to lose or gain weight?) and any special needs you might have. If you eat a special diet because of medical problems, discuss it with your healthcare provider.

While you're trying to get pregnant, don't eat more than 12 ounces of fish a week. Avoid fish not recommended during pregnancy. See the discussion in Week 26.

Exercise before Pregnancy

Exercise is good for you. Benefits may include weight control, a feeling of well-being and increased stamina or endurance, which will become important later in pregnancy.

Begin exercising regularly before you get pregnant. Make adjustments in your life so you can include regular exercise. It will help you now and make it easier to stay in shape during pregnancy.

But don't exercise to an extreme; it may cause problems. Avoid intense training. Don't increase your exercise program. Skip playing competitive sports that involve pushing yourself to the max.

Find exercise you like and will continue to do on a regular basis, in any kind of weather. Focus on improving strength in your lower back and abs to help during your pregnancy.

If you have concerns about exercise before or during pregnancy, talk to your healthcare provider. Exercise you can do easily before pregnancy may be more difficult for you during pregnancy.

The American College of Obstetricians and Gynecologists (ACOG) has proposed guidelines for exercise before and during pregnancy. Ask your healthcare provider for a copy.

Substance Use before Pregnancy

We know a lot about the effects of drugs and alcohol on pregnancy. We believe the safest approach to drug or alcohol use during pregnancy is *no use at all.*

Tell your healthcare provider about substance abuse, and deal with problems now. Your baby goes through some of its most important developmental stages in the first 13 weeks of your pregnancy. Stop using any substance you don't need at least 3 months before trying to conceive!

> **Dad Tip**
>
> If your partner is making lifestyle changes to prepare for pregnancy, such as giving up smoking or not drinking alcohol, support her in her efforts. Quit these habits if you share them.

There is help for those who use drugs—if you need to, seek help before you get pregnant. Preparing for pregnancy may be a good reason for you and your partner to change your lifestyle.

Smoking can damage your eggs and ovaries. If you stop smoking for at least 1 year before trying to get pregnant, you increase your chances of conceiving. You also reduce your odds of having a miscarriage.

Smoking cigarettes and exposure to second hand smoke deplete folic acid from your body. Mothers who smoke during pregnancy may have low-birthweight babies or babies with other problems. Ask for help to stop smoking before you become pregnant.

Most experts agree there is *no safe amount* of alcohol to drink during pregnancy. Alcohol crosses the placenta and directly affects your baby. Heavy drinking during pregnancy can cause fetal alcohol syndrome (FAS) or fetal alcohol exposure (FAE); both are discussed in Weeks 1 & 2. Stop drinking now.

If you use cocaine during the first 12 weeks of pregnancy, you run a higher risk of problems than if you don't use cocaine. Women who use cocaine throughout pregnancy also have a higher rate of problems. Stop using cocaine before you stop using birth control. Damage to a baby can occur as early as 3 days after conception!

Marijuana can cross the placenta, enter a baby's system and have long-lasting effects. If your partner smokes marijuana, encourage him to stop. One study showed the risk of SIDS was twice the average for children if their father smoked marijuana.

Work and Pregnancy

You may need to consider your job when you plan a pregnancy. Some jobs might be considered harmful during pregnancy. Some substances you might be exposed to at work, such as chemicals, inhalants, radiation or solvents, could be a problem. Consider things you're exposed to at work as part of your lifestyle. Continue reliable contraception until you know the environment at work is safe.

Check the types of benefits or insurance coverage you have and your company's maternity-leave program. Most programs allow some time off work. Prenatal care and baby's birth could cost you several thousand dollars if you don't plan ahead.

Are You in the Military?

Are you currently serving in the U.S. Armed Forces or planning to enter one of the services soon? Studies show women who get pregnant while on active duty may face many challenges, including some risks to the baby.

The pressure to meet military body-weight standards can affect your health. You may have low iron stores and lower-than-normal folic-acid levels. Some jobs may be hazardous, such as standing for a long time, heavy lifting or exposure to certain chemicals.

If you plan to get pregnant during your service commitment, work hard to reach your ideal weight a few months before you conceive, then maintain that weight. Take in enough folic acid and iron by eating well-balanced meals. You may also want to take a prenatal vitamin. If you're concerned about hazards related to your work, discuss it with a superior. Find out if you're pregnant before getting any vaccinations or inoculations.

It's important to take care of yourself and your baby. Start by making plans now to have a healthy pregnancy. Also see the discussion in Week 14.

Women who stand for long periods have smaller babies. A job that involves standing a great deal may not be a good choice during pregnancy. Talk to your healthcare provider about your work situation.

If you're stressed out, it may be harder to get pregnant. Studies show chances of getting pregnant improve when stress is lowered. Try to reduce the amount of stress in your life; you may improve your chances of getting pregnant.

Important note: If you're self-employed, you won't be qualified to receive state disability payments. You may want to think about a private disability policy to cover you for any problems before birth and for time off after baby arrives. The glitch here is that the policy must be in place *before* you get pregnant.

Sexually Transmitted Diseases

Infections or diseases passed from one person to another by sexual contact are called *sexually transmitted diseases* (STDs). These infections may affect your ability to get pregnant and can harm a growing baby. The type of contraception you use may have an effect on the likelihood of getting an STD. Condoms and spermicides can lower the risk. You're more likely to get a sexually transmitted disease if you have more than one sexual partner.

Some STD infections can cause pelvic inflammatory disease (PID). An infection can result in scarring and blockage of the tubes. This can make it difficult or impossible to get pregnant or make you more susceptible to an ectopic pregnancy. Surgery may be necessary to repair damaged tubes.

Protecting Yourself from STDs

Protect yourself against STDs. Use a condom, and limit the number of sexual partners you have. Have sexual contact only with those people you're sure don't sleep around. Get tested if you have a chance of having an infection, even if you don't have symptoms, and ask for treatment if you think you need it.

Weeks 1 & 2

Pregnancy Begins

This is an exciting time for you—having a baby growing inside you is an incredible experience! Our goal is to help you understand and enjoy your pregnancy. In this book, you will learn what is going on in your body and how your baby is growing and changing. You're not alone—millions of women successfully complete a pregnancy every year.

Material in this book is divided into weeks because this is the way healthcare providers look at pregnancy. It makes sense to look at changes in you and the baby the same way. This also lets you and your partner follow your changes and baby's growth more closely. Weekly illustrations help you see how you and baby change and grow. Weekly topics cover areas of special concern as well as how big your baby is, how big you are and how your actions affect your baby.

The information in this book is *not* meant to take the place of any discussion with your healthcare provider—discuss any and all concerns with him or her. Use this material as a starting place in your dialogue. It may help you put your concerns or interests into words.

Signs and Symptoms of Pregnancy

Many changes in your body can indicate pregnancy. If you have one or more of the following symptoms and you believe you might be pregnant, contact your healthcare provider:

- missed menstrual period
- nausea, with or without vomiting
- food aversions or food cravings

- fatigue
- frequent urination
- breast changes and breast tenderness
- new sensitivity or feelings in your pelvic area
- metallic taste in your mouth

What will you notice first? It's different for every woman. When your period doesn't begin, you may think of pregnancy.

Although this book is designed to take you through your pregnancy by examining one week at a time, you may seek specific information. Because the book cannot include *everything* you need *before* you know you're looking for it, check the index, beginning on page 653, for a particular topic. We may not cover the subject until a later week.

When Is Your Baby Due?

The beginning of a pregnancy is actually figured from the beginning of your last menstrual period. For your healthcare provider's calculations, you're pregnant 2 weeks before you actually conceive! Pregnancy lasts about 280 days, or 40 weeks, from the beginning of the last menstrual period. This can be confusing, so let's look at it more closely.

A *due date* is important in pregnancy because it helps determine when to perform certain tests or procedures. It also helps estimate the baby's growth and may indicate when you're overdue—this will be really important to you as delivery time approaches.

Your due date is only an estimate, not an exact date. Only 1 out of 20 women actually delivers on her due date. You may see your due date come and go and still not have your baby. Think of your due date as a goal—a time to look forward to and to prepare for.

Most women don't know the exact date of conception, but they usually know the beginning of their last period. This is the point from which a pregnancy is dated. Figuring a due date can be tricky because periods and menstrual histories can be uncertain.

Calculate your due date by counting 280 days from the first day of bleeding of your last period. Dating a pregnancy this way gives the gestational age (menstrual age), which is the way most healthcare providers keep track of time during pregnancy. It's different from ovulatory age (fertilization age), which is 2 weeks shorter and dates from the actual date of conception.

Some medical experts suggest instead of a "due date," women be given a "due week"—a 7-day window of time during which delivery may occur. This time period would fall between the 39th and 40th weeks. Because so few women (only 5%) deliver on their actual due date, a 7-day period could help ease a mom-to-be's anxiety about when her baby will be born.

You may hear references to your stage of pregnancy by trimester. *Trimesters* divide pregnancy into three periods, each about 13 weeks long, to help group together developmental stages.

You may even hear about lunar months, referring to a complete cycle of the moon, which is 28 days. Because pregnancy is 280 days from the beginning of your period to your due date, pregnancy lasts 10 lunar months.

Using a 40-week timetable, you actually become pregnant during the third week. Details of your pregnancy are discussed week by week beginning with Week 3. Your due date is the end of the 40th week. Each weekly discussion includes the actual age of your growing baby. For example, in Week 8, you'll see the following:

Week 8 *[gestational age]*
Age of Fetus—6 Weeks
[fertilization age]

This tells you how old your developing baby is at any point in your pregnancy.

Definitions of Time

Gestational age (menstrual age)—Begins the first day of your last period, which is actually about 2 weeks *before* you conceive. This is the age most healthcare providers use to discuss your pregnancy. The average length of pregnancy is 40 weeks.
Ovulatory age (fertilization age)—Begins the day you conceive. The average length of pregnancy is 38 weeks or 266 days.
Trimester—Each trimester lasts about 13 weeks. There are three trimesters in a pregnancy.
Lunar months—A pregnancy lasts an average of 10 lunar months (28 days each).
EDC—Estimated date of confinement or due date.

No matter how you count the time of your pregnancy, it's going to last as long as it's going to last. But a miracle is happening—a living human being is growing and developing inside you! Enjoy this wonderful time in your life.

Your Menstrual Cycle

Menstruation is the normal periodic discharge of blood, mucus and cellular debris from the cavity of the uterus. Two important cycles occur during the menstrual cycle—the ovarian cycle and the endometrial cycle. The *ovarian cycle* provides an egg for fertilization. The *endometrial cycle* provides a suitable site for implantation of the fertilized egg inside your uterus.

There are about 2 million eggs in a newborn girl at birth. This decreases to about 400,000 in girls just before puberty. The maximum number of eggs is actually present *before* birth. When a female fetus is about 5 months old (4 months before birth), she has about 6.8 million eggs!

> **Tip for Weeks 1 & 2**
>
> Over-the-counter pregnancy tests are reliable and can be positive (indicate pregnancy) as early as 10 days after conception.

About 25% of women have lower-abdominal pain or discomfort on or about the day of ovulation, called *mittelschmerz.* It may be caused by irritation from fluid or blood from the follicle when it ruptures. The presence or absence of this symptom is not considered proof ovulation did or did not occur.

Your Health Affects Your Pregnancy

Your health is one of the most important factors in your pregnancy. Good health care is important to the development and well-being of your baby. Healthy nutrition, proper exercise, sufficient rest and taking care of yourself all affect your pregnancy. Throughout this book, we provide information about medicine you may take, tests you may need, substances you might use and many other topics that may concern you. This information helps you be aware of how your actions affect your health and the health of your developing baby.

Some Information May Scare You

In an effort to give you as much information as possible about pregnancy, we do include serious discussions throughout the book that some might find "scary." The information is not included to frighten you; it's there to provide facts about particular medical situations that may occur during pregnancy.

If a woman experiences a serious problem, she and her partner will probably want to know as much about it as possible. If a woman has a friend or knows someone who has problems during pregnancy, reading about it might relieve her fears. We also hope our discussions can help you start a dialogue with your doctor, if you have questions.

Nearly all pregnancies are uneventful, and serious situations don't arise. However, please know we have tried to cover as many aspects of pregnancy as we possibly can so you'll have all the information at hand that you might need and want. Knowledge is power, so having various facts available can help you feel more in control of your own pregnancy. We hope reading information helps you relax and have a great pregnancy experience.

If you find serious discussions frighten you, don't read them! Or if the information doesn't apply to your pregnancy, just skip over it. But realize information is there if you want to know more about a particular situation.

Your Healthcare Provider

The health care you receive can affect your pregnancy and how well you tolerate being pregnant. You have many choices when it comes time to choose your doctor or other healthcare provider. An *obstetrician* is a doctor who specializes in the care of pregnant women, including delivering babies. Obstetricians are medical doctors or doctors of osteopathic medicine who have graduated from an accredited medical or osteopathic school and have fulfilled the requirements for a medical license. Both have completed further training after medical school (residency).

Dad Tip

You may find you'll need to make some changes in *your* life during your partner's pregnancy. You may have to change how often you participate in various activities or when you do them. You may not be able to travel as much for work or pleasure. But remember—pregnancy only lasts 9 months. Supporting your pregnant partner can make both of your lives better.

Perinatologists are obstetricians who specialize in high-risk pregnancies. Few women require a perinatologist (only 1 out of 10). If you're worried about past health problems, ask your healthcare provider if you need to see a specialist.

An added credential is *board certification.* Not all doctors who deliver babies are board certified. It's not a requirement. "Board certification" means your doctor has put in extra time preparing for and taking exams to qualify him or her to care for pregnant women and to deliver their babies. If your doctor has passed his or her boards, you will see the initials *F.A.C.O.G.* after the doctor's name. This means he or she is a Fellow of the American College of Obstetricians and Gynecologists. Your local medical society can also give you this information.

Some women choose a *family practitioner* for their care. In some cases, an obstetrician may not be available because a community is small or in a remote area. A family practitioner may serve as internist, pediatrician and obstetrician/gynecologist. Many family practitioners are experienced at delivering babies. If problems arise, you may be referred to an obstetrician. This may also be the case if a Cesarean section is needed to deliver your baby.

Pregnant women sometimes choose a *certified nurse-midwife,* an *advance-practice nurse* or a *physician assistant* for their prenatal care. These healthcare professionals have additional training and certification in a medical specialty. See the discussion of each and the type of care they provide that begins on page 37.

Communication Is Important

It's important to be able to communicate with your healthcare provider. You need to be able to ask any questions you have, such as those listed below.

- Do you believe in natural childbirth (if this is *your* interest)?
- Can I get an epidural?
- Are there routines you perform on every patient? Does everyone "get" an enema, fetal monitor or more?
- Who covers for you when you're away?
- Are there other healthcare providers I will meet or who will take care of me?

Your healthcare provider has experience involving many pregnancies and is drawing on this for your well-being. He or she has to consider what is best for you and your baby while trying to honor any "special" requests you may have.

You should be able to express your concerns and talk about what's important to you. Don't be afraid to ask any question; your healthcare provider has probably already heard it. A request may be unwise or risky for you, but it's important to ask about it ahead of time. If a request is possible, you can plan for it together, barring unforeseen developments.

Find the Best Caregiver for You

How do you find someone who "fits the bill"? If you already have a healthcare provider you're happy with, you may be all set. If you don't, call your local medical society. Ask for references to professionals who are taking new patients for pregnancy.

There are other ways to find a healthcare provider you'll be happy with. Ask friends who have recently had a baby to suggest someone. Ask the opinion of a labor-delivery nurse at your local hospital. Various publications, such as the *Directory of Medical Specialties* or the *Directory of the American Medical Association*, are available at most U.S. libraries. In Canada, refer to the *Canadian Medical Directory*. Another healthcare provider, such as a pediatrician or internist, may also provide a reference.

When you pick a healthcare provider, you usually also pick a hospital. Keep the following in mind when choosing where to have your baby.

- Is the facility close by?
- What are the policies regarding your partner and his participation?
- Can he be present if you have a Cesarean delivery?
- Can you have an epidural?
- Is it a birthing center (if that's what you want)?
- Does your HMO (health maintenance organization) or your insurance cover the healthcare provider *and* the hospital?

> You will find many boxes in each weekly discussion; they provide you with information you will *not* find in the text. Our boxes do not repeat information contained in a discussion. Each box is unique, so read them for specific information.

How Your Actions Affect Your Baby's Development

It's never too early to start thinking about how your activities and actions can affect your growing baby. Many substances you normally use may have negative effects on your baby. These substances include drugs, tobacco, alcohol and caffeine. Below are discussions of cigarette smoking and alcohol use. Either of these activities can harm a developing baby. Other substances are discussed throughout the book.

Cigarette Smoking

Smoking cigarettes raises your blood pressure because it narrows blood vessels, reducing the amount of oxygen and nutrients your baby receives. Smoking also causes blood to clot. These two effects are the reason smoking cigarettes is especially harmful during pregnancy.

Over 10% of all pregnant women smoke; some experts put the number at 20%. Smoking is higher among pregnant women under 20 years old and those over 35. A pregnant woman who smokes 20 cigarettes a day (one pack) inhales tobacco smoke more than 11,000 times during an average pregnancy! Cigarette smoke crosses the placenta to the baby; when you smoke, so does your baby!

Nicoderm Patch, Nicorette Gum and Zyban

You may be wondering if you can use the patch, gum or stop-smoking pill during pregnancy to help you stop smoking. We don't know specific effects on a baby if a woman uses any of these devices.

Nicotrol, available as an inhaler, nasal spray, patch or gum, is sold under the brand names *Nicoderm* and *Nicorette;* it's also sold generically. Nicotrol preparations contain nicotine and are *not* recommended for use during pregnancy.

Zyban (bupropion hydrochloride) is an oral medication that is a nonnicotine aid to help a person stop smoking. It's also sold as the antidepressant Wellbutrin or Wellbutrin SR. It's not recommended for pregnant women.

Chantix (varenicline tartrate) is a relatively new prescription medication available to help someone stop smoking. It doesn't contain nicotine, but it's not recommended for pregnant women. Studies show it may reduce a fetus's bone mass and also cause low birthweight.

Nicotine-replacement therapy may be suggested if a woman can't stop smoking on her own. Studies show the benefits of these products may outweigh the risks, but some experts disagree. They don't believe nicotine addiction can be stopped by nicotine, which is contained in sprays, inhalers, patches and gum. Discuss the situation with your healthcare provider if you have questions.

Tobacco smoke contains over 250 harmful substances. These substances may be responsible for damaging a developing baby.

Smokers may have more complications during pregnancy than nonsmokers. Infants born to mothers who smoke weigh less by nearly half a pound.

Some people believe it's OK to use smokeless tobacco during pregnancy. It's not! Use of any smokeless tobacco product contributes to nicotine in the bloodstream, which is one of the main causes of problems.

How Smoking Affects Your Baby and You. Cigarette smoking during pregnancy increases your risk of problems. Smoking also increases risks to your baby. The incidence of SIDS (sudden-infant-death syndrome) after birth may be higher, and babies may be more excitable as infants. The nicotine you take in during pregnancy could lead to nicotine withdrawal in baby after birth.

Smoking during pregnancy has been associated with overweight in the child later in life. In addition, children of smokers are more likely to suffer acute ear infections and respiratory problems. And studies show if you smoke during pregnancy, your child may be a smoker as an adult—babies born to moms who smoke during pregnancy may lean more toward nicotine addiction in the future.

Even if you don't smoke, you may be at risk. Some studies show a *nonsmoker* and her unborn baby exposed to second-hand smoke (cigarette smoke in the air) are exposed to nicotine and other harmful substances. In addition, researchers are now talking about a new threat—*third-hand smoke.* Third-hand smoke occurs when tobacco toxins stick to fabric, hair, skin and other surfaces, such as walls, carpets and floors, even after smoke has disappeared. It can be just as harmful as second-hand smoke. A clue to the presence of third-hand smoke is smell—if you can smell it, it's still there.

If baby's *dad* smoked before conception and smokes during pregnancy, the child has a higher risk of developing problems. If both parents smoke while a child is growing up, that child may have an increased risk of developing leukemia.

Stop Smoking Now. What can you do? The answer sounds simple but isn't—quit smoking. In more realistic terms, if you smoke, cut down or stop smoking before or during pregnancy. Nearly all health insurance policies provide full coverage for at least one type of stop-smoking program. Call your insurance company for further information.

Withdrawal symptoms from smoking are normal, but they're a sign your body is healing. Cravings may be strongest during withdrawal, but after a few weeks, symptoms will decrease.

Maybe your pregnancy can serve as good reason for *everyone* in the family to stop smoking!

Tips to Quit Smoking

- Make a list of things you can do instead of smoking, especially activities that involve using your hands, such as puzzles or needlework.
- List things you'd like to buy for yourself or your baby. Set aside the money you normally spend on cigarettes to buy these items.
- Identify all your "triggers"—what brings on an urge to smoke. Make plans to avoid triggers or to handle them differently.
- Instead of smoking after meals, brush your teeth, wash dishes or go for a walk.
- If you always smoke while driving, clean your car inside and out, and use an air freshener. Sing along with the radio or a CD. Listen to an audiobook. Take a bus, or carpool for a while.
- Drink lots of water.
- If you continue to have trouble stopping, one study determined that using a "quitter's hotline" for help is twice as effective as going it alone. You can talk directly to someone who has been through the same experience. If you're interested, call the National Partnership to Help Pregnant Smokers Quit at (866) 66-START.

Alcohol Use

If you drink alcohol, it carries many risks. In fact, some experts believe alcohol may be one of the worst substances a developing baby can be exposed to.

Moderate drinking has been linked to an increase in problems. Excessive drinking of alcohol during pregnancy may result in birth defects. Alcohol targets central-nervous-system development; a baby may also be born with physical defects. Babies born to mothers who drink while they're pregnant may suffer the effects of their mother's drinking for the rest of their lives.

Drinking during pregnancy has been linked with behavior problems in a child—the more alcohol a woman drinks, the more problems the child may have. Drinking during the first trimester may lead to facial disfigurement. Drinking during the second trimester can interrupt brain development. In the third trimester, drinking alcohol can interfere with development of baby's nervous system.

Taking drugs with alcohol increases the risk of damage to baby. As a safeguard, be very careful about over-the-counter cough and cold remedies. Many contain alcohol—some as much as 25%!

Some pregnant women want to know if they can drink socially. We don't know of any safe amount of alcohol a woman can drink during pregnancy. For the health and well-being of your baby, don't drink *any* alcohol.

Fetal Alcohol Disorders. Your use of alcohol in pregnancy can lead to fetal alcohol syndrome and fetal alcohol exposure in your baby. Both are discussed below. They are considered part of *fetal alcohol spectrum disorder* (FASD), which covers the range of effects that can occur.

Fetal alcohol syndrome (FAS) is characterized by smaller growth before and after birth; heart, limb and facial problems are often seen. An FAS child may also have behavior, speech and motor-function problems. Fifteen to 20% of them die soon after birth. Most studies indicate a woman would have to drink four to five drinks a day for FAS to occur.

Mild defects are the result of *fetal alcohol exposure* (FAE). This condition can result from intake of very little alcohol. The condition has led many researchers to conclude there is *no safe level of alcohol consumption* during pregnancy. For this reason, all alcoholic beverages in the United States carry warning labels similar to those on cigarette packages that advise women to avoid drinking alcohol during pregnancy.

Other Substances to Avoid

Marijuana use by you can disrupt your baby's brain development and can cause many problems. Medical marijuana use during pregnancy is not recommended. Because of known risks, pregnant women should avoid *all* marijuana use.

Cocaine can affect a fetus as early as a few days after conception. It can cause various types of deformities. *Amphetamines*, including methamphetamine, have been blamed for various birth defects. Babies born to mothers who used amphetamines experience withdrawal symptoms.

Your Nutrition

Your nutrition is very important during pregnancy. You will probably need to increase your caloric intake during pregnancy to meet demands. During the first trimester (first 13 weeks), you should eat a total of about 2200 calories a day. During the second and third trimesters, you probably need an additional 300 calories each day.

Extra calories give you energy to support your growing baby. The extra calories keep you going while your body goes through changes. Your baby uses the calories to create and to store protein, fat and carbohydrates. It needs energy for its body processes to function.

You can meet most of your nutritional needs by eating a well-balanced, varied diet. The *quality* of your calories is important. If a food grows in the ground or on a tree (meaning it's fresh), it's probably better for you than if it comes out of a box or can.

Be cautious about adding the extra 300 calories to your nutrition plan—it doesn't mean doubling your portions. A medium apple and a cup of low-fat yogurt add up to 300 calories!

Alcohol in Cooking

Most pregnant women know they should avoid alcohol during pregnancy but what about recipes that call for alcohol? A good rule of thumb is it's probably OK to eat a food that contains alcohol if it has been baked or simmered for at least 1 hour. Cooking for that length of time evaporates most of the alcohol content.

You Should Also Know

Prenatal tests are of two types—screening and diagnostic. *Screening tests* assess your risk of having a baby with a certain birth defect. These tests can provide basic information to determine if more testing is necessary. *Diagnostic testing* can provide nearly definite results. Unfortunately, some prenatal diagnostic tests carry a very small risk of miscarriage. These various tests are described in some of the following weeks.

ൟ *Healthcare Professionals Who May Care for You*

Certified Nurse-Midwives. Many doctors in the United States have certified nurse-midwives on staff. A *certified nurse-midwife* (CNM) is a registered nurse (RN) who has received additional training delivering babies and providing prenatal and postpartum care to women.

In a normal, uncomplicated pregnancy, many or most of your prenatal visits may be with a CNM, not the healthcare provider. This may include labor and delivery. Most women find this is a good thing—often these healthcare providers have more time to spend with you answering questions and addressing your concerns.

A CNM will consult with a physician about specifics of a particular pregnancy and about the labor and delivery of a woman. Most midwives can help you explore birthing methods, including natural childbirth, and pain-relief methods for labor and delivery, including the use of epidurals.

If it's important to you, a midwife may be able to help you make your baby's birth one the entire family can participate in or experience. A certified nurse-midwife can also address issues of family planning and birth-control counseling and other gynecological care, including breast exams, Pap smears and other screenings. CNMs can prescribe medications; each state has specific requirements.

A word of warning—Not all people who call themselves *midwives* are certified nurse-midwives. Some are not even registered nurses. Be sure to check the credentials of any nurse-midwife you are considering for your care.

In the United States, the profession of nurse-midwifery was established in the early 1920s. Before then, midwives had attended births; however, often they were not trained medical professionals. Nurse-midwifery in this country grew out of the Frontier Nursing Service, which provided family health services to rural areas.

The first school for nurse-midwifery graduated its first class in 1933. Today there are over 7000 certified nurse-midwives practicing in all 50 states; they attend nearly 10% of all births, mostly in hospitals. Certified nurse-midwives work in private practice (usually associated with a physician), hospitals, birthing centers and clinics.

To receive certification, a person must hold a bachelor's degree and be a registered nurse. He or she must complete a master's degree or doctorate program from an accredited institution, which usually takes 1 to 4 years. CNMs can be men or women—about 2% of all certified nurse-midwives are male.

Advance-Practice Nurses. An *advance-practice nurse,* also called a *nurse practitioner (NP),* has received postgraduate education in a medical specialty and holds either a master's degree or a doctorate. To be licensed to practice, an NP must be nationally certified in an area of specialty, such as women's health, family health, pediatrics or some other specialty. An NP is licensed through a state nursing board.

Nurse practitioners focus on individualized care, a person's condition and the effects a condition or illness may have on one's life. In a normal, uncomplicated pregnancy, many or most of your prenatal visits may be with a nurse practitioner, not the doctor. This may include labor and delivery. Most women find this is a good thing—often these healthcare providers have more time to spend with you answering questions and addressing your concerns.

Priorities of nurse practitioners include prevention, wellness and education. NPs may also be involved in research.

To be a nurse practitioner in obstetrics and gynecology, a person must be nationally certified and educated to care and treat women's health issues (WHNP). Nurses may also be certified as certified registered nurse anesthetists (CRNAs) and administer anesthetics for various procedures, including pain relief for labor and delivery.

In the United States, state regulations determine whether NPs work independently of doctors or must work with them. Some of the areas in which nurse practitioners work include providing prenatal care and family-planning services, diagnosing and treating illness and disease, doing physical exams, ordering and interpreting medical tests and prescribing medications.

A nurse practitioner may work in various institutions. Some places you may find them include private medical practices, clinics, health centers, urgent-care centers, health maintenance organizations (HMOs) and walk-in clinics.

Physician Assistants. A *physician assistant* or *physician associate (PA)* is a qualified healthcare professional who may take care of you during pregnancy. He or she is licensed to practice medicine in association with a licensed doctor. In a normal, uncomplicated pregnancy, many or most of your prenatal visits may be with a PA, not the doctor. This may include labor and delivery. Most women find this is a good thing—often these healthcare providers have more time to spend with you answering questions and addressing your concerns.

A PA's focus is to provide many health-care services traditionally done by a doctor. Most PAs work in doctors' offices, clinics, urgent care facilities and/or hospitals.

Physician assistants care for people who have conditions (pregnancy is a condition they see women for), diagnose and treat illnesses, order and interpret tests, counsel on preventive health care, perform some procedures, assist in surgery, write prescriptions and do physical exams. A PA is *not* a medical assistant, who performs administrative or simple clinical tasks.

The PA profession was created by a physician at Duke University Medical Center in the mid-1960s because of a shortage of doctors in some areas of the United States. Today, there are over 140 accredited physician-assistant programs in our country.

Physician-assistant training lasts 2 to 3 years after receiving an undergraduate degree. Many schools do not differentiate between the first-year PA students and first-year medical students; they all take classes together.

A graduate of a physician-assistant program receives a master's degree. Some programs also offer a clinical doctorate degree (Doctor of Science Physician Assistant or DScPA). There are also specialty programs or residencies some PAs choose to take to specialize in a certain area. They usually last an additional year.

A PA is licensed by the medical board of each state. After graduating from an accredited program, a PA must pass a qualifying exam-administered Physician Assistant National Certifying Exam (PANCE) before being certified.

Weekly Exercises

Each weekly discussion contains an exercise description and an illustration, if one applies, for safe exercises to do during pregnancy. If you're healthy and have no pregnancy problems, experts agree you can probably exercise moderately for at least 30 minutes three to five times a week. Studies show active pregnant women often have fewer problems during pregnancy and *don't* increase their baby's risk for problems.

If you exercised before pregnancy, continue exercising during pregnancy, at least at moderate intensity. You'll get the same benefits you did before you became pregnant.

Discuss exercising at your first prenatal appointment. Your healthcare provider may have suggestions for your particular situation. Exercises we include in this book are nonweightbearing and should cause few problems, so you can probably do them until your first prenatal visit. Be sure to discuss aerobic and weightbearing exercise with your healthcare provider at that time.

Do these exercises to condition, strengthen and tone various muscle groups, many of which you'll want to strengthen for your comfort during pregnancy. In addition, some of the exercises strengthen muscles you use during labor and delivery. It's never too early to get started!

You may decide to set up a routine of exercises to do, adding and deleting some as you get bigger. Some of the exercises are done standing, some sitting, some kneeling and some lying down. We suggest you leaf through each week and choose the exercises that appeal to you.

We advise every pregnant woman to read and practice the Kegel exercise (Week 14) to help strengthen pelvic-floor muscles. Practicing throughout pregnancy can help in lots of ways, especially with incontinence during and after pregnancy. Actually, it's an exercise *every* woman, no matter what her age, should practice every day.

Chart Your Pregnancy Weight Gain

If you want to chart your pregnancy weight gain, we've provided a chart below for that purpose. Weeks listed are selected based on when you may have a prenatal appointment. If your appointment doesn't fall on that exact week, cross out the number of the week we have listed, and mark in the number of the week you saw your healthcare provider.

Weight before pregnancy begins ____________

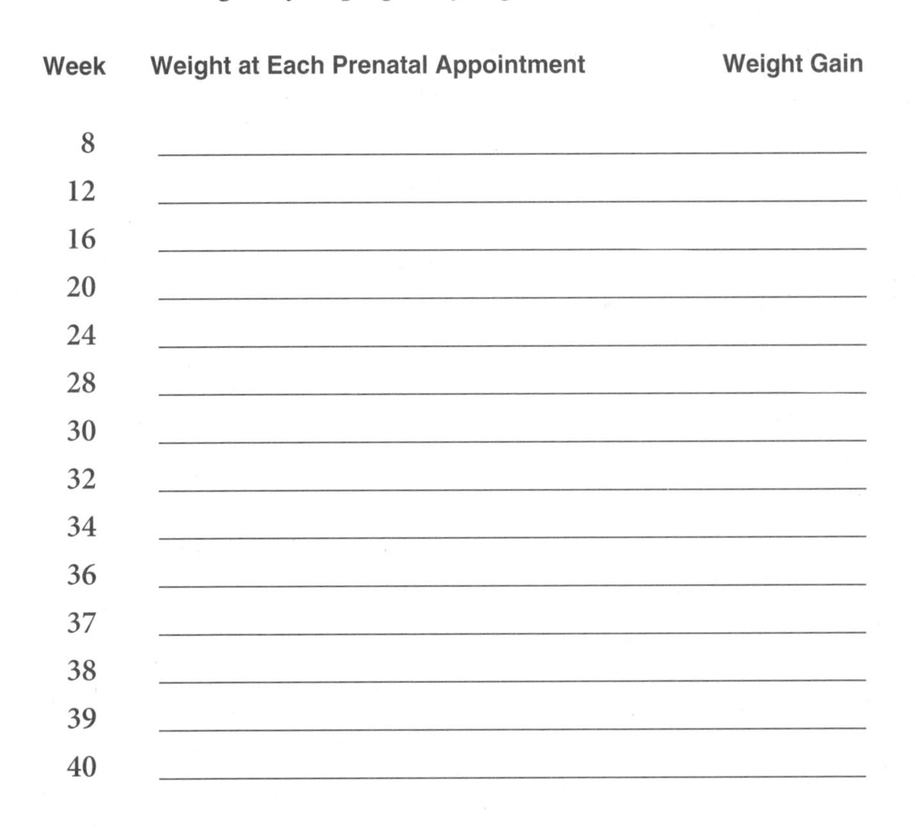

Week	Weight at Each Prenatal Appointment	Weight Gain
8		
12		
16		
20		
24		
28		
30		
32		
34		
36		
37		
38		
39		
40		

Total pregnancy weight gain ____________

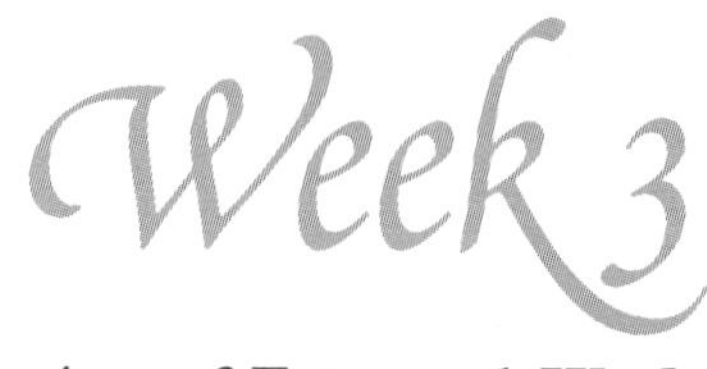

Week 3

Age of Fetus—1 Week

How Big Is Your Baby?

The embryo is very small—at this point, it's only a group of cells, but it's growing rapidly. It's the size of the head of a pin and would be visible to the naked eye if it weren't inside you. The group of cells doesn't look like a fetus or baby; it looks like the illustration on page 44. During this first week, the embryo is about 0.006 inch (0.150mm) long.

How Big Are You?

In this third week of pregnancy, it's too soon to notice any changes. Few women know they have conceived. Remember, you haven't even missed a period yet.

How Your Baby Is Growing and Developing

Fertilization is the joining together of one sperm and an egg. We believe it occurs in the middle part of the Fallopian tube, called the *ampulla,* not inside the uterus. Sperm travel through the uterine cavity and out into the tube to meet the egg.

When the sperm and egg join, the sperm passes through the outer layer of the ovum, the *corona radiata,* then digests its way through another layer of the egg, the *zona pellucida.* Although several sperm may penetrate the outer layers of the egg, usually only one sperm enters the egg and fertilizes it. The membranes of the sperm and egg unite, enclosing them in the same membrane or sac. The egg reacts by making changes in the outer layers so no other sperm can enter.

Once the sperm gets inside the egg, the head of the sperm enlarges and is called the *male pronucleus*; the egg is called the *female pronucleus*. The chromosomes of the male and female pronuclei intermingle.

When this happens, extremely small bits of information and characteristics from each partner are combined. This chromosomal information gives each of us our unique characteristics. The usual number of chromosomes in a human being is 46. Each parent supplies 23 chromosomes. Your baby is a combination of chromosomal information from you and your partner.

The developing ball of cells is called a *zygote*. The zygote passes through the uterine tube on its way to the uterus; the division of cells continues. These cells are called a *blastomere*. As the blastomere divides, a solid ball of cells is formed, called a *morula*. Gradual accumulation of fluid within the morula results in the formation of a *blastocyst*.

During the next week, the blastocyst travels through the uterine tube to the uterus (3 to 7 days after fertilization in the tube). The blastocyst lies free in the uterine cavity as it continues to grow and to develop. About a week after fertilization, it attaches to the uterine cavity (implantation), and cells burrow into the lining of the uterus.

Changes in You

Some women can tell when they ovulate. They may feel mild cramping or pain, or they may have an increased vaginal discharge. Occasionally when the fertilized egg implants in the uterine cavity, a woman may notice a small amount of bleeding.

Boy or Girl?

Your baby's sex is determined at the time of fertilization by the type of sperm (male or female) that fertilizes the egg. A Y-chromosome sperm produces a boy, and an X-chromosome sperm produces a girl.

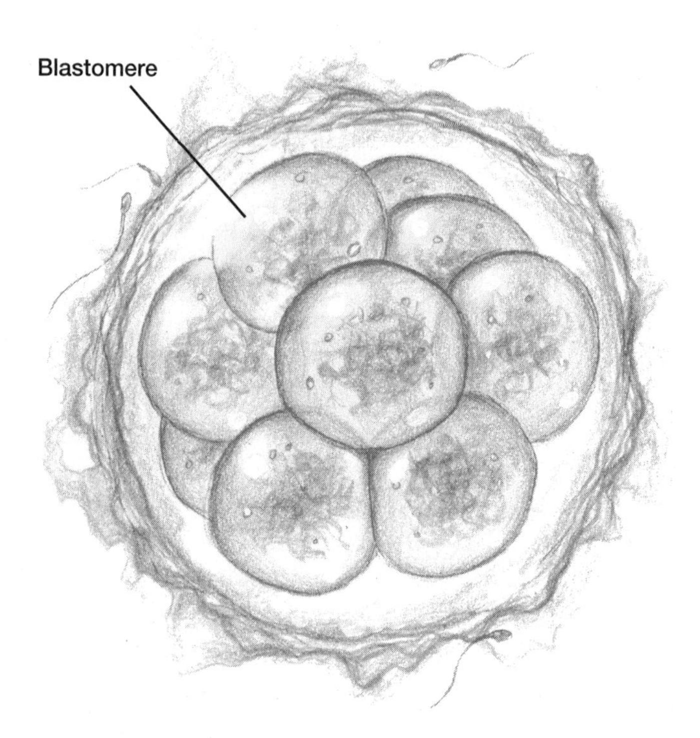

Nine-cell embryo 3 days after fertilization.
The embryo is made up of many blastomeres;
together they form a blastocyst.

It's too early for you to notice many changes. That lies ahead! (See the discussion in Weeks 1 & 2 for signs and symptoms of pregnancy.)

How Your Actions Affect Your Baby's Development

Aspirin Use

We advise caution with the use of aspirin because it can increase bleeding. If you take aspirin during pregnancy, your baby may be at higher risks for some problems.

Studies show aspirin and nonsteroidal anti-inflammatory medications (NSAIDs), such as Advil, Motrin and Aleve, may increase the risk of miscarriage. When taken soon after conception, the risk is highest. Aspirin also causes changes in blood clotting. This is important to know if you bleed during pregnancy or if you're at the end of pregnancy and close to delivery.

Read labels on any medicine you take to see if it contains aspirin. Some OTC antidiarrheal medications have it. It's also important to watch your salicylate intake. Salicylate is contained in Pepto-Bismal, Kaopectate and some skin products.

If you need a pain reliever or fever reducer and can't reach your healthcare provider for advice, acetaminophen (Tylenol) is an over-the-counter medicine you can use for a short while with little fear of problems for you or your baby.

In some cases, small doses of aspirin may be acceptable during pregnancy. However, don't take any aspirin without discussing it with your healthcare provider first!

Taking Aspirin during Pregnancy

There may be situations in which aspirin use is helpful and may be good insurance against some pregnancy problems. Talk to your healthcare provider, if you have questions.

❧ *Exercise during Pregnancy?*

Exercise is important to many pregnant women. In fact, studies show more than 60% of all pregnant women exercise. However, statistics also show that only 15% of pregnant women engage in 30 minutes of moderate exercise five or more times a week.

The aim of exercise during pregnancy is to stay fit. Women who are physically fit are better able to perform the hard work of labor and delivery.

You can benefit from exercise. Exercise can relieve back pain, increase stamina and muscle strength, and improve circulation and flexibility. You may also have less nausea and constipation; you may sleep better, feel less tired and improve your posture.

Exercise can help protect you from illness. Regular exercise may help decrease your risk of developing cardiovascular disease, osteoporosis, depression and obesity. Exercising may also help reduce your chances of having some pregnancy problems. Most pregnant women are advised to exercise moderately for 30 minutes *every* day.

Research shows healthy women who exercised during the first 20 weeks of pregnancy reduced their risk of developing pre-eclampsia by as much as 35%. It's believed exercise may increase growth of the placenta while reducing stress and blood pressure in you.

Exercise may help you control your weight during pregnancy, and you may have an easier time losing weight after pregnancy. You might even return to your prepregnancy shape faster. Research shows if *you* exercise during pregnancy, *your baby* may have a healthier start in life.

Exercise during pregnancy is not without some risk, however, so listen to your body. Risks include increased body temperature, decreased blood flow to the uterus and possible injury to the mother's abdominal area.

There are many types of exercise to choose from; each offers its own advantages. Aerobic exercise is very popular with women who want to stay in shape. Muscle-building exercises are also a popular way to tone muscles and to increase strength. Many women combine the two. Good exercise choices for pregnant women include brisk walking, stationary bicycling, swimming and aerobic exercise designed especially for pregnant women.

Aerobic Exercise. For cardiovascular fitness, aerobic exercise is the best. You must exercise 3 to 5 times a week at a sustained heart rate of 110 to 120 beats a minute, maintained for at least 15 continuous minutes. (The rate of 110 to 120 beats a minute is an approximate target for people of different ages.) Doing low-impact aerobics for at least 2 hours a week may help reduce your risk of pregnancy problems.

Tip for Week 3

Before you begin any exercise program, discuss it with your healthcare provider. Together you can develop a program that takes into account your level of conditioning and your exercise habits.

If you exercised aerobically before pregnancy, you can probably continue aerobic exercise but at a lower rate to avoid problems. Now is *not* the time to try to set new records or to train for an upcoming marathon. If you have any questions, talk them over with your healthcare provider at your first prenatal visit.

Don't start a strenuous aerobic exercise program or increase training during pregnancy. If you haven't been involved in regular, strenuous exercise before pregnancy, walking and swimming are probably about as involved as you should get with exercise.

There are some precautions to take if you exercise. Don't let your body temperature rise above 102F (38.9C). Aerobic exercise and/or dehydration can raise your body temperature higher than this, so be careful. Keep workouts short, especially during hot weather.

We used to recommend a pregnant woman keep her heart rate under 140bpm during exercise. However, today ACOG's recommendation is for a pregnant woman to exercise 30 minutes a day, without a specific heart-rate limit.

If you feel tired, *don't* skip a workout! Instead, decrease how hard you exercise or for how long. Sometimes stretching may be all you're up for. Try to stretch at least a couple of times a week. Stretching may lower stress levels and help calm you.

You will find many boxes in each weekly discussion, which will provide you with information you will *not* find in the text. Our boxes do not repeat information contained in a discussion. Each box is unique, so read them for specific information.

Muscle Strength. Some women exercise for muscle strength. To strengthen a muscle, there has to be resistance against it. There are three different kinds of muscle contractions—isotonic, isometric and isokinetic. *Isotonic exercise* involves shortening the muscle as tension is developed, such as when you lift a weight. *Isometric exercise* causes the muscle to develop tension but doesn't change its length, such as when you push against a stationary wall. *Isokinetic exercise* occurs when the muscle moves at a constant speed, such as when you swim.

Cardiac and bone muscles cannot usually be strengthened at the same time. Strengthening bone muscles requires lifting heavy weights, but you can't lift these heavy weights long enough to strengthen your heart.

If you're doing free weights, sit down when you can. Wear some type of tummy support. In your third trimester, don't lift more than 15 pounds of weight. Instead, increase the number of reps.

Weightbearing exercise is the most effective way of increasing bone density to help avoid osteoporosis. Other advantages of strengthening exercises include flexibility, coordination and improvement in mood and alertness. Stretching and warming up muscles before exercising and cooling down after exercising help you improve flexibility and avoid injury.

Other Types of Exercise. There are other types of exercise you might enjoy. A balance ball may be a good choice. Exercising on a big exercise ball is easier on your back, and it strengthens core muscles. Some women use them during labor to help relieve pain!

Pregnancy yoga or Pilates classes may be good choices during your first trimester. Ten minutes of yoga or Pilates increases your blood flow and stretches your muscles.

Try water aerobics to help relieve back and pelvic pain. Even doing it only once a week may help reduce pain.

General Exercise Guidelines. Before beginning any exercise program, consult your healthcare provider. If you get the go-ahead, begin exercising gradually. Start with 15-minute workout sessions, with 5-minute rest periods in between.

Check your heart rate every 15 minutes. Count the number of heartbeats by feeling the pulse in your neck or wrist for 15 seconds. Multiply by 4. If your pulse is too high, rest until your pulse drops below 90 bpm.

Allow enough time to warm up and to cool down. Break workouts into smaller increments to fit them into your day. Four 10-minute walks may be easier to accomplish than one 40-minute walk.

Wear comfortable clothing during exercise, including clothing that is warm enough or cool enough, and good, comfortable athletic shoes with maximum support. Drink water before, during and after exercising. Dehydration may cause contractions.

> ### Dad Tip
> **Your partner will be experiencing a lot during these next 9 months. She will experience many physical changes. A pregnant woman may have morning sickness, heartburn, indigestion, fatigue and other common discomforts. Occasionally, something serious occurs. It's helpful to know what changes *you* may be faced with. To that end, we recommend you read our book written just for you—*Your Pregnancy for the Father-to-Be*.**

You may feel better if you can remember to contract your abdomen and buttocks to help support your lower back. Never hold your breath while you exercise, and don't get overheated. Step-up the number of calories you eat.

When you're pregnant, be careful about getting up and lying down. After 16 weeks of pregnancy, don't lie on your back while exercising. This can decrease blood flow to the uterus and placenta. When you finish exercising, lie on your left side for 15 to 20 minutes.

Avoid risky sports, such as horseback riding or water skiing. Spinning—a high-intensity stationary cycling workout—may not be recommended during pregnancy because it may cause dehydration and a rapid heart rate. If you are an experienced spinner, talk to your healthcare provider about it at a prenatal visit.

Possible Problems. Stop exercising and consult your healthcare provider if you experience bleeding or loss of fluid from the vagina while exercising, shortness of breath, dizziness, severe abdominal pain or any other pain or discomfort. Consult your healthcare provider, and exercise only under his or her supervision, if you experience (or know you have) an irregular heartbeat, high blood pressure, diabetes, thyroid disease, anemia or any other chronic medical problem. Talk to your healthcare provider about exercise if you have a history of three or more miscarriages, an incompetent cervix, intrauterine-growth restriction (IUGR), premature labor or any abnormal bleeding during pregnancy.

Your Nutrition

Folic-Acid Use

Folic acid, also referred to as *folate*, *folacin* or *vitamin* B_9, is very important during pregnancy. *Folate* is the form of folic acid found in food. *Folic acid* is the synthetic version of this B vitamin. It's important to take folic acid before trying to get pregnant and during early pregnancy because this is when it is most helpful.

Taking folic acid is good for you *and* baby. We know diabetic women may benefit from taking in higher levels of folic acid. Other benefits of taking folic acid include reducing *your* risks of developing asthma and allergies.

Folic acid may help prevent problems in a baby. Neural-tube defects can occur in a baby during early pregnancy, often before you even suspect you might be pregnant. There are various types of neural-tube defects—the most common is spina bifida, when the base of the spine remains open, exposing the spinal cord and nerves.

Studies show taking folic acid before pregnancy and in early pregnancy may help prevent or decrease the incidence of neural-tube defects. Once pregnancy is confirmed, it may be too late to prevent neural-tube problems.

Your Folic-Acid Intake. A pregnant woman's body excretes four or five times the normal amount of folic acid. Folic acid isn't stored in the body for long, so you need to replace it every day. A prenatal vitamin contains 0.8mg to 1mg of folic acid. This is usually enough for a woman with a normal pregnancy. Researchers believe you can help prevent spina bifida if you take 400mcg (0.4mg) of folic acid a day, beginning before pregnancy and continuing through the first 13 weeks. This is suggested for all pregnant women.

A folic-acid deficiency can result in anemia in you. Extra folic acid may be needed with multiple fetuses or if you suffer from Crohn's disease.

Some researchers suggest a woman take 400mcg of folic acid before pregnancy and increase that amount to 600mcg when pregnancy is confirmed. Others recommend a dose of 1mg a day of folic acid, perhaps more, is necessary. Still others believe if a woman is at risk for having a baby with neural-tube defects (she had a baby before with the problem or she has epilepsy, diabetes or certain types of thrombophilia), she should take 4mg a day. Talk to your healthcare provider about it.

We know some medications interfere with folic-acid metabolism. These medicines include aminopterin, carbamazepine, methotrexate, phenytoin, phenobarbital, diphenylhydantoin and trimethoprim-sulfa (Septra, Bactrim).

Smoking cigarettes removes folic acid from the body. Second-hand smoke can also reduce folic-acid levels. In addition, drinking green tea can keep your body from absorbing folic acid, so avoid it.

Foods Supplemented with Folic Acid. Beginning in 1998, the U.S. government ordered that some grain products, including flour, breakfast cereals and pasta, be fortified with folic acid. It's made a difference! The number of babies born with neural-tube defects has decreased by nearly 20% since the program began. But many babies of Hispanic women are still at risk. Studies show nearly twice as many are born with neural-tube defects. One reason may be that many Hispanic grain foods are *not* fortified with folic acid.

Eating 1 cup of fortified breakfast cereal, with milk, and drinking a glass of orange juice supplies about half of your folic-acid requirement for one day. Folate is found naturally in many foods, such as fruits, legumes, brewer's yeast, soybeans, whole-grain products and dark, leafy vegetables. A well-balanced diet can help you reach your folic-acid-intake goal. Also see the list of foods that are good folate sources in Preparing for Pregnancy.

You Should Also Know

Bleeding and Spotting during Pregnancy

Bleeding and spotting during pregnancy cause concern. *Bleeding* is vaginal bleeding that is usually as heavy as, or heavier than, a menstrual period. *Spotting* is vaginal bleeding that is usually lighter than a regular menstrual period.

In the first trimester, bleeding or spotting can make you worry about the well-being of your baby and the possibility of miscarriage. As your uterus grows, the placenta forms and vascular connections are made, and bleeding may occur then. During the second trimester, bleeding may happen with sexual intercourse or a vaginal exam. Bleeding during the third trimester can be a sign of placenta previa or the onset of labor.

If you experience any type of bleeding during pregnancy, it is *not* unusual. Some researchers estimate 20% of all pregnant women bleed during the first trimester. But not all women who bleed have a miscarriage.

Call your healthcare provider if you experience any bleeding. If bleeding causes your healthcare provider concern, he or she may order an ultrasound exam. Sometimes ultrasound can show a reason for bleed-

> Strenuous exercise or intercourse may cause some bleeding. If this occurs, stop your activities and check with your healthcare provider.

ing, but during early pregnancy, there may be no detectable reason for it.

Most healthcare providers suggest resting, decreasing activity and avoiding intercourse if bleeding occurs. Surgery or medication are not helpful and probably won't make much difference.

Benefits of Pregnancy

- Allergy and asthma sufferers may feel better during pregnancy because the natural steroids produced during pregnancy help reduce symptoms.
- Pregnancy may help protect against ovarian cancer. The younger a woman is when she starts having babies, and the more pregnancies she has, the greater the benefit.
- Migraine headaches often disappear during the second and third trimesters.
- Menstrual cramps are a thing of the past during pregnancy. An added benefit—they may not return after baby is born!
- Endometriosis (when endometrial tissue attaches to parts of the ovaries and other sites outside the uterus) causes pelvic pain, heavy bleeding and other problems during menstruation for some women. Pregnancy can stop the growth of endometriosis.
- Having a baby may protect you against breast cancer. Researchers believe the high levels of protein secreted by the growing baby may be associated with a lower risk for younger moms. The protein may interfere with estrogen's role in causing breast cancer.

Exercise for Week 3

Stand a couple of feet away from a wall, with your hands in front of your shoulders. Place your hands on the wall, and lean forward. Bend your elbows as your body leans into the wall. Keep your heels flat on the floor. Slowly push away from the wall, and stand straight. Do 10 to 20 times. *Develops upper-back, chest and arm strength, and relieves lower-leg tension.*

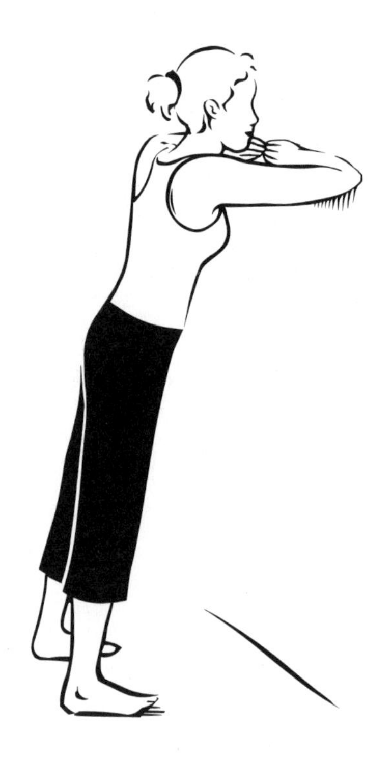

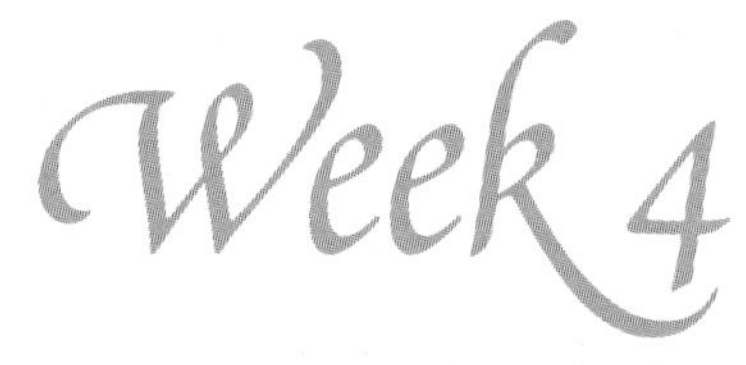

Week 4

Age of Fetus—2 Weeks

If you've just found out you're pregnant,
you might want to begin by reading the previous chapters.

How Big Is Your Baby?

Your developing baby's size varies from 0.014 inch to about 0.04 inch (0.36mm to about 1mm) in length. One millimeter is half the size of a letter "o" on this page.

How Big Are You?

At this point, your pregnancy doesn't show. The illustration on page 57 gives you an idea of how small your baby is, so you can see why you won't notice any changes yet.

How Your Baby Is Growing and Developing

Fetal development is still in the very early stages, but great changes are taking place! The blastocyst is embedded more deeply into the lining of your uterus, and the amniotic sac, which will fill with amniotic fluid, is starting to form.

The placenta is forming; it plays an important role in hormone production and transport of oxygen and nutrients. Networks that contain maternal blood are becoming established. Development of the baby's nervous system (brain and other structures, such as the spinal cord) begins.

Germ layers are developing. They develop into specialized parts of your baby's body, such as organs. The three germ layers are the *ectoderm, endoderm* and *mesoderm.*

The ectoderm becomes the nervous system (including the brain), the skin and the hair. The endoderm develops into the lining of the gastrointestinal tract, the liver, pancreas and thyroid. The mesoderm becomes the skeleton, connective tissues, blood system, urogenital system and most of the muscles.

Changes in You

You're probably expecting a period around the end of this week. When it doesn't occur, pregnancy may be one of the first things you think of.

The Corpus Luteum

The area on the ovary where the egg comes from is called the *corpus luteum.* If you become pregnant, it is called the *corpus luteum of pregnancy.* The corpus luteum forms immediately after ovulation at the site where the egg is released. It looks like a small sac of fluid. It rapidly changes in preparation for producing hormones, such as progesterone, to support a pregnancy before the placenta takes over.

We believe the corpus luteum is important in the early weeks of pregnancy because it produces progesterone. The placenta takes over this function between 8 and 12 weeks of pregnancy. Around the sixth month of pregnancy, the corpus luteum shrinks.

Tip for Week 4

Second- and third-hand smoke may harm a nonsmoking woman and her developing baby. Ask those who smoke to refrain from smoking around you during your pregnancy and avoid places where people smoke.

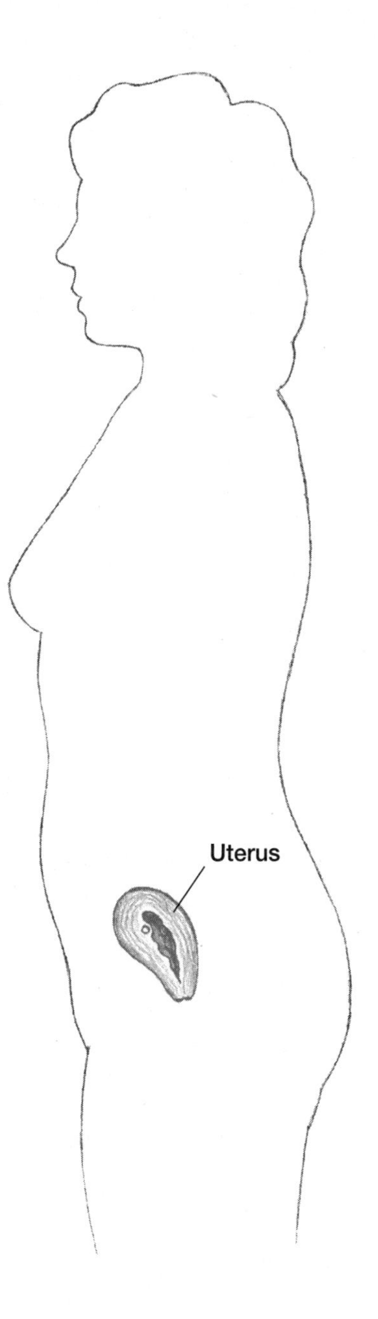

Pregnancy at around 4 weeks
(fetal age—2 weeks).

How Your Actions Affect Your Baby's Development

During pregnancy, nearly every parent worries about whether their baby will be perfect. Most parents worry unnecessarily. Major birth defects occur in few births. Most birth defects occur during the first trimester (the first 13 weeks of pregnancy).

Structural birth defects occur when some part of the baby's body is not formed correctly or is missing. Heart defects and neural-tube defects are common structural defects.

Genetic defects are caused by a mistake in a gene. Some are inherited; others occur when the egg and sperm join. *Exposure to certain chemicals*, such as medicines, alcohol, drugs or toxic agents, such as radiation, lead or mercury, account for other birth defects. Additional defects may occur if a pregnant woman is exposed to a particular infection, such as rubella (German measles).

By the time you miss a period, 80% of baby's organ development has already occurred.

Teratology is the study of abnormal fetal development. A *teratogen* is a substance that can cause birth defects. Those who care for pregnant women are often asked about substances that may be harmful.

Some substances may cause major defects if exposure occurs at a specific time in fetal development, but they may not be harmful at other times. By the 13th week, baby has completed major development. After that time, the effect of a substance may be smaller growth or smaller organ size. One example is rubella. It can cause birth defects, such as heart malformations, if the baby is infected during the first trimester. Rubella infection later in pregnancy is less serious.

Women's responses to substances, and the amount they are exposed to, vary greatly. Alcohol is a good example. Large amounts appear to have no effect on some babies, while other babies can be harmed by very low amounts.

Animal studies provide much of our information, which can be helpful but cannot always be applied to humans. Other data comes from situations in which women were exposed who didn't know they were pregnant or that a particular substance could be harmful. Information gathered from these cases is difficult to apply directly to a particular pregnancy.

Medicine and Drug Use

Information about the effects of a specific medication or drug on a pregnancy comes from cases of exposure before the pregnancy was discovered. These "case reports" help researchers understand possible harmful effects but leave gaps in our knowledge. For this reason, it can be difficult to make exact statements about a particular substance and its effect. The chart on pages 60 and 61 lists *possible effects* of drugs and other substances.

Grandma's Remedy

If you want to avoid using medication, try a folk remedy. To help relieve constipation, drink an 8-ounce glass of water with 2 teaspoons of apple-cider vinegar. Drink one glass in the morning and another at night.

If you use drugs, be honest with your healthcare provider. Tell him or her about anything you take or have taken that may affect your baby. The victim of drug use is your baby. A drug problem may have serious consequences that can be best dealt with if your healthcare provider knows about your drug use in advance.

Your Nutrition

You probably won't be able to eat all you want during pregnancy, unless you are one of the lucky women who doesn't have a problem with calories. Even then, you must pay strict attention to the types of foods you choose.

Eat nutritious foods. Avoid those with empty calories (lots of sugar and fat). Choose fresh fruits and vegetables. Avoid caffeine when possible. We discuss many of these subjects in later weeks.

Effects of Various Substances on Fetal Development

Many substances can affect your baby's early development. Below is a list of various substances and their effects on a developing fetus.

Substance	Possible Effects on Your Baby
Alcohol	fetal abnormalities, fetal alcohol disorders, intrauterine-growth restriction (IUGR)
Amphetamines	placental abruption, IUGR, fetal death
Androgens male	ambiguous genital development (depends on dose given and when given)
Angiotensin-converting enzyme (ACE) inhibitors (enalapril, captopril)	fetal and neonatal death
Anticoagulants	bone and hand abnormalities, IUGR, central-nervous-system and eye abnormalities
Antithyroid drugs (propylthiouracil, iodide, methimazole)	hypothyroidism, fetal goiter
Barbiturates	possible birth defects, withdrawal symptoms, poor eating habits, seizures
Benzodiazepines (including Valium and Librium)	increased chance of congenital malformations
Caffeine	decreased birthweight, smaller head size, breathing problems, sleeplessness, irritability, jitters, poor calcium metabolism, IUGR, mental retardation, microcephaly, various major malformations
Carbamazepine	birth defects, spina bifida
Chemotherapeutic drugs (methotrexate, aminopterin)	increased risk of miscarriage
Cocaine/crack	miscarriage, stillbirth, congenital defects, severe deformities in a fetus, long-term mental deficiencies, sudden infant death syndrome (SIDS)
Coumadin derivatives (warfarin)	hemorrhage (bleeding), birth defects, an increase in miscarriage and stillbirth
Cyclophosphomide	transient sterility
Diethylstilbestrol (DES)	abnormalities of reproductive organs (females and males), infertility
Ecstasy	long-term learning problems, memory problems
Folic-acid antagonists (methotrexate, aminopterin)	fetal death and birth defects
Glues and solvents	birth defects, including shortened stature, low birthweight, small head, joint and limb problems, abnormal facial features, heart defects

(continues)

Substance	Possible Effects on Your Baby
Iodine-131 (after 10 weeks)	adverse effects of radiation, growth restriction, birth defects
Isotretinoin (Accutane)	increased miscarriage rate, nervous-system defects, facial defects, cleft palate
Ketamine	behavioral problems, learning problems
Lead	increased miscarriage and stillbirth rates
Lithium	congenital heart disease
Marijuana and hashish	attention-deficit disorder (ADD), attention-deficit hyperactivity disorder (ADHD), memory problems, impaired decision-making ability
Methamphetamines	IUGR, difficulty bonding, tremors, extreme fussiness
Misoprostol	skull defects, cranial-nerve palsies, facial malformations, limb defects
Nicotine	miscarriage, stillbirth, neural-tube defects, low birthweight, lower IQ, reading disorders, minimal-brain dysfunction syndrome (hyperactivity)
Opioids (morphine, heroin, Demerol)	congenital abnormalities, premature birth, IUGR, withdrawal symptoms in baby
Organic mercury	cerebral atrophy, mental retardation, spasticity, seizures, blindness
PCBs	possible neurological problems
Phenytoin (Dilantin)	IUGR, microcephaly
Progestins (high dose)	masculinization of female fetus
Streptomycin	hearing loss, cranial-nerve damage
Tetracycline	hypoplasia of tooth enamel, discoloration of permanent teeth
Thalidomide	severe limb defects
Trimethadione	cleft lip, cleft palate, IUGR, miscarriage
Valproic acid	neural-tube defects
Vitamin A and derivatives (isotretinoin, etritinate, retinoids)	fetal death and birth defects
X-ray therapy	microcephaly, mental retardation, leukemia

(Modified from A.C.O.G. Technical Bulletin 236, Teratology, American College of Obstetricians and Gynecologists)

You Should Also Know

Weight Gain

You must be prepared to gain weight. It's necessary for your health and the health of your growing baby. Getting on the scale and seeing your weight rise may be very hard for you. Recognize now it's OK to gain weight. You don't have to let yourself go; control your weight by eating

You may be eating for two during pregnancy, but you don't have to eat twice as much, just twice as smart!

carefully and nutritiously. But you *need* to gain enough weight to meet the needs of your pregnancy.

Many years ago, women were not allowed to gain much weight—sometimes only 12 to 15 pounds for their entire pregnancy! Today, we know restricting weight gain to this extent is not healthy for the baby or the mother-to-be.

However, you shouldn't gain too much weight. Researchers have found that normal-weight women who gained more than 38 pounds during pregnancy with one baby were at higher risk for developing breast cancer after menopause. Not shedding those extra pounds after pregnancy also contributed to a higher risk.

Dad Tip

Make it a habit to pull out your favorite pregnancy book, such as *Your Pregnancy Week by Week*, and read together about what is happening each week in your pregnancy.

The amount of weight you gain during the first trimester has been tied to the size of your baby at birth. If you gain a lot of weight during the first trimester, your baby may be big. On the other hand, if you don't gain very much weight in early pregnancy, you may have a smaller baby.

Environmental Pollutants and Pregnancy

An environment that is healthful for you will be healthy for your developing baby. Some environmental pollutants may be harmful to you and baby. It's important to avoid exposure to them. The box on page 63 lists specific pollutants to avoid.

There isn't much clear information on the safety of many chemicals. It's best to avoid exposure when possible, but it may not be possible to keep away from every chemical. If you know you'll be around various chemicals, wash your hands well before eating. Not smoking cigarettes also helps. If you have a dog or cat that wears a flea collar, don't touch the collar.

Some latex paints contain lead. You may not want to use some oil-based paints and some solvents. Solvents are chemicals that dissolve other substances. Read labels.

Drinking water may contain lead if your home has brass faucets, lead pipes or lead solder on copper pipes. You can call your state health department and ask them to test your water. Run water for 30 seconds before you use it to reduce levels of lead; cold water contains less lead than hot water.

If you use crystal goblets, they contain lead. Some scented candles have wicks that contain lead. You could increase your exposure to lead with either.

Arsenic may be hiding outdoors in your back yard—furniture, decks and play sets made from pressure-treated lumber may be preserved

Some Pollutants to Avoid during Pregnancy

The toxicity of *lead* has been known for centuries. In the past, most lead exposure came from the atmosphere. Today, exposure comes from many sources, including water pipes, solders, storage batteries, construction materials, paints, dyes and wood preservatives.

Lead is easily transported across the placenta to the baby. Toxicity can occur as early as the 12th week of pregnancy, which could result in lead poisoning in the baby. If you might be exposed to lead in your workplace, discuss it with your physician.

Mercury has a long history as a potential poison to a pregnant woman. Reports of fish contaminated with mercury have been linked to cerebral palsy and microcephaly.

Our environment has been significantly contaminated with *PCBs* (polychlorinated biphenyls). PCBs are mixtures of several chemical compounds. Most fish, birds and humans now have measurable amounts of PCB in their tissues. This is one reason to limit your intake of fish during pregnancy.

Pesticides cover a large number of agents used to control unwanted plants and animals. Human exposure is common because pesticides are used extensively. Those of most concern contain several agents—DDT, chlordane, heptachlor, lindane and others.

with chromated copper arsenate. Wash your hands thoroughly after you've been outside, and cover picnic tables with tablecloths when you eat on them. Apply a polyurethane sealant once a year.

Do You Take Paxil?

If you take the antidepressant Paxil, discuss its use with your healthcare provider immediately. You may need to start other treatment options early in pregnancy. But ***don't stop*** taking any antidepressant medication without consulting your healthcare provider.

Paxil belongs to a class of medications called *selective serotonin reuptake inhibitors,* sometimes abbreviated as SSRIs. There is continued concern about the safety of Paxil during pregnancy. Paxil use in the first and third trimesters may put your baby at risk.

Certified Nurse-Midwives, Advance-Practice Nurses and Physician Assistants

In today's obstetric-and-gynecology medical practices, you may find many types of highly qualified people taking care of you. These people—mostly women, but not all!—are on the forefront in guiding couples through pregnancy to delivery.

In a normal, uncomplicated pregnancy, many or most of your prenatal visits may be with a certified nurse-midwife, advance-practice nurse or physician assistant, not the doctor. This may include labor and delivery. Most women find this is a good thing—often these healthcare providers have more time to spend with you answering questions and addressing your concerns.

A *certified nurse-midwife (CNM)* is an advance-practice registered nurse (RN). He or she has received additional training delivering babies and providing prenatal and postpartum care to women. A CNM works closely with a doctor or team of healthcare providers to address specifics about a particular pregnancy, and labor and delivery. Often a CNM delivers babies.

A certified midwife can provide many types of information to a pregnant woman, such as guidance with nutrition and exercise, ways to deal with pregnancy discomforts, tips for managing weight gain, dealing with various pregnancy problems and discussions of different methods of pain relief for

(continues)

labor and delivery. A CNM can also address issues of family planning and birth-control and other gynecological care, including breast exams, Pap smears and other screenings. In some cases, a CNM may prescribe medications.

An *advance-practice nurse (APN)* is an advance-practice registered nurse (RN). He or she has received additional training providing prenatal and post-partum care to women. An advance-practice nurse may work with a doctor or work independently to address specifics about a woman's pregnancy, and labor and delivery.

An APN can provide many types of information to a pregnant woman, such as guidance with nutrition and exercise, ways to deal with pregnancy discomforts, tips for managing weight gain, dealing with various pregnancy problems and discussions of different methods of pain-relief for labor and delivery. He or she can also address issues of family planning and birth-control and other gynecological care, including breast exams, Pap smears and other screenings. A nurse practitioner may prescribe medications or provide pain relief during labor and delivery (as a certified registered nurse anesthetist [CRNA]).

A *physician assistant* or *physician associate (PA)* is licensed to practice medicine with the supervision of a licensed doctor. A PA's focus is to provide many health-care services traditionally done by a doctor. Most PAs work in doctors' offices, clinics or hospitals.

Physician assistants care for people who have conditions (pregnancy is a condition they see women for), diagnose and treat illnesses, order and interpret tests, counsel on preventive health care, assist in surgery, write prescriptions and do physical exams. A PA is *not* a medical assistant, who performs administrative or simple clinical tasks.

We are fortunate to have these dedicated professionals working in OB/GYN practices and clinics. The care they provide is crucial to the medical community and makes quality medical care for women something every woman can look forward to.

Exercise for Week 4

Sit on the floor, bring your feet close to your body and cross your ankles. Apply gentle pressure to your knees or the inside of your thighs. See illustration. Hold for a count of 10, relax and repeat. Do this exercise 4 or 5 times. Then place your hands under your knees, and gently press down with your knees while resisting the pressure with your hands. See illustration. Count to 5, then relax. Increase the number of presses until you can do 10 presses twice a day. *Develops pelvic-floor strength and quadricep strength.*

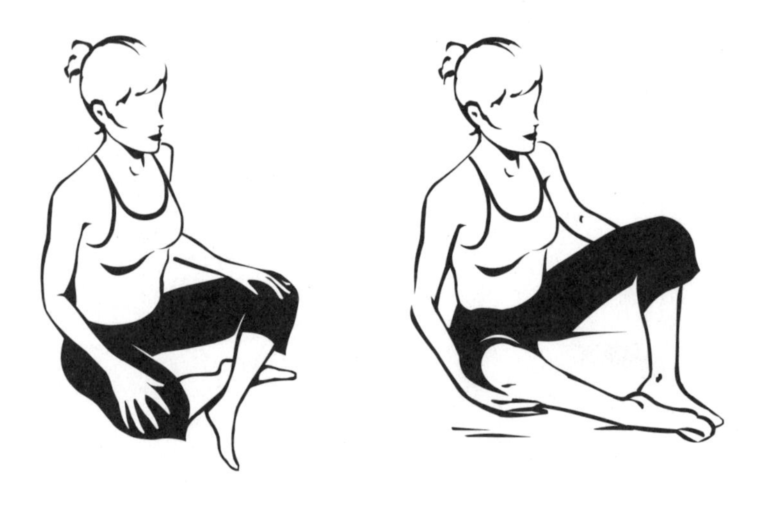

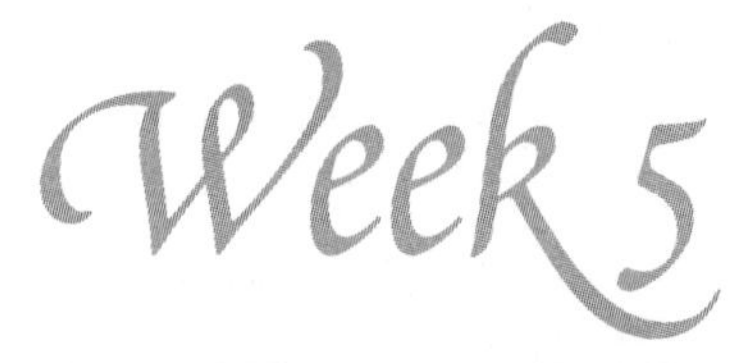

Week 5

Age of Fetus—3 Weeks

If you've just found out you're pregnant, you might want to begin by reading the previous chapters.

How Big Is Your Baby?

Your developing baby hasn't grown a lot. By this week, it's about 0.05 inch (1.25mm) long.

How Big Are You?

At this point, there are still no big changes in you. Even if you are aware you're pregnant, it will be a while before others notice your changing figure.

How Your Baby Is Growing and Developing

As early as this week, a plate that will become the heart has developed. Two tubes join to form the heart, and it begins to contract by day 22 of development. A beating heart is visible as early as 5 to 6 weeks of pregnancy during an ultrasound examination.

Eyes first appear around this time and look like a pair of shallow grooves on each side of the developing brain. These grooves continue to develop and eventually turn into pockets called *optical vesicles.* Early in development, eyes are on the side of the head.

The central nervous system (brain and spinal cord) and muscle and bone formation continue. During this time, baby's skeleton is starting to form.

Changes in You

Home pregnancy tests are very sensitive, which makes early diagnosis of pregnancy possible. Tests detect the presence of *human chorionic gonadotropin* (HCG), a hormone of early pregnancy. A pregnancy test can be positive before you have even missed a period! Some brands of at-home pregnancy tests can pick up lower levels of HCG than others. A couple of at-home pregnancy tests, *First Response* and *Early Result Pregnancy Test,* may be more sensitive than others. For women who want to test early, these products may be good choices.

Many tests can provide positive results (you're pregnant) 10 days after you conceive. You might want to wait until you miss a period before investing money and emotional energy in any pregnancy test.

The best time to take a home pregnancy test is the first day after your missed period or any time thereafter. If you take the test too early, you may get a result that says you aren't pregnant when you really are! This happens for about 50% of the women who take the test *very early.*

Nausea and Vomiting

An early symptom of pregnancy for some women is nausea, with or without vomiting; it is often called *morning sickness.* About half of all pregnant women experience nausea and vomiting, about 25% of pregnant women have nausea only and 25% experience no symptoms. You may get morning sickness if you suffer from motion sickness or migraines before pregnancy. If you're going to get morning sickness, it usually appears before the 12th week of pregnancy.

> If your sense of smell becomes more intense during pregnancy, it may add to the problem of morning sickness.

There is good news about morning sickness—women with nausea and vomiting in pregnancy have a lower incidence of miscarriage. The sicker you are, the less chance you will miscarry.

Morning sickness can occur in the morning or later in the day. It often starts early and improves during the day as you become active. The condition may begin around the 6th week of pregnancy.

Take heart—morning sickness usually improves and disappears around the end of the first trimester (week 13). Hang in there, and keep in mind that this is all temporary.

Morning sickness can affect your pregnancy weight gain. For many women with morning sickness, weight gain may not begin until the beginning of the second trimester, when nausea and vomiting often pass.

If morning sickness is wearing you down, call your healthcare provider. Ask about different ways to deal with it. Reassurances that this situation is normal and your baby is OK can be comforting.

Hyperemesis Gravidarum. Nausea doesn't usually cause enough trouble to require medical attention. However, a condition called *hyperemesis gravidarum* (severe nausea and vomiting) causes a lot of vomiting, which results in loss of nutrients and fluid.

You have hyperemesis gravidarum if you're unable to keep down 80 ounces of fluid in 24 hours, if you lose more than 2 pounds a week or 5% of your prepregnancy weight, or if you vomit blood or bile. Contact your healthcare provider immediately!

Only 1 to 2% of all pregnant women experience hyperemesis gravidarum. Very high levels of nausea-inducing hormones may be one cause.

If symptoms are severe, call your healthcare provider's office as soon as possible. Even though your first prenatal appointment may not be scheduled for a while, there's no reason to suffer. Your healthcare provider will want to know about the problem. You may have to ask to be seen sooner than a normal first prenatal appointment so you can find some relief.

Studies show if you experience hyperemesis gravidarum, your chance of having a daughter increases by more than 75%. Experts believe the cause may be an overabundance of female hormones produced by the baby and mom-to-be in the first trimester.

If you experience severe nausea and vomiting, if you cannot eat or drink anything or if you feel so ill you can't carry on your daily activities, call your healthcare provider. Call if your urine is dark, you produce little urine, you feel dizzy when you stand up, your heart races or pounds, or you vomit blood or bile.

In severe cases, a woman may need to be treated in the hospital with intravenous fluids and medications. Hypnosis has also been used successfully in treating the problem.

Hyperemesis after Pregnancy? It has been commonly believed that symptoms associated with hyperemesis gravidarum disappear after pregnancy. This is the case for most women, but a few women will have problems even after baby's birth.

Studies show some women with severe hyperemesis gravidarum can experience symptoms well beyond delivery that can take months to overcome. Symptoms include food aversions, gastroesophageal reflux (GERD), digestive problems, nausea, gallbladder issues, fatigue and muscle weakness. Women who received I.V. feedings during pregnancy because they couldn't eat had the highest rate of symptoms.

Recovery can take a few months to as long as 2 years. Some believe it takes 1 to 2 months of recovery for *every month* you were ill. Women who have nausea and/or vomiting into late pregnancy find it usually takes several months to regain their energy and restore nutritional reserves.

If your hyperemesis gravidarum persists after baby's birth, you may need to see a nutritionist. Talk to your healthcare provider about it. It is especially important to seek help before you plan another pregnancy.

Tip for Week 5

Pregnancy may affect your sense of smell. You may smell odors more intensely; odors that do not normally affect you may now smell bad. If you're sensitive to the smell of food, try eating a piece of cheddar, cottage cheese, dry-roasted nuts or cold chicken.

A *ReliefBand* may help relieve morning sickness. It's worn like a wrist watch on the inside of your wrist and stimulates nerves with gentle electric signals. This stimulation is believed to interfere with messages between the brain and stomach that cause nausea. It has various stimulation levels so you can adjust signals to control your comfort. It can be used when nausea begins, or you can wear it before you feel ill. This device does not interfere with eating or drinking. It's water resistant and shock resistant, so you can wear it just about any time!

Treating Morning Sickness. There is no completely successful treatment for normal nausea and vomiting. Research has found some women find relief by taking vitamin B_6 supplements. It's a good therapy to try because it's readily available and inexpensive. Ask your healthcare provider about taking PremesisRx, a once-a-day tablet. If vitamin B_6 alone doesn't work, your healthcare provider might want to add an antihistamine.

You can ask your healthcare provider about taking over-the-counter antinausea medication, such as Emetrol. In addition, ask about using a different prenatal vitamin that might be easier on your stomach. You might ask about taking a regular multivitamin—not a prenatal vitamin—or a folic-acid supplement during the first trimester.

Acupressure, acupuncture and massage may prove helpful in dealing with nausea and vomiting. Acupressure wristbands, worn for motion and seasickness, and other devices help some women feel better.

This is an extremely important period in the development of your baby. Don't expose baby to herbs, over-the-counter treatments or any other "remedies" for nausea that are not known to be safe during pregnancy.

Some Actions You Can Take. Eat small meals more frequently. Experts agree you should eat what appeals to you—these foods may be the ones you can keep down more easily right now. If that means sourdough bread and lemon-lime soda, go for it! Some women find protein foods settle more easily in their stomachs; these foods include cheese, eggs,

Some Interesting Facts about Morning Sickness

- Nausea and vomiting are uncommon in Asia and Africa.
- Morning sickness is more common in women carrying multiples.
- Heartburn and reflux can make morning sickness worse.
- Other conditions can cause nausea and vomiting in early pregnancy, including pancreatitis, gastroenteritis, appendicitis and pyelonephritis, as well as some metabolic disorders.
- If you don't have morning sickness in early pregnancy, then experience nausea and vomiting later in pregnancy, it's *not* morning sickness.

peanut butter and nonfatty meats. A 2-ounce bar of *dark* chocolate may also help relieve nausea.

Ginger may help reduce vomiting. Make tea from fresh ginger, and drink it to calm your stomach. Taking about 350mg of ginger supplements may also help. Be careful when choosing ginger-root supplements. There's a difference in quality of ginger from different manufacturers. Buy from a reliable company.

If you've heard about *Nzu* to treat morning sickness, *don't* use it. It is a traditional remedy from Africa that looks like balls of mud or clay. However, it's dangerous to use because it contains high levels of lead and arsenic.

Keep up your fluid intake, even if you can't keep food down. Dehydration is more serious than not eating for a while. If you vomit a lot, you may want to choose fluids that contain electrolytes to help replace those you lose when you vomit. Ask your healthcare provider what fluids he or she recommends.

Other Changes You May Notice

In early pregnancy, you may need to go to the bathroom a lot. This can continue during most of your pregnancy. It may really get annoying near delivery because your uterus gets bigger and puts pressure on your bladder.

You may also notice breast changes. Tingling or soreness in the breasts or nipples is common. You may see a darkening of the areola or a lifting of the glands around the nipple. See Week 13 for more information on how breasts are affected by pregnancy.

Another early symptom of pregnancy is tiring easily, which may continue through pregnancy. See the discussion below. Take your prenatal vitamins and any other medications prescribed by your healthcare provider. Get enough rest. If you're tired, stay away from sugar and caffeine; either can make the problem worse.

Fatigue in Pregnancy

You may feel exhausted early in pregnancy. It may be hard to get out of bed in the morning, or you may find yourself falling asleep in the middle of the afternoon. Don't worry—this is normal, especially in early pregnancy. Your body uses a lot of energy as your baby grows.

Take time to deal with your fatigue. Do what you can. Rest during the day, if possible. To help fight fatigue, follow the 45-second rule—*if it takes 45 seconds or less to take care of something, do it.* This helps reduce fatigue *and* stress.

You may want to try some other things to help you feel better. Lavender can help you feel calm. One whiff may do the trick. Experts believe the smell helps you feel calmer. You may feel less stress if you keep a bouquet of pretty flowers on your desk or at home.

Nearly 80% of all pregnant women have trouble sleeping at some time in pregnancy. Some reasons include hormone changes and the size of your tummy. A short nap in the middle of the afternoon can pep you up and help make up for lost sleep.

If You're Absent from Work with Morning Sickness

If morning sickness causes you to be absent from your job, you may be interested to know the Family and Medical Leave Act (FMLA) states you do *not* need a healthcare provider's note verifying the problem. Nausea and vomiting of pregnancy is classified as a "chronic condition" and may require you to be out occasionally, but you don't need treatment.

Many moms-to-be wake up five or more times a night, which can cause fatigue during the day. Baby's movements, leg cramps and shortness of breath may also keep you up later in pregnancy. It's important to get enough rest during the night, especially late in pregnancy. Research shows women who slept fewer than 6 hours at night were four times more likely to have a Cesarean delivery.

How Your Actions Affect Your Baby's Development

When Should You Visit the Healthcare Provider?

One of the first questions you may ask when you suspect you're pregnant is, "When should I see my healthcare provider?" Good prenatal care is necessary for the health of the baby and mother-to-be. Make an appointment for your first prenatal visit as soon as you're reasonably sure you're pregnant. This could be as early as a few days after a missed period.

Getting Pregnant while Using Birth Control

If you've been using some type of birth control, tell your healthcare provider. No method is 100% effective. Occasionally a method fails, even oral contraceptives. Don't panic if this happens to you. If you're sure you're pregnant, stop taking the pill and make an appointment as soon as possible.

Pregnancy can also occur with an intrauterine device (IUD). If this happens, see your healthcare provider immediately. Discuss whether the IUD should be removed or left in place. In most cases, an attempt

> Home pregnancy-test kits were first introduced in 1976; in 1999 the average price for an at-home pregnancy kit was between $15 and $20. Today, a test averages $6 to $10. Some even cost as little as $1—and they're accurate. A study compared pregnancy tests from dollar stores with tests used in doctors' offices and clinics. The study found the dollar-store tests were just as sensitive as more expensive tests.

is made to remove the IUD. If left in place, the risk of miscarriage increases slightly.

You may be using a spermicide, sponge or diaphragm when pregnancy occurs. They have not been shown to be harmful to a developing baby.

Your Nutrition

As discussed above, you may have to deal with nausea and vomiting during pregnancy. If you experience morning sickness, try some of the following suggestions.

- Eat small meals frequently to keep your stomach from being overfull.
- Drink lots of fluid.
- Find out what foods, smells or situations nauseate you. Avoid them when possible.
- Avoid coffee because it stimulates stomach acid.
- A high-protein or high-carbohydrate snack before bed may help.
- Ask your partner to make you some dry toast in the morning before you get up; eat it in bed. Or keep crackers or dry cereal near you to nibble on before you get up in the morning to help absorb stomach acid.
- Keep your bedroom cool at night, and air it out often. Cool, fresh air may help you feel better.
- Get out of bed slowly.
- If you take an iron supplement, take it an hour before meals or 2 hours after a meal.
- When you feel queasy, eat some soda crackers, cold chicken, pretzels or ginger snaps.
- Nibble on raw ginger, or pour boiling water over it and sip the "tea."
- Salty foods help some women with nausea.
- Lemonade and watermelon may also relieve symptoms.

You Should Also Know

Weight Gain during Pregnancy

The amount of weight women gain during pregnancy varies greatly. It may range from weight loss to a total gain of 50 pounds or more, so it's difficult to set one figure as an "ideal" weight gain during pregnancy. But experts agree—gain the recommended weight during pregnancy to have a healthier pregnancy.

Pregnancy Weight Gain

Weight before Pregnancy	Recommended Gain (pounds)
Underweight	28 to 40
Normal weight	25 to 35
Overweight	15 to 25
Obese	11 to 20
Morbidly obese	Your healthcare provider will determine weight gain

Another way to figure how much weight you should gain during pregnancy is to look at your BMI (body mass index). BMI guidelines for weight gain during pregnancy include the following:

- BMI of less than 18.5—gain between 28 and 40 pounds
- BMI of 18.5 to 25—gain between 25 and 35 pounds
- BMI of 26 to 29—gain between 15 and 25 pounds
- BMI of 30 or more—gain between 11 and 20 pounds
- BMI of 40 and over—healthcare provider will determine weight gain

How much weight you gain is influenced by your prepregnancy weight. Experts agree that what you weigh *before* pregnancy is the best indicator of how much weight you should gain *during* pregnancy. In addition, if you're shorter than 5'2" tall, try to gain at the *lower* end of your weight range.

Statistics show nearly 45% of all pregnant women gain more weight than they should. If you do, your risk of problems goes up. You also put your baby at risk. And your child has a much higher risk of being overweight by age 7.

Many experts call for a weight-gain figure of ⅔ of a pound (10 ounces) a week until 20 weeks, then 1 pound a week from 20 to 40 weeks. Other researchers have set up weight-gain guidelines for underweight, normal weight, overweight and obese women. See the box on this page.

Nearly half of all women who get pregnant have had a weight problem before pregnancy. You shouldn't diet while you're pregnant, but that doesn't mean you shouldn't watch what you eat. You should! Your baby will get proper nutrition from the foods you eat.

Research shows if you dieted a lot before pregnancy, you may gain more weight than recommended during pregnancy, so pay strict attention to your eating plan. Choose foods for the nutrition they provide for you and your growing baby. Watch your stress levels, and try not to get too tired. If you're stressed, fatigued or anxious, you may eat more fats, sweets and junk-food snacks. This can lead to an unhealthy amount of weight gain during pregnancy.

If you want to breastfeed, gaining more weight than you should may contribute to breastfeeding problems. The extra weight may also delay your milk from coming in.

If you have any questions, discuss them with your healthcare provider. He or she can advise you on how much weight you should gain during your pregnancy.

Ectopic (Tubal) Pregnancy

In a normal pregnancy, fertilization occurs in the Fallopian tube and the fertilized egg travels through the tube to the uterus. There it implants on the cavity wall.

An *ectopic pregnancy* occurs in the first 12 weeks of pregnancy when the egg implants *outside* the uterine cavity, usually in the tube. Ninety-five percent of all ectopic pregnancies occur in the Fallopian tube (hence the term *tubal pregnancy*). The illustration on page 79 shows some possible locations of an ectopic pregnancy.

We have seen the number of ectopic pregnancies almost triple since 1985. Today about 7 in every 1000 pregnancies is ectopic. The reason for the increase? Researchers believe STDs (sexually transmitted diseases) are the cause, especially chlamydia and gonorrhea. If you have had an STD, tell your healthcare provider at your first prenatal visit. And be sure to tell him or her if you have had a previous ectopic pregnancy; there's a 12% chance it will happen again.

Chances of having an ectopic pregnancy increase with damage to the Fallopian tubes from pelvic inflammatory disease (PID), other infections, infertility, endometriosis and tubal or abdominal surgery. Smoking, exposure to DES (diethylstilbestrol) during your mother's pregnancy and being older may also increase your risk. Use of an IUD also increases the chance of ectopic pregnancy.

Symptoms of ectopic pregnancy include:

- cramps or low-back pain
- tenderness in the lower abdomen
- bleeding or brown spotting
- shoulder pain
- weakness, dizziness or fainting caused by blood loss
- nausea
- low blood pressure

Diagnosing Ectopic Pregnancy. To test for ectopic pregnancy, human chorionic gonadotropin is measured. The test is called a *quantitative HCG.* The level of HCG increases rapidly in a normal pregnancy and doubles in value about every 2 days. If HCG levels do not increase as they should, an ectopic pregnancy is suspected.

Ultrasound testing is helpful. An ectopic pregnancy may be visible in the tube. Blood may be seen in the abdomen.

We are better able to diagnose ectopic pregnancy with laparoscopy. Tiny incisions are made in the area of the bellybutton and in the lower-abdomen area. Healthcare providers look inside the abdomen at the pelvic organs with a small instrument called a *laparoscope.* They can see an ectopic pregnancy if one is present.

It's best to diagnose a tubal pregnancy before it ruptures and damages the tube. This could make it necessary to remove the entire tube. Early diagnosis also tries to avoid the risk of internal bleeding from a ruptured tube.

Dad Tip

You may be a happier camper if you help out around the house more during your partner's pregnancy. It can make your life and hers easier if you pitch in to do some of the shopping and household chores. Making your home safe for her also makes it safe for your baby.

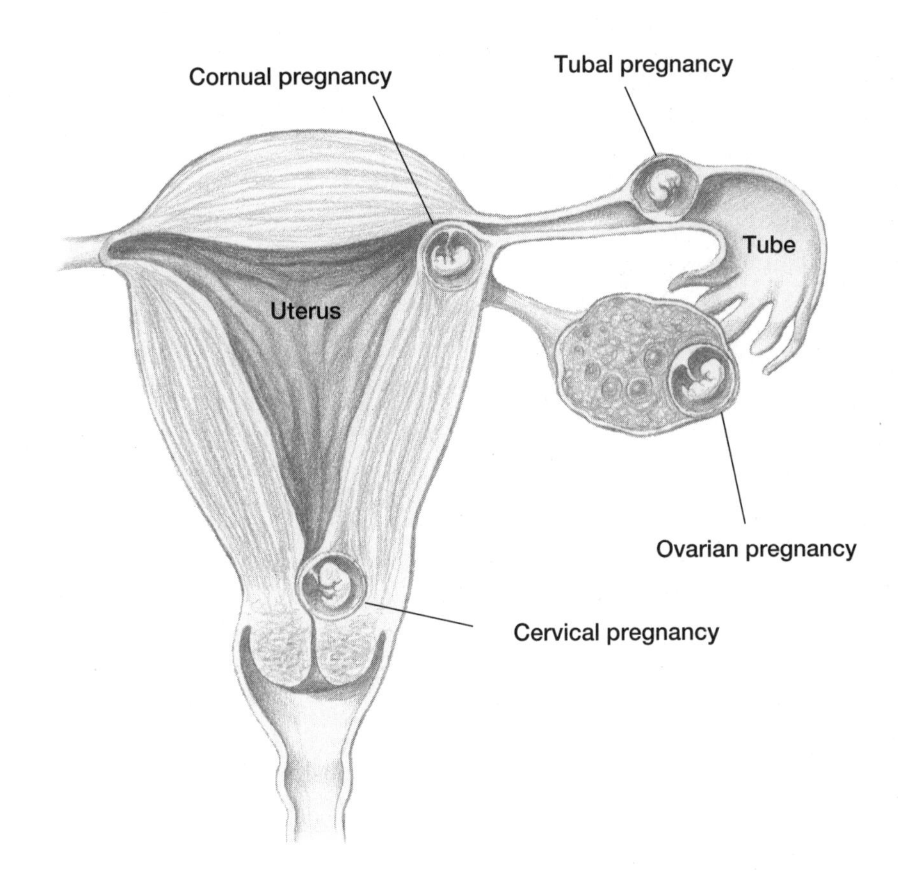

Possible locations of an ectopic pregnancy.

Most ectopic pregnancies are detected around 6 to 8 weeks of pregnancy. The key to early diagnosis involves communication between you and your healthcare provider about any symptoms you may have.

Treatment for Ectopic Pregnancy. The goal is to remove the pregnancy while maintaining fertility. Surgery requires general anesthesia, laparoscopy or laparotomy (a larger incision and no scope) and recovery from surgery. In many instances, the Fallopian tube may need to be removed, which may affect future fertility.

A nonsurgical treatment involves the use of a cancer drug, methotrexate. It is given by I.V. in the hospital or at an outpatient clinic. Methotrexate ends the pregnancy. HCG levels should decrease after this treatment, and symptoms should improve. If methotrexate is used to treat an ectopic pregnancy, a couple should wait at least 3 months before trying to conceive again.

Exercise for Week 5

Lightly grasp the back of a chair or a counter for balance. Stand with your feet shoulder-width apart. Keep your body weight over your heels and your torso erect. Bend your knees, and lower your torso in a squatting position. Don't round your back. Hold the squatting position for 5 seconds, then straighten to starting position. Start with 5 repetitions and work up to 10. *Strengthens hip, thigh and buttocks muscles.*

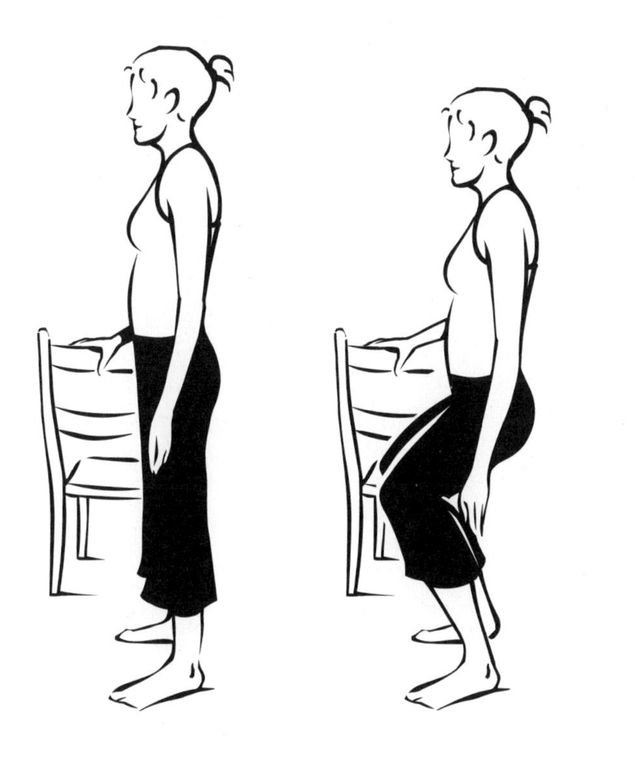

Week 6

Age of Fetus—4 Weeks

If you've just found out you're pregnant,
you might want to begin by reading the previous chapters.

How Big Is Your Baby?

Crown-to-rump is the sitting height or distance from the top of the baby's head to its rump or buttocks. The crown-to-rump length of your baby by this week is 0.08 to 0.16 inch (2 to 4mm).

How Big Are You?

You've been pregnant for 1 month, so you should have noticed some changes in your body by now. You may have gained a few pounds. Or you may have lost weight. If this is your first pregnancy, your abdomen probably hasn't changed much. You may be gaining weight in your breasts or other places. If you have a pelvic exam, your healthcare provider can usually feel your uterus and note some change in its size.

How Your Baby Is Growing and Developing

This is the *embryonic period* (from conception to week 10 of pregnancy, or from conception to week 8 of fetal development). During this time, the embryo is most susceptible to things that can interfere with its development. Most birth defects happen during this critical period.

As the illustration on page 84 shows, baby's body has a head and tail area. Around this time, early brain chambers form. The forebrain, midbrain, hindbrain and spinal cord are established.

The heart tube divides into bulges, which develop into heart chambers, called *ventricles* (left and right) and *atria* (left atrium and right atrium). They form between weeks 6 and 7. Occasionally, with the proper equipment, a heartbeat can be seen on ultrasound by the 6th week. Eyes are also forming, and limb buds appear.

Changes in You

Heartburn

Heartburn discomfort *(pyrosis)* is one of the most common discomforts of pregnancy. Heartburn is defined as a burning sensation in the middle of your chest; it often occurs soon after eating. You may also experience an acid or bitter taste in your mouth and increased pain when you bend over or lie down.

During the first trimester, nearly 25% of all pregnant women have heartburn. It may become more severe later, when your growing baby compresses your digestive tract. See the box on page 86 for a comparison of heartburn and indigestion.

Heartburn occurs when your digestive tract relaxes and stomach acid creeps back into the esophagus. It occurs more frequently during pregnancy for two reasons—food moves more slowly through the intestines and the stomach is squeezed a bit as the uterus gets bigger and moves up into the abdomen.

Symptoms are not severe for most women. Eat small, frequent meals, and avoid some positions, such as bending over or lying flat. One sure way to get heartburn is to eat a large meal, then lie down! (This is true for anyone, not just pregnant women.)

Some antacids offer relief, including aluminum hydroxide, magnesium trisilicate and magnesium hydroxide (Amphojel, Gelusil, milk of

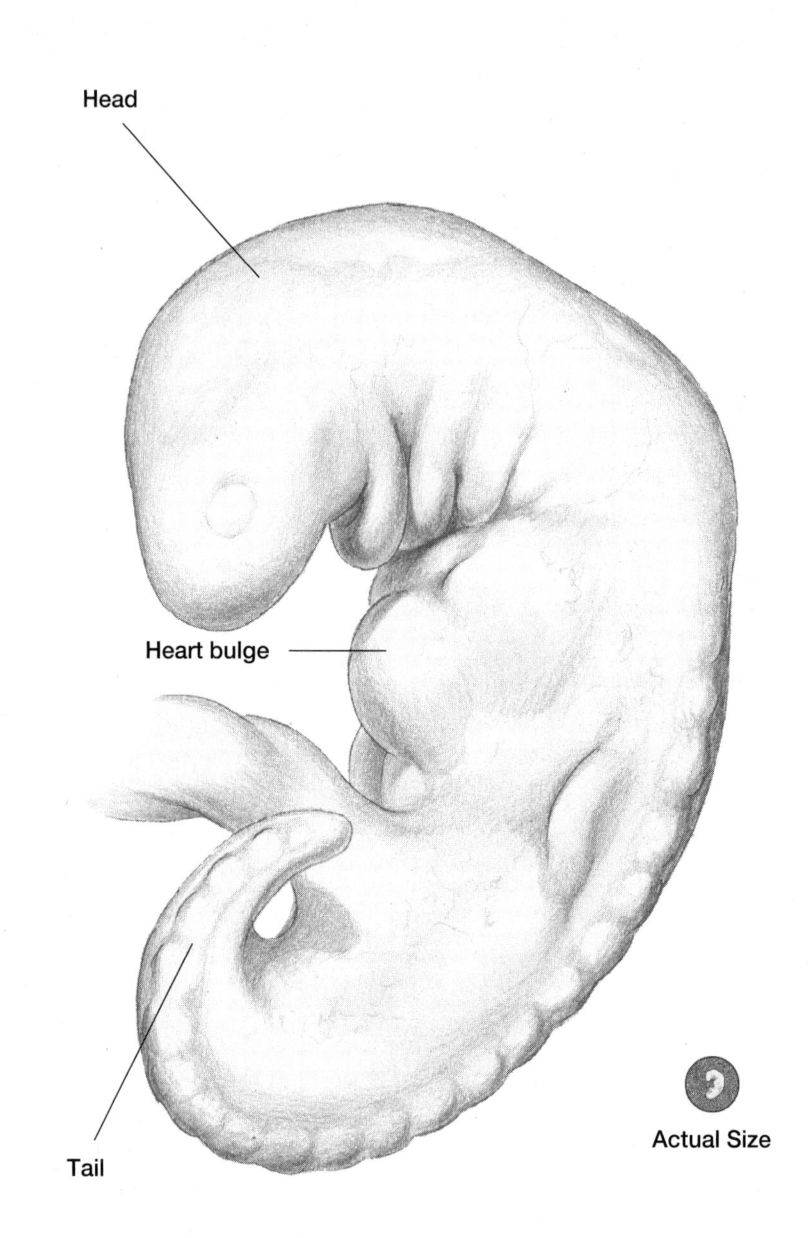

Embryo at 6 weeks of pregnancy (fetal age—4 weeks).
It is growing rapidly.

magnesia, Maalox). Follow your healthcare provider's advice or package instructions relating to pregnancy. Don't take too much antacid! Avoid sodium bicarbonate because it contains a lot of sodium, which may cause you to retain water.

Other actions you take may help with heartburn. Try some of the following, and use what works for you.

- Don't overeat.
- Avoid foods that trigger your heartburn.
- Don't eat late at night.
- Be careful with carbonated drinks.
- Use less fat when cooking.
- Wear loose clothing.
- Stay upright after meals, especially in late pregnancy.
- Chew gum for 30 minutes after meals and when heartburn strikes.
- Suck on hard candy.
- Get some exercise, but don't eat for 2 hours *before* you begin. Use smooth moves to avoid pushing acids into your esophagus.
- Reduce stress in your life.

Another way to help relieve heartburn is to mix the juice of ½ lemon and a pinch of salt in 8 ounces of water, and drink it before meals. After meals, 1 teaspoon of honey may help ease discomfort.

GERD. *GERD (gastroesophageal reflux disease)* or *acid-reflux disease* may be mistaken for heartburn during pregnancy. It's very common but often overlooked. The three most common symptoms include heartburn, sour or bitter taste, and difficulty swallowing. Other symptoms may include persistent cough, hoarseness, upset stomach and chest pain.

Be careful with the foods you eat. Eating too much food that is spicy, highly acidic or high in fat may aggravate acid reflux.

Only your healthcare provider can determine if you have acid reflux or GERD, so talk to him or her at a prenatal appointment if it bothers you. He or she may prescribe a medication that is safe to use during pregnancy. If you are now taking prescription or over-the-counter medicines to treat your problem, check with your healthcare provider before continuing their use.

Constipation

Your bowel habits will probably change during pregnancy. Most women notice some constipation. Two things add to the problem in pregnancy—increased hormones and blood-volume increase. You may not be drinking enough fluid, which can cause dehydration (and constipation) in you.

Increase your fluid intake. Foods that contain a lot of water include frozen juice treats, watermelon or a slush made with fresh fruit juice and water. In addition, foods with lots of fiber hold onto water longer, which helps soften your stools.

Exercise may help. It shifts body position, which may stimulate your bowels and increase muscle contractions to help move food through your intestines.

The Difference between Indigestion and Heartburn

Some people who suffer from heartburn say they are suffering from indigestion, but indigestion isn't the same thing as heartburn. Although they have similar triggers, and treatment may be the same in many instances, they are different. *Indigestion* is a condition; *heartburn* may be a symptom of indigestion.

Indigestion is a vague feeling of discomfort and pain in the upper abdomen and chest. It includes a feeling of fullness and bloating, accompanied by belching and nausea. Occasionally, heartburn is a symptom.

Several things can trigger indigestion, including overeating, eating a particular food, drinking alcohol or carbonated beverages, eating too fast or too much, eating fatty or spicy foods, drinking too much caffeine, smoking or eating too much high-fiber foods. Anxiety and depression can worsen symptoms.

Many healthcare providers suggest a mild laxative, such as milk of magnesia or prune juice, if you have problems. Certain foods, such as bran and prunes, can increase the bulk in your diet, which may help relieve constipation.

Don't use laxatives without your healthcare provider's OK. If constipation is a continuing problem, discuss treatment at a prenatal visit. Try not to strain when you have a bowel movement; straining can lead to hemorrhoids. See Week 14 for information on hemorrhoids.

How Your Actions Affect Your Baby's Development

Infections or diseases passed from one person to another by sexual contact are called *sexually transmitted diseases (STDs)*. These infections can affect your ability to get pregnant. During pregnancy, a sexually transmitted disease can harm your growing baby. Take care of any STD as soon as possible!

About 2 million pregnant women have an STD. That's over 40%! Many don't even know they have one. Ask for a test or treatment if you think you have an STD. Your healthcare provider routinely offers tests for hepatitis B, HIV and syphilis.

Genital Herpes

More than 45 million people in the United States over the age of 12 have had active cases of *genital herpes* (HSV type 2); 1 million new cases are reported every year. It's not uncommon for a woman to have this problem during pregnancy. In fact, 2% of all pregnant women who do not have the disease when they get pregnant get it during pregnancy. Of those women who have herpes, 75% will have an outbreak during pregnancy.

Herpes can be dangerous for your baby. If you contract herpes *during* pregnancy, your baby is at highest risk. If your first outbreak is near delivery, your baby has a higher chance of having problems.

There's no safe treatment during pregnancy for genital herpes. Some women are given valacyclovir during the last month of pregnancy in an attempt to suppress an outbreak. One study found this decreases the chances of an outbreak by nearly 70%. If a woman has a herpes outbreak late in pregnancy, she may have a Cesarean delivery.

Yeast Infections

Monilial (yeast) infections are more common in pregnant women. They have no major effect on pregnancy, but they may cause you discomfort and anxiety.

Yeast infections are sometimes harder to control and may require frequent retreatment or longer treatment during pregnancy. Creams used for treatment are usually safe during pregnancy. Avoid fluconazole (Diflucan); it may not be safe to use during pregnancy. Your partner does not need to be treated.

A newborn infant can get thrush after passing through a birth canal infected with monilial vulvovaginitis. Treatment with nystatin is effective.

Vaginitis

Vaginitis, also called *trichomonal vaginitis* or *trichomoniasis,* is the most common STD among women. It has no major effects on a pregnancy.

Treatment includes metronidazole (Flagyl) for you and your partner. A problem in treatment may arise because some experts believe metronidazole shouldn't be taken in the first trimester of pregnancy. Most healthcare providers will prescribe metronidazole for a bad infection *after* the first trimester.

Human Papillomavirus (HPV; Genital Warts)

There are over 100 different viruses included under the umbrella term *human papillomavirus* (HPV)—30 of them are transmitted sexually. In some people, this virus causes venereal (genital) warts, also called *condyloma acuminata.* Genital warts may grow faster during pregnancy because of lowered immunity, pregnancy hormones and increased blood flow to the pelvic area.

HPV is one of the most common STDs in the United States—20 million Americans have it. HPV can affect your vagina, cervix and rectum, and your partner's penis.

The Pap smear done at one of your first prenatal visits can reassure you that you do not have this problem. HPV is one of the main causes of abnormal Pap smears. If you have genital warts, tell your healthcare provider at your first prenatal appointment. During pregnancy, certain treatments should be avoided.

Warty skin tags may enlarge during pregnancy; in rare instances, they have blocked the vagina at the time of delivery. If you have many venereal warts, a Cesarean delivery may be necessary. Babies have also been known to get small benign tumors on the vocal cords after delivery.

HPV vaccines are recommended for all females between the ages of 9 and 26. They are not recommended during pregnancy. However, they are considered safe during breastfeeding.

Gonorrhea

Gonorrhea presents risks to a woman and her partner, and to her baby when it passes through the birth canal. The baby may contract gonorrheal ophthalmia, a severe eye infection. Eye drops are used in newborns to prevent this problem. Other infections may result in the mother, which are treated with penicillin or other medications that are safe during pregnancy.

Syphilis

Detection of a *syphilis* infection is important for you, your partner and your growing baby. Fortunately this rare infection is also treatable. Screening tests for syphilis during pregnancy have reduced the rate of syphilis in babies.

If you notice any open sore on your genitals, have your healthcare provider check it. Syphilis can be treated with penicillin and other safe medications.

Chlamydia

Chlamydia is a common sexually transmitted disease; between 3 and 5 million people are infected every year. Infection is caused by a germ that invades certain types of healthy cells; it may be passed through sexual activity, including oral sex. Between 20 and 40% of all sexually active women have probably been exposed to chlamydia. In fact, over 200,000 pregnant women are infected every year.

Chlamydial infection may be linked to ectopic pregnancy. In one study, 70% of the women studied who had an ectopic pregnancy also had chlamydia.

Chlamydia is most likely to occur in people who have more than one sexual partner. It may also occur in women who have other sexually transmitted diseases.

Some healthcare providers believe chlamydia occurs more commonly in women who take oral contraceptives. Barrier methods of contraception, such as diaphragms and condoms used with spermicides, may offer some protection from infection.

During pregnancy, a mother-to-be can pass the infection to her baby as it comes through the birth canal. The baby has a 20 to 50% chance of getting chlamydia if the mother has it. It may cause an eye infection in baby, but that's easily treated. A baby may also get a chylamdial infection during birth and develop pneumonia, which can be fatal.

Pelvic inflammatory disease (PID) can result from an untreated chlamydia infection. Chlamydia is one of the main causes of PID. See the discussion of PID on page 91.

You may not have symptoms of chlamydia—75% of those infected do not. Symptoms include burning or itching in the genital area, discharge from the vagina, painful or frequent urination, or pain in the pelvic area. Men may also have symptoms.

Chlamydia can be detected by a cell culture. Rapid diagnostic tests done in the doctor's office can provide a result quickly, possibly even before you go home.

Chlamydia is usually treated with tetracycline, but it shouldn't be given to a pregnant woman. During pregnancy, erythromycin may be the drug of choice, or Zithromax may be prescribed for you and your partner.

After treatment, your healthcare provider may want to do another culture to make sure the infection is gone. The test may be repeated late in pregnancy to be sure you don't have the disease when you deliver.

Pelvic inflammatory disease

Pelvic inflammatory disease (PID) is a severe infection of the upper genital organs involving the uterus, the Fallopian tubes and even the ovaries. There may be pelvic pain, or there may be no symptoms at all.

Infection can result in scarring and blockage of the tubes, making it difficult or impossible to get pregnant or making you more susceptible to an ectopic pregnancy. Surgery may be required to repair damage.

HIV and AIDS

HIV. *HIV (human immunodeficiency virus)* is the virus that causes *AIDS (acquired immune deficiency syndrome)*. More than 1 million people in the United States are HIV-positive or have AIDS. Nearly 56,000 new HIV infections occur every year—20% do not even know they are infected.

About 2 out of every 1000 women who enter pregnancy are HIV-positive, and the number of cases among women is rising. It's estimated that 6000 babies are born every year to mothers infected with HIV. In fact, the CDC now recommends that all pregnant women be offered HIV testing. Home testing kits are available; most are very reliable.

After HIV enters a person's bloodstream, the body begins to produce antibodies to fight the disease. A blood test can detect these antibodies. When detected, a person is considered "HIV-positive" and can pass the virus to others. This is not the same as having AIDS.

The virus weakens the immune system and makes it difficult for the body to fight off disease. Gynecological problems can be an early sign of an HIV infection, including ulcers in the vagina, yeast infections that won't go away and severe pelvic inflammatory disease. If you have any of these problems, discuss them with your healthcare provider. Early diagnosis and treatment are crucial.

There may be a period of weeks or months when tests don't reveal the virus. In most cases, antibodies can be detected 6 to 12 weeks after exposure. In some cases, it can take as long as 18 months before antibodies are found.

Once a test is positive, a person may be free of symptoms for some time. Studies indicate taking over-the-counter multivitamins containing vitamins B, C and E every day may delay the progression of HIV and delay the need to start antiretroviral medications.

Two tests are used to determine if someone has HIV—the ELISA test and the Western Blot test. The ELISA is a screening test. If positive, it should be confirmed by the Western Blot test. Both tests involve testing blood to measure antibodies to the virus. The Western Blot test is believed to be more than 99% sensitive and specific.

Before testing, a woman is advised she will be tested for HIV unless she declines—this is called *opt-out testing*. For those at high risk of HIV, experts suggest testing before pregnancy or as early in pregnancy as possible and testing again in the third trimester. Rapid HIV testing during labor is recommended if a woman's HIV status is unknown.

With rapid HIV testing, results are available within 30 minutes. This test has the same sensitivity and specificity as the ELISA test. Positive results require confirmation with Western Blot testing.

We know 90% of all cases of HIV in children are related to pregnancy—mother to baby during pregnancy, childbirth or breastfeeding. Research has shown an infected woman can pass the virus to her baby as early as 8 weeks of pregnancy. A mother can also pass HIV to her baby during its birth. Breastfeeding is not recommended for women who are HIV-positive.

Research shows the chance of a woman infected with HIV passing the virus to her baby can be nearly eliminated with some medications. However, if an infection is not treated, there's a 25% chance a baby will be born with the virus. If a woman takes AZT during pregnancy and has a Cesarean delivery, she reduces the risk of passing the virus to about 2%! Studies have found no birth defects linked to the use of AZT. Other HIV medications have also been proved safe for use during pregnancy.

If you are HIV-positive, expect more blood tests during pregnancy. These tests help your healthcare provider assess how well you are doing.

AIDS. A person is HIV-positive before developing AIDS. This process can take 10 or more years, due to the medications in use at this time.

The rate of AIDS among women has grown to 20% of all reported cases. AIDS can leave a person prone to, and unable to fight, various infections. If you are unsure about your risk, seek counseling about testing for the AIDS virus. Pregnancy may hide some AIDS symptoms, which makes the disease harder to discover.

There is some positive news for women who suffer from AIDS. We know if a woman is in the early course of the illness, she can usually have an uneventful pregnancy, labor and delivery.

Your Nutrition

During your pregnancy, you need to be selective in the foods you choose. Eating the right foods, in the correct amounts, takes planning. Eat foods high in vitamins and minerals, especially iron, calcium, magnesium, folate and zinc. You also need fiber.

Some of the foods you should eat, and the amounts of each, are listed below. Try to eat these foods every day. We discuss food groups in the following weeks. Check weekly discussions for nutrition tips. Foods to help your baby grow and develop include:

- bread, cereal, pasta and rice—at least 6 servings/day
- fruits—3 to 4 servings/day
- vegetables—4 servings/day
- meat and other protein sources—2 to 3 servings/day
- dairy products—3 to 4 servings/day
- fats, sweets and other "empty" calorie foods—2 to 3 servings/day

You Should Also Know

Your First Visit to Your Healthcare Provider

Your first prenatal visit may be one of your longest. There's a lot to do. If you saw your healthcare provider before you got pregnant, you may have already discussed some of your concerns.

Understanding Serving Portions

You may believe it will be difficult for you to eat all the portions you need for the health of your growing baby. However, many people overeat because they don't understand what a "portion" or "serving" really is.

Supersizing in fast-food restaurants and huge meal portions at other restaurants have skewed our idea of what a normal portion size really is. For example, a blueberry muffin is now about 500 calories. Twenty-five years ago, it was about 200 calories. Look for the following serving sizes when you eat—they're what a "normal" portion size is.

- cup of vegetables—the size of a lightbulb
- 1 serving of juice—a champagne flute
- 1 pancake—the size of a CD
- 1 teaspoon of peanut butter—the end of your thumb
- 3 ounces of fish—an eyeglass case
- 3 ounces of meat—a deck of playing cards
- 1 small potato—a 3x5 index card

Read labels for portion sizes; a common mistake is to read the calorie/nutrient information on a label and not take into account the *number of servings* each package contains. Even a very small package may contain two or more servings, doubling or tripling the calories if you eat the whole thing.

To learn the *correct* serving size for each of the food groups, check out the USDA's website www.cnpp.usda.gov; it lists actual serving portions. For example, a large bagel may be *four* to *five* grain servings! If you don't have access to a computer, ask your healthcare provider for some guidelines or nutrition handouts.

Feel free to ask questions to get an idea of how your healthcare provider will relate to you and your needs. During pregnancy, there should be an exchange of ideas. Consider what your healthcare provider suggests and why. It's important to share your feelings and ideas. Your healthcare provider has experience that can be valuable to you during pregnancy.

At this first visit, you will be asked for a history of your medical health. This includes general medical problems and any problems relating to your gynecological and obstetrical history. You will be asked about your periods and recent birth-control methods. If you've had an abortion or a miscarriage, or if you've been in the hospital for surgery or for some other reason, it's important information. If you have old medical records, bring them with you.

Your healthcare provider needs to know about medicine you take or medication you are allergic to. Your family's medical history may also be important.

Various tests may be done at this first visit or on a subsequent visit. If you have questions, ask them. If you think you may have a "high-risk" pregnancy, discuss it with your healthcare provider.

Tip for Week 6

If you have questions between prenatal visits, call the office. It's OK; your healthcare provider wants you to call to get correct medical information. You'll probably feel more comfortable when your questions are answered.

In most cases, you will be asked to return every 4 weeks for the first 7 months, then every 2 weeks until the last month, then every week. If problems arise, you may be scheduled for more frequent visits.

Ways to Have a Great Pregnancy

Every woman wants to have a happy, healthy pregnancy. Start now to help ensure that yours will be the best it can be! Try the following.

- Prioritize—Examine what you need to do to help yourself and your growing baby. Do what you need to do, decide what else you can do and let the rest go.
- Involve others in your pregnancy—When you include your partner, other family members and friends in your pregnancy, it helps them understand what you're going through so they can be more understanding and supportive.
- Treat others with respect and love—You may be having a hard time, especially at the beginning of pregnancy. You may have morning sickness. You may find adjusting to the role of "mom-to-be" difficult. People will understand if you take the time to let them know how you feel. Show respect for their concern, treat them with kindness and love, and they will respond in kind.

- Create memories—It takes some planning, but it's definitely worth it. When you're pregnant, it seems like it will go on forever. However, speaking from experience, we can tell you it passes very quickly and is soon a memory. Take steps to document the many changes occurring in your life right now. Include your partner. Have him jot down some of his thoughts and feelings. Take his picture, too! You'll be able to look back and share the highs and lows with him, and, in the years ahead, you and your kids will be glad you did.
- Relax when you can—Easing the stress in your life is important. Do things that help you relax and focus on what is important in your lives right now.
- Enjoy this time of preparation—All too soon your pregnancy will be over, and you'll be a new mother, with all the responsibilities of being a mom and a partner! You may also have other responsibilities in your professional or personal life. Concentrate on your couple relationship and on the many changes you will be experiencing in the near future.
- Focus on the positive—You may hear negative things from friends or family members, such as scary stories or sad tales. Ignore them. Most pregnancies work out great!
- Don't be afraid to ask for help—Your pregnancy is important to others. Friends and family will be pleased if you ask them to be involved.
- Get information—There are many sources today, such as our books, various magazine articles, television programs, radio interviews and the Internet.
- Smile—You're part of a very special miracle that is happening to you and your partner!

Dad Tip

Is your partner suffering from morning sickness? If so, cooking can be a real chore for her. Just looking at food or smelling it can make her feel sick. To help out, bring home your dinner, or cook it yourself. Sometimes it's the only way you'll get any food!

Exercise for Week 6

Stand with your left side next to the sofa or a sturdy chair. Hold onto the back with your left hand. Standing with your feet shoulder-width apart, step back about 3 feet with your right foot. Bend your leg until your thigh is parallel to the floor. Keep your knee over your toes. Hold for 3 seconds, then as you return to standing position, lift your right leg and squeeze your buttocks muscles for 1 second. Start with 3 repetitions and work up to 6. Repeat for your other leg. *Strengthens hip, thigh and buttocks muscles.*

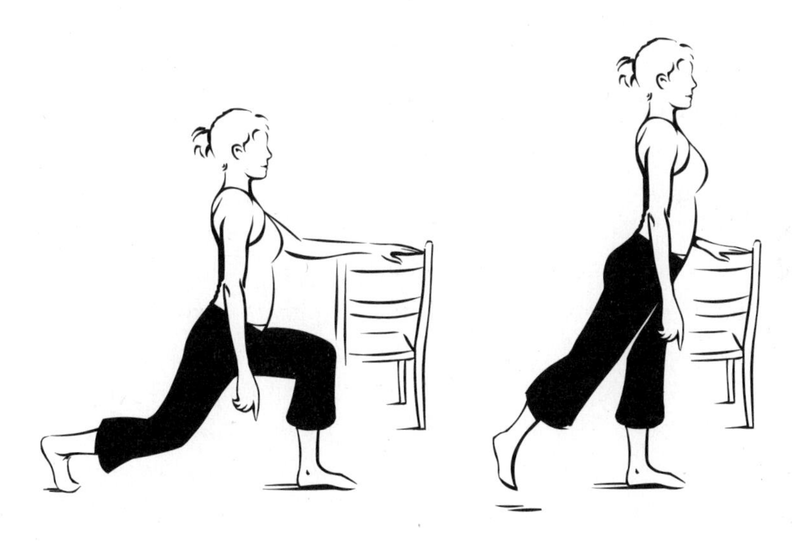

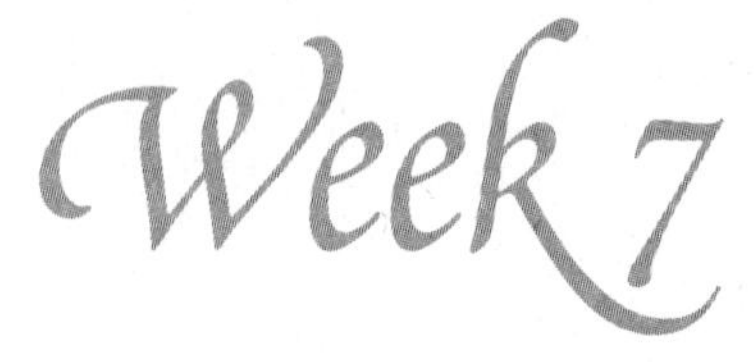

Age of Fetus—5 Weeks

If you've just found out you're pregnant,
you might want to begin by reading the previous chapters.

How Big Is Your Baby?

Your baby goes through an incredible growth spurt around this time! At the beginning of this week, the crown-to-rump length is 0.16 to 0.2 inch (4 to 5mm), about the size of a BB pellet. By the end of the week, your baby has more than doubled in size, to about ½ inch (1.1 to 1.3cm).

How Big Are You?

Although you are probably quite anxious to show the world you're pregnant, there still may be little noticeable change. Changes will come soon.

How Your Baby Is Growing and Developing

Leg buds are beginning to appear as short fins. As you can see on page 100, arm buds have grown and divided into a hand segment and an arm-shoulder segment. The hand and foot have a plate where the fingers and toes will develop.

The heart has divided into right and left chambers. An opening between the chambers called the *foramen ovale* appears. This opening lets blood pass from one chamber to the other, allowing it to bypass the lungs. At birth, the opening closes.

The primary *bronchi* (air passages in the lungs) are present. The brain is growing; the forebrain divides into two parts. Eyes and nostrils are developing.

Intestines are forming, and the appendix and pancreas are present. Part of the intestine bulges into the umbilical cord. Later in development, it returns to the abdomen.

Changes in You

Changes occur gradually. You should have gained only a couple of pounds by this time. If you haven't gained weight or if you have lost a couple of pounds, it's OK. It will go the other direction in the weeks to come. You may still have morning sickness and other symptoms of early pregnancy.

How Your Actions Affect Your Baby's Development

Jewish Genetic Disorders

A group of medical conditions considered genetic disorders occur more commonly among Ashkenazi Jews, who are of eastern European descent. About 95% of the Jewish population in North America is of Ashkenazi heritage. Some of the diseases found in this group also affect Sephardi Jews and non-Jews; however, the conditions are more common among Ashkenazi Jews—sometimes 20 to 100 times more common.

> Although this book is designed to take you through pregnancy by examining one week at a time, you may want specific information. Because the book can't include *everything* you need *before* you know you're looking for it, check the index, beginning on page 655, for a particular topic. We may not cover the subject until a later week.

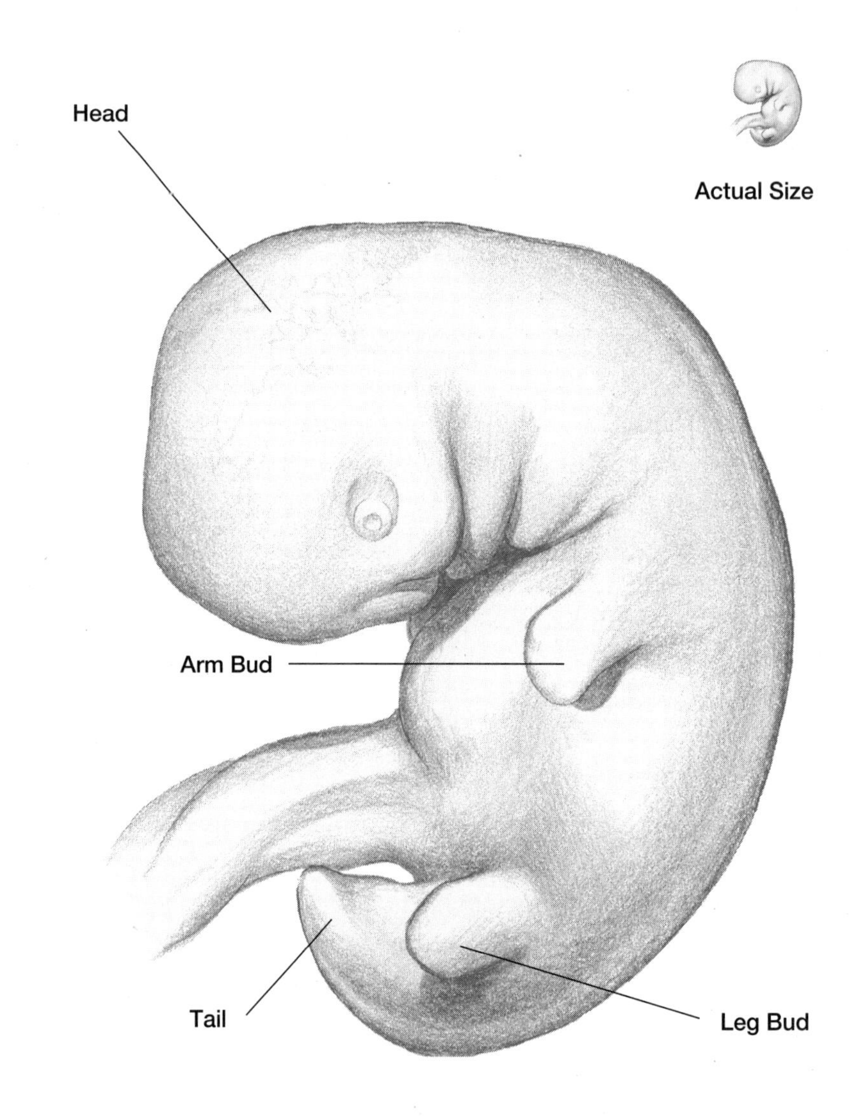

Your baby's brain is growing and developing.
The heart has divided into right and left chambers.

A great deal of research has been done to determine why these disorders occur more frequently in the Ashkenazi Jewish population. Researchers believe two processes are at work—the founder effect and genetic drift.

With the *founder effect*, genes that cause certain problems just happened to occur among the founders of the Ashkenazi Jews. They emigrated to eastern Europe around 70 A.D. Before they left Palestine, these disorders were probably as common among all other groups in the area. When the Ashkenazi Jews settled together in Europe, they carried these genes.

Because Ashkenazi Jews do not often marry outside their faith or community, the genes were not spread among other communities. This is called *genetic drift*. The presence of the genes was not decreased by introducing genes from outside the community, so many of the problems remained within this group.

Some diseases and conditions occur within other Jewish groups, such as Sephardi Jews. Sephardi Jews are of Spanish or Portuguese descent, and particular disorders occur within this group, probably for the same reasons they occur among Ashkenazi Jews.

Today, various conditions are considered "Jewish genetic disorders." However, we know people of other ethnic backgrounds can inherit some of these diseases. Some diseases and conditions are not usually found outside the various Jewish populations and are rare in the general population. These disorders include:

- Bloom syndrome
- factor-XI deficiency
- familial dysautonomia (Riley-Day syndrome)
- Fanconi anemia (Group C)
- Gaucher disease
- glucose-6 phosphate dehydrogenase deficiency (G6PD)
- glycogen storage disease, type III
- mucolipidosis IV
- Niemann-Pick disease (Type A)
- nonclassical adrenal hyperplasia

- nonsyndromic hearing loss
- torsion dystonia

Some very good resources are available to anyone who wants to learn more about Jewish genetic disorders. Two we have contacted for information include:

The Chicago Center for Genetic Disorders
Ben Gurion Way
One S. Franklin Street, 4th Floor
Chicago, IL 60606
312-357-4718
Email: jewishgeneticsctr@juf.org
www.jewishgeneticscenter.org

Center for Jewish Genetic Diseases
Mount Sinai School of Medicine
Box 1497
One Gustave L. Levy Place
New York, NY 10029
212-659-6774 (Main)
212-241-6947 (Consultation/Screening)
www.mssm.edu/jewish_genetics/

Screening tests are available for some of the diseases listed above. One test targets 11 genetic diseases and is designed for couples in which one or both members are of Ashkenazi or Sephardi Jewish descent. Many diseases can be identified before pregnancy or in early pregnancy. Discuss testing with your healthcare provider, if you're interested.

Using Over-the-Counter (OTC) Medicines

Nearly 65% of all pregnant women use some sort of medicine during pregnancy, including nonprescription medicine, also called *over-the-counter* medication. Often, it is used to treat pain and discomfort.

Facts about OTC Medicines

Below are some interesting facts about over-the-counter medicines and how they can affect you. Be careful with any medications you take during pregnancy.

- Avoid sudafed during the first trimester.
- Avoid cold remedies that contain iodine. Iodine can cause problems in baby.
- Claritin and Zyrtec are believed to be safe during pregnancy.
- Primatene Mist is not recommended for use when you're pregnant.
- If you regularly take Airborne to prevent colds when you aren't pregnant, it may be a good idea to skip it during pregnancy. It hasn't been tested on pregnant women.
- Be careful with antacid use—it can interfere with iron absorption.
- If you have a yeast infection, ask your healthcare provider about using an over-the-counter treatment, such as Terazol or Monistat.

Many people don't think of OTC products as medications, and they take them willy nilly, pregnant or not. Some researchers believe over-the-counter medication use actually *increases* during pregnancy.

Some OTC products may not be safe during pregnancy. See the box above. Use them with as much caution as any other drug! Many products are combinations of medicines. For example, pain medicine can contain aspirin, caffeine and phenacetin. Cough syrups or sleep medications can contain alcohol.

Tip for Week 7

Don't take any over-the-counter medicines for longer than 48 hours without talking to your healthcare provider. If a problem doesn't get better, your healthcare provider may have another treatment plan for you.

Read package labels and package inserts about safety during pregnancy—nearly all medicines contain this information. For example, some antacids can cause constipation and gas.

Some OTC products can be used safely during pregnancy, if you use them wisely. Check the list below:

- analgesics and pain relievers—acetaminophen (Tylenol)
- decongestants—chlorpheniramine (Chlor-Trimeton)
- nasal spray decongestants—oxymetazoline (Afrin, Dristan Long-Lasting)
- cough medicine—dextromethorphan (Robitussin; Vicks Formula 44)
- stomach relief—antacids (Amphojel, Gelusil, Maalox, milk of magnesia)
- throat relief—throat lozenges (Sucrets)
- laxatives—bulk-fiber laxatives (Metamucil, Fiberall)

If you think your symptoms or discomfort are more severe than they should be, call your healthcare provider. Follow his or her advice, and take good care of yourself.

Using Acetaminophen

Most experts believe acetaminophen is OK to use during pregnancy—it's hard to avoid because it's in over 200 products! Studies show it's easy to overdose on the medication because it *is* in so many preparations. You may not be aware it is contained in various products you may take to treat a single problem. Taking more than one product to treat a condition or illness could be dangerous. *Always read labels!* For example, take only *one* medication to treat a cold or flu symptoms, and always take the correct dose!

Your Nutrition

Dairy products can be very important during pregnancy. They contain calcium and vitamin D; both are important to you and baby. Calcium helps keep your bones healthy; baby needs it to develop strong bones and teeth.

A pregnant woman should take in 1200mg of calcium a day (1½ times the recommended amount for nonpregnant women). Your prenatal vitamin supplies about 300mg, so be sure you eat enough of the right foods to get the other 900mg.

Read food labels to find out how much calcium per serving is in a packaged food. Every day, write down the amount of calcium in each food you eat, and keep a running total to be sure you're getting 1200mg. Also see the box on page 106 to find out how to figure your daily calcium intake.

Some Good Sources of Calcium. Milk, cheese, yogurt and ice cream are good calcium sources. Other foods that contain calcium include broccoli, bok choy, collards, spinach, salmon, sardines, garbanzo beans (chickpeas), sesame seeds, almonds, cooked dried beans, tofu and trout. Some foods are fortified with calcium, such as some orange juice, breads, cereals and grains. Check your grocery shelves.

Some dairy foods you may choose, and their serving sizes, include the following:

- cottage cheese—¾ cup
- processed cheese (American)—2 ounces
- hard cheese (Parmesan or Romano)—1 ounce
- custard or pudding—1 cup
- milk (whole, 2%, 1%, skim)—8 ounces
- natural cheese (cheddar)—1½ ounces
- yogurt (plain or flavored)—1 cup

If you want to lower calories, choose low-fat dairy products. Calcium content is unaffected in low-fat dairy products. Good choices include skim milk, low-fat yogurt and low-fat cheese.

Increase the amount of calcium you get by adding powdered nonfat milk to recipes, such as mashed potatoes and meat loaf. Make fruit shakes with fresh fruit and milk; add a scoop of ice milk, frozen yogurt or ice cream. Cook rice and oatmeal in skim or low-fat milk. When you make canned soups, substitute milk for water. Have a smoothie instead of plain orange juice.

Some foods interfere with calcium absorption. Salt, tea, coffee, protein and unleavened bread lower the amount of calcium absorbed.

If you take antibiotics, read the label on your prescription. If it says not to take it with calcium-containing foods, take the antibiotic 1 hour before or 2 hours after meals.

If you're having trouble getting enough calcium into your diet, ask your healthcare provider about taking a calcium supplement. He or she can advise you.

Lactose Intolerance. When lactose is not properly digested, it can cause gas, bloating, cramps and diarrhea; a person with this problem is referred to as *lactose intolerant.* If you're lactose intolerant, there are many sources of calcium available to you. Look for calcium-fortified products. Try rice milk and soy milk fortified with calcium and vitamin D. You may be able to buy lactose-free milk at your grocery store. If you like cheese, there are lactose-free brands you can buy. Ask your grocer about them.

The OTC medicine *Lactaid* helps the body break down lactose. There are no warnings or precautions about it for use in pregnancy, but check with your healthcare provider *before* you use it.

How Much Calcium?

It may be a little difficult to determine how much calcium you're getting in foods you eat. Package labeling usually lists the *percentage* of calcium in a food. This may be confusing because it's hard to know how much that is.

The solution is to understand that labeling is based on the RDA recommendation for a nonpregnant woman, which is 800mg a day. If a package states "calcium 20%," just multiply 800 times 0.2, which gives you the amount of 160mg. Keep a written record of how much calcium you take in every day. You need a total of about 1200mg of calcium a day.

Listeriosis

Every year about 1500 cases of listeriosis, a form of food poisoning, are reported in the United States. About 500 of these cases occur in pregnant women, who are more susceptible to infection. Babies born to moms who had listeriosis are at higher risk of developing problems.

> Your body can't absorb more than 500mg of calcium at a time, so spread your intake out every day. At breakfast, if you have calcium-fortified orange juice, calcium-fortified bread, cereal with milk and a carton of yogurt, you may be taking in a lot more than 500mg, but your body won't be able to absorb it!

To prevent listeriosis, avoid unpasteurized milk and any foods made from unpasteurized milk. Avoid unpasteurized soft cheeses such as Camembert, Brie, feta, Gorgonzola, bleu cheese and Roquefort. ***If they have been made with pasteurized milk,*** soft cheeses are OK during pregnancy. Read labels very carefully.

You also need to be careful of other products that are not pasteurized, such as some juices. Use caution when buying fruit juice at a farmers' market or a farm stand. It may not be pasteurized. Unpasteurized fresh juice can contain a lot of germs.

Undercooked poultry, red meat, seafood and hot dogs can also contain listeriosis. Cook all meat and seafood thoroughly. Be careful about cross-contamination of foods. If you put raw seafood or hot dogs on a counter or cutting board, thoroughly wash the area with soap and hot water or a disinfectant *before* you put other food on that surface.

You Should Also Know

Sexual Intimacy During Pregnancy

Many couples want to know if it's all right to have sexual intercourse during pregnancy. Many men wonder if sex can harm a growing baby. Sexual relations are usually OK for a healthy pregnant woman and her partner.

Frequent sexual activity shouldn't hurt a healthy pregnancy. Neither intercourse nor orgasm should be a problem if you have a low-risk pregnancy. The baby is well protected inside the amniotic sac.

If you have questions, bring them up at a prenatal visit. If your partner goes with you to your appointments, he may benefit from hearing your healthcare provider's advice. If he doesn't go with you, assure him there should be no problems if your healthcare provider gives you the go-ahead.

Sex doesn't just mean sexual intercourse. There are other ways for couples to be sensual together, including giving each other a massage, bathing together and talking about sex. Whatever you do, be honest with your partner about how you feel—and keep a sense of humor!

Dad Tip

It's important to know what your partner is talking about when she talks to you about her pregnancy. If she uses terms you don't understand, ask her to explain them. Or take a quick look in our Glossary for a definition, page 620. It helps to become familiar with all the technical pregnancy terms you'll be hearing in the months that lie ahead.

Your Prenatal Vitamin

Taking a prenatal vitamin can be very important for you and your baby. Be sure your prenatal vitamin contains iodine—it's important for baby's brain development. A recent study showed only about half of all prenatal vitamins have it.

Don't drink coffee or tea for 1 hour after taking your prenatal vitamin. These drinks prevent iron absorption.

Omega-3 fatty acids and DHA are good for baby's brain development. Ask your pharmacist or healthcare provider about whether your prenatal vitamin contains them.

Do You Need Extra Iron?

Nearly all diets that supply enough calories for you to gain weight during pregnancy have enough minerals to prevent mineral deficiency. However, few women have iron stores to meet pregnancy demands. The recommended dose is 27mg a day.

A Look at Prenatal Vitamins

Prenatal vitamins contain many needed substances for you and baby. That's why you should take them every day until baby is born. A typical prenatal vitamin contains the following:

- calcium to build baby's teeth and bones, and to help strengthen your own
- copper to help prevent anemia and to help in bone formation
- folic acid to reduce the risk of neural-tube defects and to help in blood-cell production
- iodine to help control metabolism
- iron to prevent anemia and to help baby's blood development
- vitamin A for general health and body metabolism
- vitamin B_1 for general health and body metabolism
- vitamin B_2 for general health and body metabolism
- vitamin B_3 for general health and body metabolism
- vitamin B_6 for general health and body metabolism
- vitamin B_{12} to promote blood formation
- vitamin C to aid in your body's absorption of iron
- vitamin D to strengthen baby's bones and teeth, and to help your body use phosphorus and calcium
- vitamin E for general health and body metabolism
- zinc to help balance fluids in your body, and to aid nerve and muscle function

During pregnancy, your iron needs increase. Iron intake is most important in the second half of pregnancy. Most women don't need iron supplements during the first trimester. If you take iron then, it can worsen symptoms of nausea and vomiting. In addition, iron can irritate your stomach and may cause constipation.

Other Supplementation

Zinc may help you if you are thin or underweight. We believe zinc helps a thin woman increase her chances of giving birth to a bigger, healthier baby. Recent reports have tied the use of zinc to reducing the length and severity of a cold. You may even have used some of these cold remedies in the past. However, we recommend you talk to your healthcare provider before using any zinc product for a cold. We don't have information on how using zinc to help fight a cold could affect a pregnant woman. Better to be safe than sorry.

The value of fluoride and fluoride supplementation in a pregnant woman is unclear. Some researchers believe fluoride supplementation during pregnancy results in improved teeth in the child, but not everyone agrees. Fluoride supplementation in a pregnant woman has not been proved harmful to her baby. Some prenatal vitamins contain fluoride.

Overactive Bladder and Incontinence Medications

Do you take medicine to treat an overactive bladder? If you do, you need to talk to your healthcare provider before pregnancy or as soon as you find out you're pregnant. He or she can advise you about continued use of your medicine during pregnancy.

The problem of overactive bladder occurs when the brain tells nerves in the bladder there's a need to urinate, even if the bladder isn't full.

Some Information May Scare You

In an effort to give you as much information as possible about pregnancy, we do include serious discussions throughout the book that some might find "scary." The information is not included to frighten you; it's there to provide facts about particular medical situations that may occur during pregnancy.

If a woman experiences a serious problem, she and her partner will probably want to know as much about it as possible. If a woman has a friend or knows someone who has problems during pregnancy, reading about it might relieve her fears. We also hope our discussions can help you start a dialogue with your doctor, if you have questions.

Nearly all pregnancies are uneventful, and serious situations don't arise. However, please know we have tried to cover as many aspects of pregnancy as we possibly can so you'll have all the information at hand that you might need and want. Knowledge is power, so having various facts available can help you feel more in control of your own pregnancy. We hope reading information helps you relax and have a great pregnancy experience.

If you find serious discussions frighten you, don't read them! Or if the information doesn't apply to your pregnancy, just skip over it. But realize information is there if you want to know more about a particular situation.

Symptoms include going to the bathroom more than 12 times a day, getting up two or more times at night and a sudden, immediate need to go. You may also leak urine.

Medicines to treat the problem work by relaxing muscles. Some commonly prescribed medications include Ditropan, Detrol LA, Sanctura and Enablex.

Exercise for Week 7

Stand with your right side next to the sofa or a sturdy chair. Holding onto the sofa or chair with your right hand, lift your right foot and place it on the arm of the piece of furniture. Bend forward until you feel a stretch in your leg. Hold for 10 seconds. Repeat for your left leg. *Stretches hamstrings, and strengthens thigh muscles.*

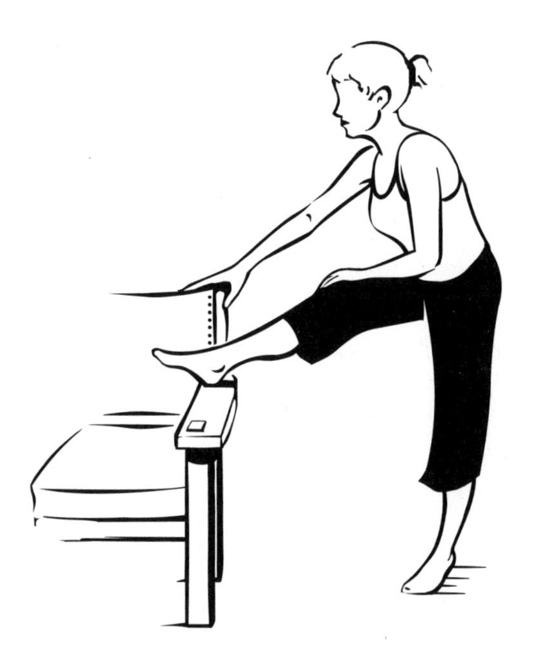

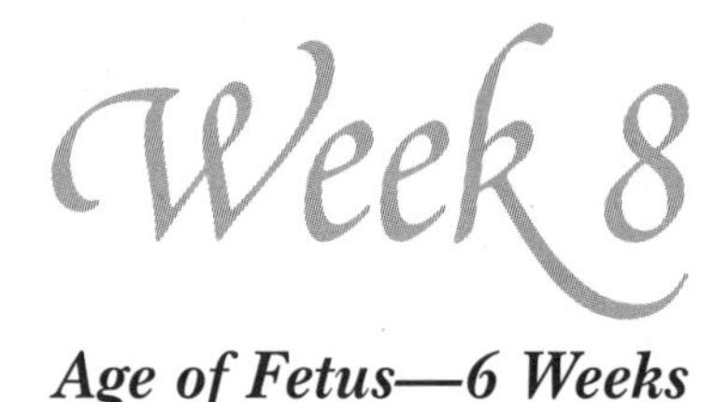

Age of Fetus—6 Weeks

If you've just found out you're pregnant,
you might want to begin by reading the previous chapters.

How Big Is Your Baby?

By this week of pregnancy, the crown-to-rump length of baby is ½ to ¾ inch (1.4 to 2cm). This is about the size of a pinto bean.

How Big Are You?

Your uterus is getting bigger, so you should be noticing a change in your waistline and the fit of your clothes. Your healthcare provider will see that your uterus is enlarged, if you have a pelvic exam.

How Your Baby Is Growing and Developing

Your baby is continuing to grow and to change. Compare the illustration on page 114 with previous illustrations. Can you see the changes?

Eyes are moving toward the middle of the face. Eyelid folds appear on the face, and nerve cells in the eye are beginning to develop.

The tip of the nose is present. Internal and external ears are forming. The body's trunk area is getting longer and straightening out.

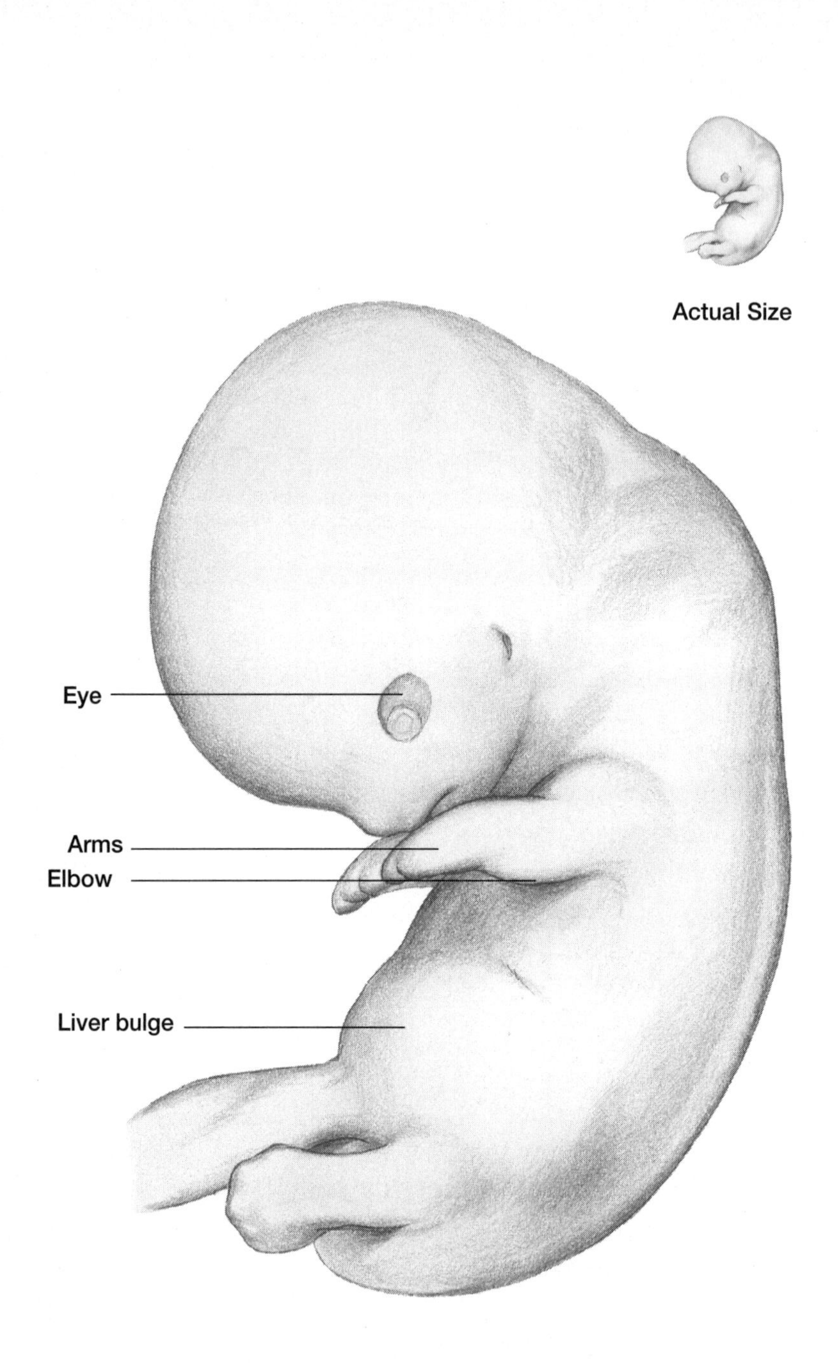

Embryo at 8 weeks (fetal age—6 weeks).
Crown-to-rump length is about ¾ inch (20mm).
Arms are longer and bend at the elbows.

Arms are longer. Elbows are present, and arms now bend at the elbows and curve slightly over the heart. Arms and legs extend forward. The beginning of fingers and toes can be seen.

Changes in You

As your uterus grows, you may feel cramping or even pain in your lower abdomen or at your sides. Some women feel tightening of the uterus throughout pregnancy. If you don't feel it, don't worry. But if you also have bleeding from the vagina, call your healthcare provider immediately.

Headaches and Migraines

Some pregnant women have headaches during pregnancy. *Tension headaches* can be caused by stress, fatigue, heat, noise, thirst, hunger, loud music and bright lights. Be careful what you eat. Some foods can trigger a headache, including peanuts, chocolate, cheese and some meats. If your sinuses are clogged, that may also increase headaches.

> A headache or migraine that doesn't go away in late pregnancy could signal problems. Call your healthcare provider immediately!

Cluster headaches come in groups, last about an hour and can continue for weeks or months. Acetaminophen is OK to use for these types of headaches.

Don't want to take medicine for a pounding headache? There are other things you can try. Exercise may help. Massage your neck and shoulders to help relax tight muscles. If you have a sinus headache, put a warm wash cloth over your nose and eyes. Or put a cold pack on the base of your neck. Fold a scarf lengthwise to make a 2-inch-wide band, tie it around your head and knot it at the point where pain is most intense. It can help.

Migraines. Migraine headaches are often an inherited problem. Nearly 20% of all pregnant women have a migraine at some point in pregnancy.

Tip for Week 8

Wash your hands thoroughly throughout the day, especially after handling raw meat or using the bathroom. This simple act can help prevent the spread of many bacteria and viruses that cause infection.

A migraine can last for a few hours up to 3 days. Some women suffer more during pregnancy because of their changing hormone levels.

Ginger may help with migraines—a pinch of powdered ginger in water may be as good as prescription medicine. When you first feel symptoms, mix ⅓ teaspoon of powdered ginger in a cup of water. Drink this three or four times a day for 3 days.

Sciatic-Nerve Pain and Sacroiliac-Joint Pain

Many women experience an occasional excruciating pain in their buttocks and down the back or side of their legs as pregnancy progresses. It is called *sciatic-nerve pain* or *sciatica*. Some people may mistakenly refer to it as sacroiliac pain. However, sciatica pain and sacroiliac pain are not the same thing.

Sciatica is a sharp, searing pain that travels down your buttocks, legs and thighs. The best treatment is to lie on your opposite side to help relieve pressure on the nerve. Sitting on a tennis ball on a hard surface may also help.

Sacroiliac joint pain (SJP) is joint related and feels like a sharp jolt of pain on either side of the back or hips. It may extend down your legs. Warm baths (not hot) and acetaminophen may help.

How Your Actions Affect Your Baby's Development

Acne during Pregnancy

Some women notice an improvement in their acne during pregnancy, but it doesn't happen for everyone. Some women find that acne becomes a problem for them during pregnancy, even if they haven't been bothered by it in the past.

Acne can range from whiteheads and blackheads to inflamed red bumps. Flare-ups in the first trimester are fairly common because hormones change rapidly. Pimples can appear on your neck, shoulders, back and face.

To treat acne, use a mild cleanser, followed by a mild, nonclogging moisturizer with sunscreen. Don't use products that contain salicylic acid; we don't know about their safety during pregnancy. Drinking lots of water also seems to help.

Talk to your healthcare provider before using over-the-counter acne treatments. Avoid *any* prepregnancy prescription skin products until you talk to your healthcare provider about them. It's safe to use azelaic acid gel 15% (Finacea) twice a day.

Accutane (isotretinoin) is commonly prescribed to treat acne. Do *not* take Accutane during pregnancy! If taken during the first trimester, it may increase your chances of miscarriage and birth defects in baby.

Miscarriage and Stillbirth

Nearly every pregnant woman thinks about miscarriage during pregnancy, but it occurs in only about 20% of all pregnancies. *Miscarriage* occurs when a pregnancy ends before the embryo or fetus can survive on its own outside the uterus, usually within the first 3 months. After 20 weeks, loss of a pregnancy is called a *stillbirth*. Many causes of miscarriage also apply to stillbirth, and in this discussion, we will use the term "miscarriage" to apply to both. A discussion of stillbirth follows.

> *Screening* tests provide odds of a problem occurring. *Diagnostic* tests determine if a problem is present.

Some signs of miscarriage include vaginal bleeding, cramps, pain that comes and goes, pain that begins in the small of the back and moves to the lower abdomen and loss of tissue. If you experience any of these symptoms, call your healthcare provider immediately.

What Causes a Miscarriage? We don't usually know, and are often unable to find out, what causes a miscarriage. The most common reason in early miscarriages is abnormal development of the embryo. Experts believe there are many reasons miscarriage occurs, including:

- chromosome problems
- hormone problems
- problems with the uterus
- chronic health conditions
- a high fever in early pregnancy
- autoimmune disorders
- unusual infections
- mother-to-be's age
- obesity, especially in women with a BMI higher than 35
- cigarette smoking
- drinking alcohol
- trauma from an accident or major surgery
- an incompetent cervix after the first trimester

Use of aspirin and nonsteroidal anti-inflammatories (NSAIDs) may increase the risk of miscarriage. Caffeine use before and during pregnancy may increase your risk. Some experts believe a father-to-be's age may play a role in the risk of miscarriage. When a man is over age 35, there may be a greater risk of miscarriage than for younger men, no matter what the woman's age is.

Below is a discussion of different types and causes of miscarriage. It is included to alert you about what to watch for if you have any symptoms of a miscarriage. If you have questions, discuss them with your healthcare provider.

Different Types of Miscarriage. If you have a *threatened miscarriage,* it appears as a bloody discharge from the vagina during the first half of pregnancy. Bleeding may last for days or even weeks. There may not be any cramping or pain. If there is pain, it may feel like a menstrual cramp or a mild backache. Resting in bed is about all you can do, but being active does not cause miscarriage. No procedure or medication can keep a woman from miscarrying.

An *inevitable miscarriage* occurs when the bag of water breaks (rupture of membranes), the cervix dilates and you pass blood clots and/or tissue. Miscarriage is almost certain under these circumstances. The uterus usually expels the fetus or products of conception.

With an *incomplete miscarriage*, the entire pregnancy may not be passed at once. Part is passed while part of it remains in the uterus. Bleeding may be heavy and continues until the uterus is empty.

A *missed miscarriage* can occur if the body retains an embryo that died earlier. There may be no symptoms or bleeding. The time period from when the pregnancy failed to the time the miscarriage is discovered is usually weeks.

If you suffer a miscarriage, research shows you have a 90% chance of having a healthy pregnancy the next time you get pregnant.

About 1 to 2% of all couples will experience a *recurrent* or *habitual miscarriage*. This usually refers to three or more consecutive miscarriages. Studies show that 60 to 70% of couples who have recurrent or habitual miscarriages eventually have a successful pregnancy.

A *chemical pregnancy* occurs when tissue forms that produces the hormone (HCG) that makes a pregnancy test positive. However, the tissue embryo dies very soon, so there actually is no pregnancy.

If You Have Problems. If you have problems, notify your healthcare provider immediately! Bleeding often appears first, followed by cramping. Ectopic pregnancy must also be considered. A quantitative-HCG test may be useful in identifying a normal pregnancy, but a single test report doesn't usually help. Your healthcare provider needs to repeat the test over a period of several days.

Ultrasound may help if you are more than 5 gestational weeks into your pregnancy. You may continue to bleed, but seeing your baby's heartbeat may be reassuring. If the first ultrasound is not reassuring, you may be asked to wait a week or 10 days, then repeat the test.

The longer you bleed and cramp, the more likely you are having a miscarriage. If you pass all of the pregnancy, bleeding stops and cramping goes away, you may be done with it. However, if everything is not expelled, it may be necessary to perform a *dilatation and curettage (D&C)* to empty the uterus. It's better to do this so you won't bleed for a long time, risking anemia and infection.

Some women are given progesterone in an effort to help them keep a pregnancy. Medical experts do not agree on its use or its effectiveness.

Dad Tip

If you have pets, take over their care during your partner's pregnancy. Change the cat's litter box (she shouldn't do this while pregnant). Walk the dog (the pull on the leash might hurt her back). Buy food and other pet supplies (to save her back from the strain of lifting big food bags). Make and keep vet appointments.

Rh-Sensitivity and Miscarriage. If you're Rh-negative and you have a miscarriage, you will need to receive RhoGAM. This applies *only* if you are Rh-negative. RhoGAM is given to protect you from making antibodies to Rh-positive blood.

Stillbirth. Stillbirth is the death of a fetus after 20 weeks of pregnancy. Various reasons are cited for stillbirth, including being older, having had more children and carrying more than one baby. Nearly 50% of all unexplained stillbirths may be related to problems in the fetus.

If you're obese before pregnancy, it increases your risk of stillbirth. Other causes may include high blood pressure, diabetes, lupus, renal disease, thrombophilia, multiples, some infections and placenta and cord accidents.

Having a stillborn baby can be a traumatic experience for you, and it can take time to recover from it. You and your partner will probably have many questions and concerns. To help you find answers to your questions, discuss them with your healthcare provider.

If You Have a Miscarriage or Stillbirth. Having a miscarriage or stillbirth can be difficult. Some couples experience more than one miscarriage, which can be very difficult to deal with. In most cases, repeated miscarriages occur due to chance or "bad luck." Most healthcare providers don't recommend testing to find a reason for miscarriage unless you have three or more pregnancy losses in a row.

Don't blame yourself or your partner for the loss of a pregnancy. It's usually impossible to look back at everything you've done, eaten or been exposed to and find the cause.

If a miscarriage or stillbirth occurs, give yourself plenty of time to recover physically and emotionally. In the past, we have advised a couple not to try to get pregnant immediately and to allow 3 or 4 months for a woman's body to return to its normal cycle and for hormone levels to return to normal. However, some experts now believe a couple doesn't have to wait a few months to try again. They believe it's safe for a woman to try to get pregnant again as soon as she has a menstrual period. Talk to your healthcare provider if you have questions.

As a couple, you might want to allow yourselves time to recover emotionally. This may take longer than the actual physical recovery.

Your Nutrition

It's hard to eat nutritiously for *every* meal. You may not always get the nutrients you need, in the amounts you need. On page 122 is a chart showing where you can get the various nutrients you should be eating every day. In each meal during pregnancy, try to include a whole-grain product, fruits and/or veggies, a lean protein and a healthy fat.

Your prenatal vitamin is *not* a substitute for food, so don't count on it to supply you with all the essential vitamins and minerals you need. Food is your most important source of nutrients!

You Should Also Know

Braces during Pregnancy?

It seems people of all ages are getting braces these days. We've been asked by women about braces for their teeth during pregnancy. They want to know if it's OK to continue wearing braces during pregnancy,

Sources of Food Nutrients

Nutrient (Daily Requirement)	***Food Sources***
Calcium (1200mg)	dairy products, dark leafy vegetables, dried beans and peas, tofu
Folic acid (0.4mg)	liver, dried beans and peas, eggs, broccoli, whole-grain products, oranges, orange juice
Iron (30mg)	fish, liver, meat, poultry, egg yolks, nuts, dried beans and peas, dark leafy vegetables, dried fruit
Magnesium (320mg)	dried beans and peas, cocoa, seafood, whole-grain products, nuts
Vitamin B_6 (2.2mg)	whole-grain products, liver, meat
Vitamin E (10mg)	milk, eggs, meat, fish, cereals, dark leafy vegetables, vegetable oils
Zinc (15mg)	seafood, meat, nuts, milk, dried beans and peas

and they want to know if they can have braces put on when they're pregnant.

If you already have braces, some things could make treatment a bit more taxing for you. If you have morning sickness and vomit a lot, you'll need to take very good care of your teeth. Brushing is important to clean acid off teeth. When your braces are tightened, you may want to eat soft foods, but that's acceptable for a few days. You can take acetaminophen for any discomfort.

If you're scheduled to have your braces put on then discover you're pregnant, don't panic. Contact your orthodontist, and tell him or her you're pregnant. Discuss any plans regarding braces with your pregnancy healthcare provider *and* your orthodontist *before* any action is taken!

Concern comes if you need dental X-rays; they may be an essential part of the treatment plan. However, with modern equipment and use of digital radiography, these risks can be reduced.

You may need to have one or more teeth pulled. Tooth extraction by itself may not be dangerous, but the anesthesia necessary to pull a tooth may not be good for you or baby. Your treatment plan must be discussed and agreed upon by your pregnancy healthcare provider and your orthodontist before your begin.

If you get the go ahead to put your braces on, you may want to eat soft foods for a few days after you get them. You may also have some soreness when braces are put on or tightened. It's OK to take acetaminophen for any discomfort.

Lab Tests Your Healthcare Provider May Order

When you go for your first or second prenatal visit, your healthcare provider may order a lot of tests, including blood tests. You may also have a urinalysis and urine culture, and cervical cultures to test for STDs. A Pap smear may also be done. Other tests are done as required.

Most of the tests are done on your blood—usually only a vial or two is needed to perform all the tests. If you have difficulty having your blood drawn or you get lightheaded or faint after blood is taken, you might want to ask your partner to accompany you to the test. Blood tests that may be ordered include:

- complete blood count (CBC) to check your iron stores and to check for infections
- rubella titer to see if you have immunity against rubella (German measles)
- blood type to determine what your blood type is (A, B, AB or O)
- an Rh-factor test to determine if you are Rh-negative
- a blood-sugar-level test to look for diabetes
- test for varicella (chicken pox) to see if you have had this disease in the past
- test for hepatitis-B antibodies to determine whether you have ever been exposed to hepatitis-B
- screening test for syphilis (VDRL or ART)
- test for thrombophilia
- an HIV/AIDS test to see if you have been infected with the AIDS virus

It is not routine to screen all women for HIV during pregnancy. It may be offered to you; you must decide whether you should be tested. Some experts recommend all women undergo screening during pregnancy. Discuss it with your healthcare provider.

Ask your healthcare provider about a test for hypothyroidism. Researchers believe women should be tested for thyroid-stimulating hormone (TSH) at the beginning of pregnancy. One study showed that after 16 weeks, pregnant women who had higher-than-normal levels of TSH had 4 times the chance of having a miscarriage or stillbirth than women with normal levels.

Toxoplasmosis

If you have a cat, you may be concerned about *toxoplasmosis*. The disease is spread by eating raw, infected meat or by contact with infected

Medical Conditions and "Safe" Medications to Use during Pregnancy

Condition	Drugs of Choice that Are Safe to Use
Acne	benzoyl peroxide, clindamycin, erythromycin
Asthma	inhalers—beta-adrenergic antagonists, corticosteroids, cromolyn, ipratropium
Bacterial infection	cephalosporins, clindamycin, cotrimoxazole, erythromycin, nitrofurantoin, penicillin
Bipolar disorder	chlorpromazine, haloperidol
Coughs	cough lozenges, dextromethorphan, diphenhydramine, codeine (short term)
Depression	fluoxetine, tricyclic antidepressants
Headache	acetaminophen
Hypertension	hydralazine, methyldopa
Hyperthyroidism	propylthiouracil
Migraines	codeine, dimenhydrinate
Nausea and vomiting	doxylamine plus pyridoxine
Peptic ulcer disease	antacids, rantidine

cat feces. Usually an infection in the mother-to-be has no symptoms but can cross the placenta to the baby.

Infection during pregnancy can lead to miscarriage or an infected infant at birth. Toxoplasmosis in a mother-to-be can cause serious problems in her baby. Antibiotics can be used to treat toxoplasmosis, but the best plan is prevention. Sanitary measures prevent transmission of the disease.

Get someone else to change the kitty litter. Wash your hands thoroughly after petting your cat, and keep your cat off counters and tables. Wash your hands after contact with meat and soil. Cook all meat thoroughly. Avoid cross-contamination of foods while preparing and cooking them.

Exercise for Week 8

Sit on the floor in a comfortable position. Inhale as you raise your right arm over your head. Reach as high as you can, while stretching from the waist. Bend your elbow, and pull your arm back down to your side as you exhale. Repeat for your left side. Do 4 or 5 times on each side. *Relieves upper backache and tension in shoulders, neck and back.*

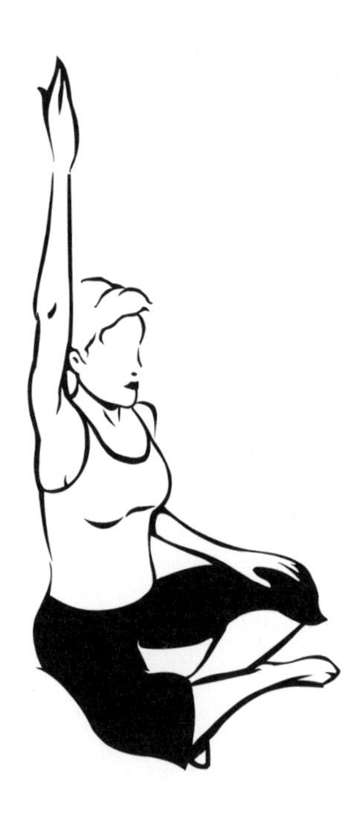

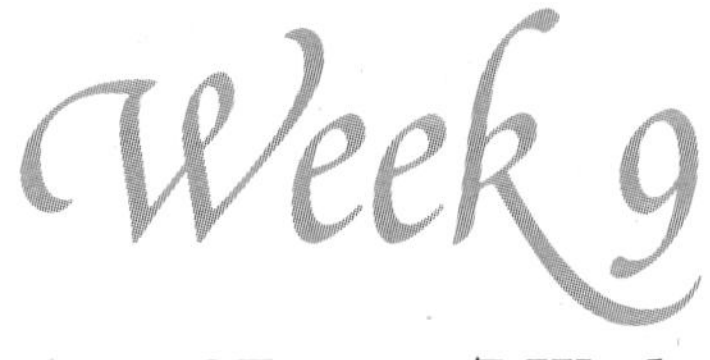

Age of Fetus—7 Weeks

If you've just found out you're pregnant, you might want to begin by reading the previous chapters.

How Big Is Your Baby?

The crown-to-rump length of the embryo is 1 to 1¼ inches (2.2 to 3cm). This is close to the size of a medium green olive.

How Big Are You?

Your waistline may be growing thicker. This occurs as your uterus fills your pelvic area and starts to grow up into the tummy area.

How Your Baby Is Growing and Developing

If you could look inside your uterus, you'd see many changes in your baby. The illustration on page 128 shows some of them.

Baby's arms and legs are longer. Fingers are longer, and the tips are slightly enlarged where touch pads are developing. The feet are approaching the midline of the body and may meet in front of the torso.

The head is more erect, and the neck is more developed. The pupil forms this week, and the optic nerve begins to form. Eyelids almost cover the eyes; up to this time, eyes have been uncovered. External ears

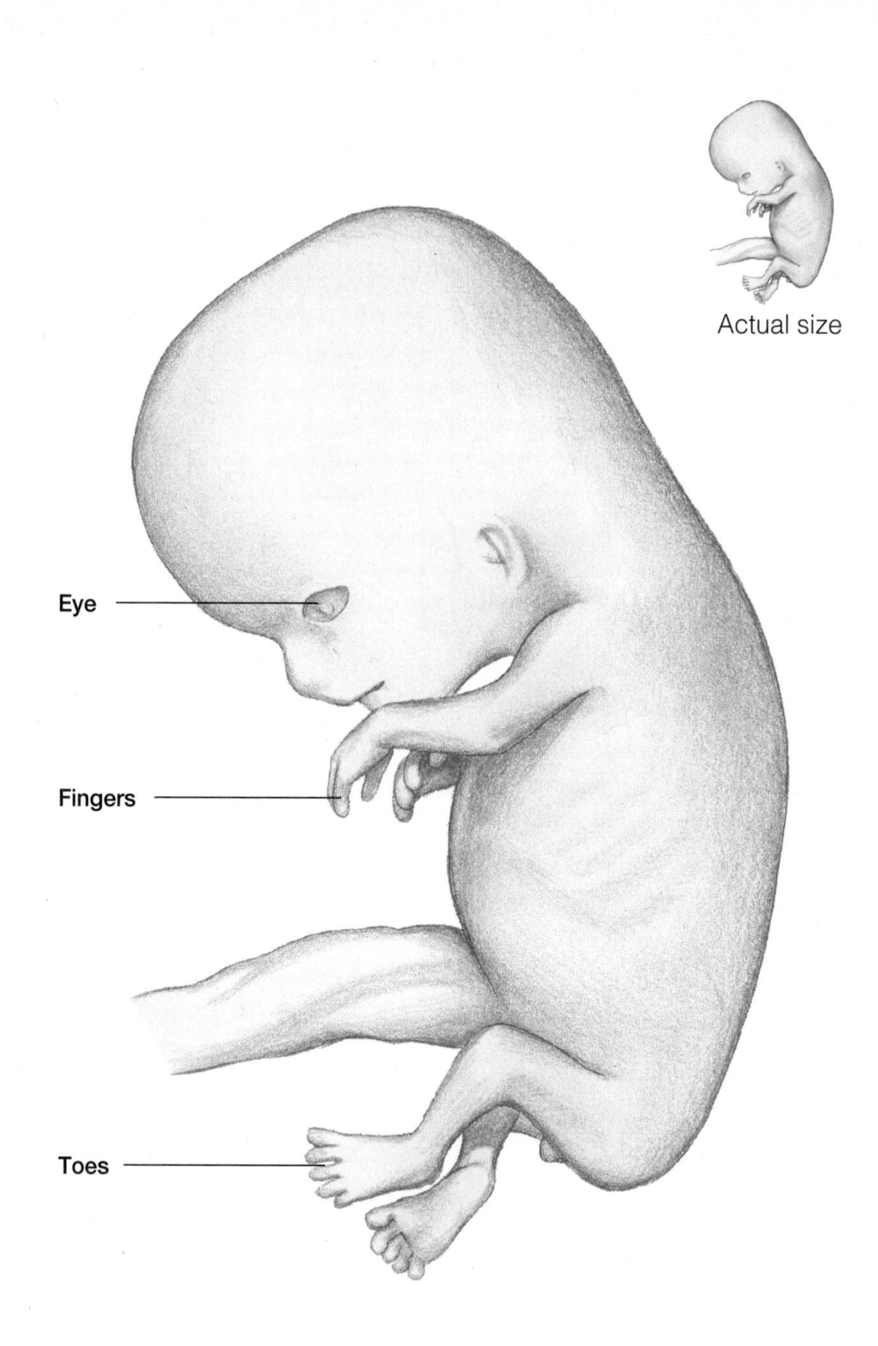

Embryo at 9 weeks of pregnancy (fetal age—46 to 49 days).
Toes are formed and feet are more recognizable.
Crown-to-rump length is about 1 inch (25mm).

are evident and well formed. Your baby now moves its body and limbs. This movement may be seen during an ultrasound exam.

The baby looks more recognizable as a human being, although it is still extremely small. But you still can't tell the difference between a boy and a girl. You won't be able to do that for another few weeks.

Changes in You

Your blood system changes a lot during pregnancy, and the amount of blood in your body, called *blood volume,* increases as much as 50%. Higher blood volume helps meet the demands of your growing baby and helps protect you both. It's also important during labor and delivery, when some blood is lost.

Increased blood volume begins during the first trimester. The greatest increase occurs in the second trimester. It continues to increase but at a slower rate during the third trimester.

The increase in red blood cells increases your body's need for iron and can cause anemia. If you're anemic during pregnancy, you may get tired easily or feel ill.

> *Dad Tip*
>
> Ask your partner which prenatal visits she'd like you to attend. Some couples attend every visit together, when possible. Ask her to let you know the date and time of each appointment.

How Your Actions Affect Your Baby's Development

Celiac Disease

Celiac disease, also called *celiac sprue, nontropical sprue* and *gluten-sensitive enteropathy,* is a digestive disease that affects the small intestine. If you have celiac disease, you have an allergy to gluten, which is found in wheat, oats, rye and barley. This allergy causes your immune system to attack your intestines so you absorb fewer nutrients. Symptoms include diarrhea, abdominal pain, bloating, irritability and depression.

How Is Pregnancy Weight Distributed?

When a baby is born, an average-weight mother should have gained between 25 and 35 pounds. A woman who has gained 30 pounds may see her weight distributed as shown below.

11 pounds	Fat, protein and other nutrients in mom
4 pounds	Increased fluid volume
2 pounds	Breast enlargement
2 pounds	Uterus
7½ pounds	Baby
2 pounds	Amniotic fluid
1½ pounds	Placenta

The condition is hereditary and occurs more often in women than men. It's most common in Western Europeans and rare in Africans and Asians. We believe celiac disease affects 1 in 100 people worldwide and 1 in every 133 Americans. It may be overlooked during pregnancy because symptoms can be the same as for other problems. Many healthcare providers don't know much about the disease, and it can be difficult to diagnose.

A blood test can determine if you may have a problem with celiac disease. A biopsy of the small intestine can confirm it.

If you have celiac disease, it's important to have it under control before pregnancy by eating a gluten-free diet. You can learn whether a food contains gluten by reading labels because manufacturers are required by law to list this information. Many foods are now gluten-free. Because folic acid is found in many fortified grain products, you will probably need supplements to ensure you receive enough folic acid.

Tip for Week 9

It's an old wives' tale that your hair won't curl if you have a permanent during pregnancy. Our only precaution is that if odors affect you, the fumes from a permanent or hair coloring could make you feel ill.

Celiac disease may appear for the first time during pregnancy or after childbirth. If you have symptoms, talk to your healthcare provider. You may need to meet with a dietician to develop a nutritional meal plan.

Some General Lifestyle Precautions

Some women are concerned about using *saunas, hot tubs* and *spas* during pregnancy. They want to know if it is OK to relax in this way.

We recommend you don't take a chance with a sauna, hot tub or spa. Your baby relies on you to maintain correct body temperature. If your body temperature gets high enough, and stays there for a while, it may hurt the baby.

There is disagreement about using *electric blankets* and *electric warming pads* to keep you warm in bed. Some experts question whether they can cause health problems.

Electric blankets and warming pads produce a low-level electromagnetic field. The growing baby may be more sensitive than an adult to these electromagnetic fields. Because we have no "acceptable level" of exposure for you and baby, it's probably best not to use them during pregnancy. There are other ways to keep warm, such as down comforters and wool blankets or snuggling with your partner. Any of these may be a better choice.

Your Nutrition

Fruits and vegetables are important during pregnancy. Because different kinds of produce are available in different seasons, they are a great

> The FDA is updating labels on prescription medicine to include a *fetal-risk summary.* This will tell you the possible drug effects on a fetus. It is also updating labels to include information on the amount of a medicine that may be present in breast milk after you take it. Ask your pharmacist about it if you're interested.

When buying vitamins, look for the *U.S.P. verified* symbol, which means the vitamins are usually good quality.

way to add variety to your diet. They are excellent sources of vitamins, minerals and fiber. Eating a variety of fruits and vegetables can supply you with iron, folate, calcium and vitamin C.

When you eat raw veggies, include a little fat to help absorb nutrients from the vegetables. A little salad dressing, a piece of avocado or some nuts may also enhance the flavor. When you don't feel like eating your vegetables, soups can add variety and substance to your meal plan. Broth-based vegetable soups may provide more nutrients and fewer calories than a sandwich or a plate of pasta. To add veggies to your meal plan, try grilling, baking or broiling them. Stir-fry veggies with a little bit of meat, or add beans to stews and soups. Make tabbouleh, and flavor it with herbs.

Tasty, Low-Cal Sources of Vitamin C

Five excellent sources of vitamin C are easy to add to your diet, and if you're watching your weight, they're also low in calories! Try the following:

- strawberries—94 mg in 1 cup
- orange juice—82 mg in 1 cup
- kiwi fruit—74 mg in 1 medium kiwi fruit
- broccoli—58mg in ½ cup, cooked
- red peppers—57mg in ¼ of a medium red pepper

Vitamin C Is Important

Vitamin C can be very important during pregnancy. It can help you and baby in many different ways.

The recommended daily dose of vitamin C is 85mg—a bit more than what is contained in a prenatal vitamin. You can get some of the extra vitamin C you need by eating fruits and vegetables rich in the vitamin.

Each day, eat one or two servings of fruit high in vitamin C and at least one dark-green or deep-yellow vegetable for extra iron, fiber and folate. Fruits and vegetables you may choose, and their serving sizes, include the following:

- grapes—¾ cup
- banana, orange, apple—1 medium
- dried fruit—¼ cup
- fruit juice—½ cup
- canned or cooked fruit—½ cup
- broccoli, carrots or other vegetables—½ cup
- potato—1 medium
- leafy green vegetables—1 cup
- vegetable juice—¼ cup

Don't take in more than the recommended dose of vitamin C; too much may cause stomach cramps and diarrhea. It can also negatively affect baby's metabolism.

You Should Also Know

Avoid Anxiety-Producing TV Programs

Some women get very anxious after watching television programs dealing with labor and delivery. These programs may be interesting to watch, but we want you to be aware they may be "worst-case scenarios." By that we mean they may deal with situations that are not the norm for a large percentage of deliveries in the United States.

Most labor/delivery experiences are not as critical or as sensational as what is shown on TV. Think about it—who wants to watch an ordinary labor and delivery? There's no real drama in it, so these programs often focus on some kind of unusual problem a woman could face.

Even when the content is not sensational, we have found pregnant women who watch these programs often get anxious. If you haven't experienced labor and delivery before, you may be a little scared about what will happen during your own labor and delivery. That's normal.

Labor and delivery is an unknown—no one can tell you what will happen to *you* until it happens. When your labor begins, your healthcare team will take care of you, in the best way they can, to ensure the safe delivery of your baby and your good health.

Be Careful of What You Read on the Internet

We have had pregnant women ask us the most bizarre questions or present us with information that is totally incorrect or only partially correct. When we ask them where they found these facts, they often tell us "the Internet."

Just because you read it on the Internet does *not* make it true. Some people think if they find it on the Internet, it's a fact. That's often not the case.

We know you can find a lot of good information on the Internet, but then again, you can also find a lot of misinformation. If you're searching for advice or facts about something, read what you find *very* carefully. If you have questions about something you find, print out the piece and take it with you to a prenatal visit so you can discuss it with your healthcare provider.

Grandma's Remedy

If you want to avoid using medication, try a folk remedy. Chew a combination of fresh mint and parsley leaves to help deal with bad breath and intestinal gas.

Do *not* change anything your healthcare provider has told you. *Do* address your questions and concerns at a prenatal appointment. Your healthcare provider knows about your unique pregnancy situation. If you disagree or question what you're told, ask for a second opinion.

Tuberculosis (TB)

Tuberculosis occurs more often in the United States today than it did in the past. In our country, the disease primarily affects the elderly, the poor, minority groups and those with AIDS. The immigration of women from Asia, Africa, Mexico and Central America has resulted in an increase of

Eyelash-Growth Enhancers

Prescription eyelash-growth enhancers, such as Latisse, and over-the-counter products, such as Revitalash, are used to help make eyelashes grow longer and thicker. If you normally use these products, it's best to stop using them during pregnancy. We don't have enough information to know if they're safe during pregnancy. Better to be safe than sorry.

TB in pregnant women. In addition, women who are HIV-positive are at greater risk for tuberculosis because of decreased immunity.

Worldwide attention has been directed toward rare, serious cases of TB. But relax—it's highly unlikely tuberculosis will be a problem for you or your baby. Even with an increase in the number of TB cases, the risk to most women is very low.

Tuberculosis is caused by the bacteria *Mycobacterium tuberculosis.* The most common site of tuberculosis infection is the lungs, but infection can also occur in other parts of the body. You get it by breathing in the bacteria; it's passed to others through coughing and sneezing.

Tuberculosis is diagnosed with skin testing; the TB skin test is safe during pregnancy. If the skin test is negative, no further testing is done. If it is positive, a chest X-ray is usually done. If you have been vaccinated with the TB vaccine, BCG, it can make diagnosis more difficult.

The infection can be active or lie dormant (inactive) for a long time. Active TB usually shows up on a chest X-ray. Latent TB often has no symptoms; if you have a chest X-ray, it will be normal. Most people infected with tuberculosis have latent TB. Latent tuberculosis can become active and cause a cough, with or without sputum production, fever, night sweats, bloody sputum (hemoptysis), fatigue and weight loss.

Medication is used to treat TB. Many of the drugs used to treat tuberculosis are safe during pregnancy.

A baby can become infected with active or latent TB from its mother's blood or from breathing the bacteria after birth. If you have tuberculosis, baby's pediatrician should be involved immediately after birth. If you're contagious, baby may need to be separated from you for a short time. Most people aren't contagious after 2 weeks of treatment. After that time, it's safe to breastfeed.

Having a Baby Costs Money!

Every couple wants to know what it will cost to have a baby. There are really two answers to that question—it costs a lot, and cost varies from one part of the country to another. From prenatal care to baby's birth, the average cost of having a baby today is around $8000 in the United States.

Insurance makes a big difference in the cost to you. If you don't have it, you'll pay for everything. If you do have insurance, you need to check out some things. Ask your employer or insurance agent the following questions.

- What type of coverage do I have?
- Are there maternity benefits? What are they?
- What percentage of my costs are covered?
- Do I have to pay a deductible? If so, how much is it?
- Is there a cap (limit) on total coverage?
- If my pregnancy lasts into a new year, will I have to pay 2 years' worth of deductibles?
- How do I submit claims?
- Do maternity benefits cover Cesarean deliveries?
- What kind of coverage is there for a high-risk pregnancy?
- Is the cost of taking childbirth-education classes covered?
- Does my coverage restrict the kind of hospital accommodations I may choose, such as a birthing center or a birthing room?
- What procedures must I follow before entering the hospital?
- Does my policy cover a nurse-midwife (if this is of interest to you)?
- Does coverage include medications?
- What tests during pregnancy are covered?
- What tests during labor and delivery are covered?
- What types of anesthesia are covered during labor and delivery?
- How long can I stay in the hospital?
- Does payment go directly to my healthcare provider or to me?

- What conditions or services are not covered?
- What kind of coverage is there for the baby after it is born?
- How long can the baby stay in the hospital?
- Is there an additional cost to add the baby to the policy?
- How do I add the baby to the policy?
- How soon do we need to add the baby to the policy?
- Can we collect a percentage of a fee from my husband's policy and the rest from mine?

Having a baby involves different costs. Much of the covered cost for the hospital is determined by how long you stay and the "services" you use. Having an epidural or Cesarean delivery may add to the bill. Your healthcare provider's bill is separate, except under some plans. Another cost is the pediatrician, who usually examines the baby, does a physical and sees baby each day in the hospital.

It would be nice to think about costs before pregnancy and be sure to have insurance to help out. However, about half of all pregnancies are surprises. What can you do? First, find the answers to your questions. Talk to your insurance carrier, then talk to someone in your healthcare provider's office who handles insurance claims. This person may have answers or know of resources you haven't thought about. Don't be embarrassed to ask questions. You'll be happier if you get answers.

Pregnancy is not the time to cut corners to save money. Call around so you can compare hospitals and prices. Sometimes it's worth spending a little more to get what you want. When you call, ask for specifics about what is included in the prices they quote you. You may get a price that seems lower and better than others but really doesn't cover everything you'll want and need.

Some hospitals and medical centers offer "pregnancy packages." A package can cover many services for one fee. Ask about it in your area.

Costs of Having a Baby in Canada. The Canadian healthcare system is different from that in the United States. Canadians pay a premium on a monthly basis. Maternity costs vary, depending on which province you live in. The healthcare provider who delivers your baby is paid by the government. He or she submits the bill to the government, not you.

Certified Nurse-Midwives, Advance-Practice Nurses and Physician Assistants

In today's obstetric-and-gynecology medical practices, you may find many types of highly qualified people helping to take care of you. These people—mostly women, but not all!—are on the forefront in guiding women through pregnancy to delivery. They may even help deliver their babies!

A *certified nurse-midwife* (CNM) is an advance-practice registered nurse (RN). He or she has received additional training delivering babies and providing prenatal and postpartum care to women. A CNM works closely with a doctor or team of doctors to address specifics about a particular pregnancy, and labor and delivery. Often a CNM delivers babies.

A certified midwife can provide many types of information to a pregnant woman, such as guidance with nutrition and exercise, ways to deal with pregnancy discomforts, tips for managing weight gain, dealing with various pregnancy problems and discussions of different methods of pain relief for labor and delivery. A CNM can also address issues of family planning and birth-control and other gynecological care, including breast exams, Pap smears and other screenings. A CNM can prescribe medications; each state has their own specific requirements.

A *nurse practitioner (NP)* is also an advance-practice registered nurse (RN). He or she has received additional training providing prenatal and postpartum care to women. A nurse practitioner may work with a doctor or work independently to address specifics about a woman's pregnancy, and labor and delivery.

An NP can provide many types of information to a pregnant woman, such as guidance with nutrition and exercise, ways to deal with pregnancy discomforts, tips for managing weight gain, dealing with various pregnancy problems and discussions of different methods of pain relief for labor and delivery. He or she can also address issues of family planning and birth control and other gynecological care, including breast exams, Pap smears and other screenings. In some cases, a nurse practitioner may prescribe medications or provide pain relief during labor and delivery (as a certified registered nurse anesthetist [CRNA]).

A *physician assistant (PA)* is a qualified healthcare professional who may take care of you during pregnancy. He or she is licensed to practice medicine in association with a licensed doctor. In a normal, uncomplicated pregnancy, many or most of your prenatal visits may be with a PA, not the doctor. This may include labor and delivery. Most women find this is a good thing—often

(continues)

these healthcare providers have more time to spend with you answering questions and addressing your concerns.

A PA's focus is to provide many health-care services traditionally done by a doctor. They care for people who have conditions (pregnancy is a condition they see women for), diagnose and treat illnesses, order and interpret tests, counsel on preventive health care, perform some procedures, assist in surgery, write prescriptions and do physical exams. A PA is *not* a medical assistant, who performs administrative or simple clinical tasks.

We are fortunate to have these dedicated professionals working in OB/GYN practices and clinics. The care they provide is crucial to the medical community and makes quality medical care for women something every woman can look forward to.

Exercise for Week 9

Hold onto a door jamb or the back of a sturdy chair. Beginning with your right leg, point your toe and lift your leg forward to 90°, then lower it to the floor. Without stopping, lift the same leg to the side, as far as you can but not beyond 90°. Return to the starting position. Repeat 10 times for each leg. *Tones leg muscles and buttocks muscles.*

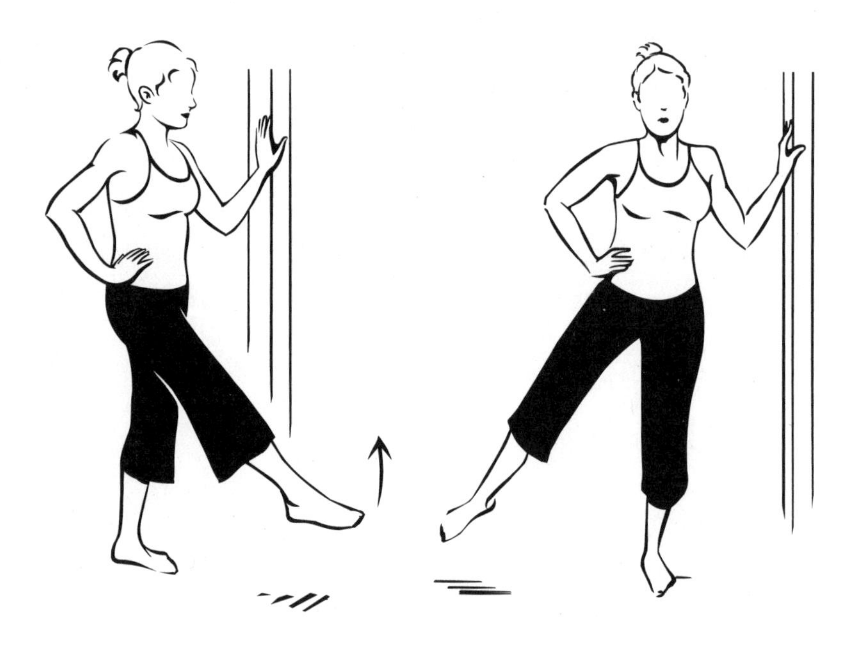

Week 10

Age of Fetus—8 Weeks

If you've just found out you're pregnant, you might want to begin by reading the previous chapters.

How Big Is Your Baby?

By this week, crown-to-rump length of baby is about 1¼ to 1¾ inches (3.1 to 4.2cm). Now we can also start measuring how much baby weighs. Before this week, weight was too small to measure weekly differences. Now baby is starting to put on a little weight, so we'll add weight in this section. The baby weighs close to 0.18 ounce (5g) and is the size of a small plum.

How Big Are You?

A condition that can make you grow too big too fast is a molar pregnancy, sometimes called *gestational trophoblastic neoplasia* (GTN) or *hydatidiform mole.* A molar pregnancy develops from an abnormally fertilized egg.

When a molar pregnancy occurs, an embryo does not usually develop. Abnormal placental tissue grows instead. The most common symptom is bleeding during the first trimester. A woman may have a lot of nausea and vomiting. Another symptom is the size of the mother-to-be and how far along she is supposed to be in pregnancy. Half the time, a woman is too large. Twenty-five percent of the time, she is too small.

The most effective way to diagnose molar pregnancy is by ultrasound. The ultrasound picture has a "snowflake" appearance. The problem is usually found when the test is done to find the cause of bleeding or rapid growth of the uterus.

A molar pregnancy can become cancerous. When it is diagnosed, surgery (dilatation and curettage [D&C]) is usually done as soon as possible.

After a molar pregnancy, effective birth control is important to be sure the molar pregnancy is completely gone. Most healthcare providers recommend using reliable birth control for at least 1 year before trying to get pregnant again.

How Your Baby Is Growing and Developing

The end of this week is the end of the embryonic period. During the embryonic period, the baby has been most susceptible to things that could harm it. Most birth defects occur then. It's good to know a vital part of your baby's development is behind you.

Few birth defects happen after this time. However, drugs and other harmful exposures, such as severe stress or radiation (X-ray), can hurt the baby at any time during pregnancy. Continue to avoid them.

Changes in You

Emotional Changes

When pregnancy is confirmed, it can affect you in many ways. Some women see pregnancy as a sign of womanhood. Some consider it a blessing. Still others feel it's a problem. If you aren't excited about pregnancy, don't feel alone. It's common.

When and how you begin to regard the fetus as a person is different for everyone. Some women say it's when their pregnancy test is positive. Others say it occurs when they hear the fetal heartbeat, usually around 12 weeks. For still others, it happens when they first feel their baby move, at between 16 and 20 weeks.

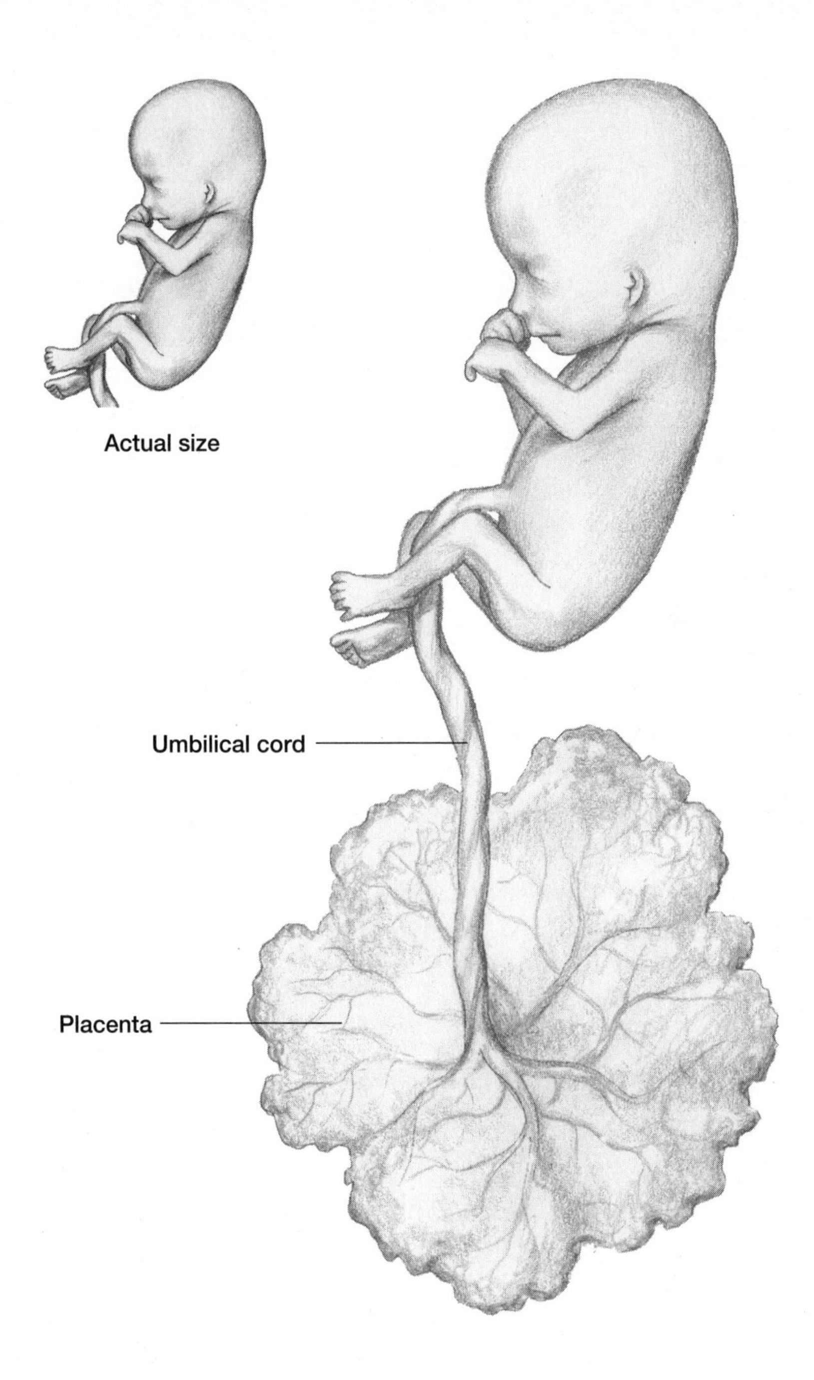

Baby is shown attached to the placenta by its umbilical cord. Eyelids are fused and remain closed until week 27 (fetal age—25 weeks).

You may find you are emotional about many things. You may feel moody, cry at the slightest thing or drift off in daydreams. Emotional swings are normal and continue to some degree throughout your pregnancy.

Many pregnant women wonder why these emotional changes happen. Most of the time, people tell them "it's just part of being pregnant." But most often, it's the hormones your body makes during pregnancy. The changes can really affect your moods and lead to forgetfulness and cloudy thinking.

Tip for Week 10

It's common for your breasts to tingle and to feel sore early in pregnancy. In fact, it may be one of the first signs of pregnancy.

Some emotions you feel may be caused by other things. For example, if you cry and feel down for longer than 2 weeks, feel worthless or hopeless, or don't take pleasure in most things, you may be depressed. Be sure you discuss how you feel emotionally with your healthcare provider.

You can help yourself by getting good prenatal care, and following your healthcare provider's advice. Keep all your prenatal appointments. Establish good communication with your healthcare provider and the office staff. Ask questions. If something bothers you or worries you, discuss it with someone reliable.

How Your Actions Affect Your Baby's Development

When You're Underweight

If you are underweight when you begin pregnancy, you face special challenges. You may need to gain between 28 and 40 pounds during your pregnancy. However, studies show that 20% of all pregnant women fail to gain the amount of weight their healthcare provider recommends.

Weight loss during the first trimester can happen if you have morning sickness. If you're underweight and lose weight because of morning sickness or other problems, talk to your healthcare provider.

Gaining weight gives your baby the nutrients it needs to grow and to develop. If you need to gain extra weight during pregnancy, use the tips below to help you reach that goal.

- Don't drink diet sodas or eat low-calorie foods.
- Choose nutritious foods to help you gain weight, such as cheeses, dried fruits, nuts, avocados, whole milk and ice cream.
- Eat higher-calorie foods.
- Add nutritious, calorie-rich snacks to your daily menu.
- Avoid junk food with lots of empty calories.
- You may need to exercise *less*, if you burn too many calories when you work out.
- Eating small, frequent meals may help.

Make a good nutrition plan at the beginning of pregnancy. Ask your healthcare provider about seeing a dietician to help you.

Vaccinations and Immunizations

Immunizations and vaccinations protect you from diseases. A vaccine is usually given by injection or taken orally. Each vaccine dose contains a very small amount of a weakened form of the disease. When you receive a vaccine, your immune system makes antibodies to fight the disease in the future. In most cases, this is enough to keep you from getting a disease. However, in some cases, it doesn't prevent the disease entirely but lessens the symptoms.

Vaccines come in three forms—live virus, killed (dead) virus and toxoids (chemically altered proteins from bacteria that are harmless). Most vaccines are made from killed viruses; it's nearly impossible to get the disease after receiving this type of vaccine. With a live-virus vaccine, the virus is so weakened that if your immune system is normal, you probably won't get sick from it.

Many women of childbearing age in the United States and Canada have been immunized against measles, mumps, rubella, tetanus and diphtheria. A blood test for measles and rubella is necessary to determine immunity. Physician-diagnosed mumps or a mumps vaccination is necessary to know you're immune.

Risk of Exposure. During pregnancy, try to reduce your chance of exposure to disease and illness. Avoid visiting areas known to have diseases. Avoid people (usually children) who are sick. But it's just about impossible to avoid all exposure to all diseases. If you're exposed, or if exposure is unavoidable, the risk of the disease must be balanced against the likely effects of vaccination.

The vaccine must also be measured in terms of its effectiveness and its expected effect on a pregnancy. There's not a lot of information on harmful effects of a vaccine on the developing baby. However, live-measles vaccine should *never* be given to a pregnant woman.

Vaccinations You Should Have during Pregnancy. The only immunizing agents recommended for use during pregnancy are the *Tdap* (or DPT) vaccine and the *flu vaccine*. The Tdap vaccine (tetanus, diphtheria, pertussis) can help you avoid whooping cough. Be sure to get a Tdap booster if it's been 10 years since your last one. If you work in the garden, with your hands in dirt, you need a booster.

If you get the flu during pregnancy, you may have complications, such as pneumonia. Pregnancy can alter your immune system, which can increase your risk.

It is recommended that *all* women who will be pregnant during flu season get a flu shot. A flu shot can protect you against three strains of influenza. Flu shots can be given safely during all three trimesters. Talk to your healthcare provider about it.

Other Vaccines during Pregnancy. As many as 35% of all pregnant women are at risk of getting measles, mumps or rubella because they haven't been vaccinated or they have been vaccinated but their immunity has weakened. The *MMR vaccine* should be given before pregnancy or after delivery. The Centers for Disease Control and Prevention (CDC) recommends a woman should wait at least 1 month to get pregnant after receiving the MMR vaccine.

A pregnant woman should receive a vaccination against *polio* only if her risk of exposure to the disease is high. Only inactivated polio vaccine should be used.

If your healthcare provider believes you may be at risk for getting *hepatitis B*, it's safe to take the vaccine during pregnancy. Talk to your healthcare provider if you have concerns.

Ask about receiving the pneumococcal vaccine if you have a chronic medical condition, such as lung problems, asthma or heart problems. This vaccine protects you against bacteria that can cause pneumonia, meningitis and ear infections. A plus to taking this vaccine is that antibodies you make after taking the vaccine pass to your baby and may protect him or her from ear infections for up to 6 months!

Human papillomavirus (HPV) vaccine is a series of shots over 6 months to protect against HPV. HPV is responsible for 70% of cervical cancers and 90% of genital warts cases. Don't have this vaccine during pregnancy; it's not recommended. If a woman discovers she is pregnant while she is receiving the vaccine, she should delay finishing the series until after she gives birth. Women who are breastfeeding can receive the vaccine.

Thimerosal Use during Pregnancy. *Thimerosal* is a preservative used in vaccines that contains ethyl mercury. It was barred from childhood vaccines several years ago but is still used in most flu vaccines. Some experts recommend pregnant women ask for a thimerosal-free flu vaccine.

The Centers for Disease Control and Prevention (CDC) believes it's OK for pregnant women to receive flu vaccine that contains thimerosal. They state the benefits of flu vaccine with thimerosal outweigh the risk. The American College of Obstetricians and Gynecologists (ACOG) has issued a similar statement.

Until 2001, thimerosal was used in RhoGAM preparations. However, thimerosal is no longer used in RhoGAM in this country. (For more on RhoGAM, see Week 16.)

Influenza (Flu)

The flu seems to be a problem every year because different flu viruses come and go. In 2009 and 2010, the H1N1 flu affected many people. When an outbreak of H1N1 or other type of influenza occurs, it can impact a pregnant woman more greatly because of her altered immune system.

If you are pregnant when a breakout occurs, you should receive the specific flu vaccine *and* the seasonal flu vaccine. You can be vaccinated any time during pregnancy. There are ways to protect yourself in addition to getting a seasonal flu shot. Use "social distancing" to protect yourself. Avoid crowded areas, use a mask and wash your hands frequently (flu virus can live up to 2 hours on surfaces like doorknobs and telephones).

Before you get a flu shot, go to bed extra early the night before. When you're well rested, your body produces twice as many infection-fighting antibodies.

Follow your healthcare provider's guidelines about using medicine you are advised to take. The benefits of taking a medicine outweigh any risk to the baby. Treatment should begin as soon as possible; don't wait for lab results to confirm the type of flu.

Rubella Immunity

It's a good idea to get checked to see if you are immune to rubella before you get pregnant. Rubella (German measles) during pregnancy can be responsible for various pregnancy problems. Because there's no known treatment for rubella, the best approach is prevention.

If you're not immune, you can receive a vaccination after delivery, while you take reliable birth control. Don't have a vaccination shortly before or during pregnancy because of the possibility of exposing baby to the rubella virus.

Chicken Pox during Pregnancy

Did you have chicken pox when you were a child? Ninety percent of women today are immune to chicken pox. If you didn't have chicken pox, you may be one of the 1 in 2000 women who will develop it during pregnancy. Chicken pox is more serious during the first 10 weeks of pregnancy. If you get it during the third trimester, it could affect baby's brain development.

Effects of Infections on Your Baby

Some infections and illnesses a woman contracts can affect her baby's development. The chart below cites a type of infection or disease and the effects each may have on a developing baby.

Infections	Effects on Fetus
Cytomegalovirus (CMV)	microcephaly, brain damage, hearing loss
Rubella (German measles)	cataracts, deafness, heart lesions, can involve all organs
Syphilis	fetal death, skin defects
Toxoplasmosis	possible effects on all organs
Varicella	possible effects on all organs

Chicken pox usually affects kids; only 2% of all cases occur in the 15-to-49 age group. The CDC, the American Academy of Pediatrics and the American Academy of Family Physicians all recommend healthy children age 1 year and older receive the chicken-pox vaccine; it is usually given at 12 to 18 months of age.

If you get chicken pox during pregnancy, take good care of yourself. About 15% of those who get chicken pox also develop a form of pneumonia, which can be very serious for a pregnant woman. If you get chicken pox 5 days before or 2 days after delivery, baby can also develop a severe chicken-pox infection.

If you're exposed to chicken pox, contact your healthcare provider immediately! A pregnant woman should receive varicella-zoster immune globulin (VZIG). If you receive it within 72 hours of exposure, it can help prevent infection or lessen symptoms. If you do get chicken pox, you will probably be treated with acyclovir.

Your Nutrition

Pregnancy increases your protein needs. It's important for you and baby. Try to eat 6 ounces of protein each day during the first trimester and

8 ounces a day during the second and third trimesters. Don't eat too much protein; it should only make up about 15% of your total calorie intake.

Many protein sources are high in fat. If you need to watch your calories, choose low-fat protein sources. Some protein foods you may choose, and their serving sizes, include the following:

- chickpeas (garbanzo beans)—1 cup
- cheese, mozzarella—1 ounce
- chicken, roasted, skinless—½ breast (about 4 ounces)
- eggs—1
- hamburger, broiled, lean—3½ ounces
- milk—8 ounces
- peanut butter—2 tablespoons
- tuna, canned in water—3 ounces
- yogurt—8 ounces

When you eat eggs or dairy products for protein, be sure to add a complementary plant protein source for a complete protein. Rice and beans, tofu and sesame seeds or green beans with almonds are good choices. If eating protein makes you ill, look for a carbohydrate food (like crackers, cereal, pretzels) that contains protein.

Brain Builders

Choline and docosahexaenoic acid (DHA) can help build baby's brain cells. Choline is found in milk, egg yolks, chicken liver, wheat germ,

Stay Healthy!

Studies suggest eating 2 cups of fresh fruit a day may help reduce your risk of getting a cold or the flu by nearly 35%. Fresh fruit helps your body increase virus-fighting cells found in the throat and nose. Bright-colored fruit is your best bet, such as oranges, kiwi, red grapes, strawberries and pineapple. If you do get a cold, eating nutrient-rich foods may help your body produce more white blood cells to help fight it. Eat ½ cup pineapple or ½ cup sweet potatoes to increase your resistance.

cod, cooked broccoli, peanuts and peanut butter, whole-wheat bread and beef. You need at least 450mg of choline a day during pregnancy. DHA is found in fish, egg yolks, poultry, meat, canola oil, walnuts and wheat germ.

Some pregnancy nutrition bars contain DHA; others have added vitamins and minerals. If you eat a variety of foods that contain choline and DHA during pregnancy and while breastfeeding, you can help your baby obtain important nutrients.

You Need to Gain Weight

You should be gaining weight slowly; it can be harmful to your baby if you don't. To an extent, your weight gain lets your healthcare provider know how you're doing.

Pregnancy is not a time to experiment with different diets or cut down on calories. However, this doesn't mean you have the go-ahead to eat anything you want, any time you want. Exercise and a proper nutrition plan, without junk food, will help you manage your weight. Be smart about food choices.

You Should Also Know

Down Syndrome

Nearly every pregnant woman receives information on Down syndrome. Older women have traditionally been offered various tests to determine whether their fetus is affected by the condition.

Down syndrome was given its name by British physician J. Langdon Down in the 19th century. He found babies born with the syndrome have an extra chromosome 21; this is called *aneuploidy*. The normal number of chromosomes in humans is 46. With Down syndrome, an individual has 47 chromosomes.

Down syndrome is the most common chromosome abnormality and the most common cause of mental retardation. It occurs in about 1 in 800 births. Those born with Down syndrome today can live fairly long lives. Some women are at higher risk of giving birth to a child with Down syndrome, including older women, those who have given birth previously to a child with Down syndrome and those who have Down syndrome.

Many tests are available that screen for Down syndrome in a developing fetus. Tests include:

- maternal alpha-fetoprotein test
- triple-screen test
- quad-screen test
- nuchal translucency screening
- ultrasound

Tests to diagnose Down syndrome include amniocentesis and chorionic villus sampling (CVS).

ACOG Recommendations. The American College of Obstetricians and Gynecologists recommends *all* pregnant women be offered screening for Down syndrome, regardless of their age. In the past, testing for Down syndrome was usually offered mainly to women over age 35 and others who were at risk. Even though many women would not consider terminating a pregnancy with a Down-syndrome child, it's important to know this information before baby's birth so specialized care can be planned for delivery.

Although the condition occurs at a higher frequency in older mothers, the majority of babies born with Down syndrome are born to younger women. Younger women give birth to a larger number of babies, therefore, a larger number of babies with Down syndrome are delivered to younger women. Eighty percent of babies born with Down syndrome are born to women *under* age 35.

If your healthcare provider offers you this screening test, consider it. Ask any questions you may have about the condition, and, together with your partner, decide whether to have the test. This information is most useful when screening is done during the first trimester.

Down Syndrome Children Are Special. People want to know if there are any positive aspects of giving birth to a child with Down syndrome. The answer is "Yes!"

A child born with Down syndrome can bring a special, valuable quality of life into the world. Down children are well known for the love and joy they bring to their families and friends. They remind us of the pleasure in doing simple tasks when they learn new skills. They embody the concept of unconditional love, and we can often learn how to cope and to grow as we interact with them. Many families are on waiting lists to adopt children with Down syndrome.

Rearing a child with Down syndrome can be challenging, but many who have faced this challenge are positive about it. If you have a child with Down syndrome, you may work harder for every small advance in your child's life. You may experience frustration and feelings of helplessness at times, but every parent has these feelings at some time.

All parents-to-be should know the following facts about children born with Down syndrome. The average IQ for a child with Down syndrome is between 60 and 70. Most are in the mildly retarded range. Some children with Down syndrome have normal IQs. IQ scores for those with Down syndrome have risen steadily in the last 100 years. Less than 5% of those with Down syndrome are severely to profoundly retarded.

The reading levels of those with Down syndrome who are in special-education programs in public schools range from kindergarten to 12th grade. The average is about 3rd grade.

Nearly 90% of all those with Down syndrome are employable as adults. Most adults with Down syndrome are capable of living independently or in group homes. People with Down syndrome have an average life expectancy of about 55 years, if they survive infancy.

Fetoscopy

Fetoscopy provides a view of the baby and placenta inside your uterus. In some cases, abnormalities and problems can be detected and corrected.

The goal of fetoscopy is to correct a problem before it worsens, which could keep a baby from developing normally. A physician can see some problems more clearly with fetoscopy than with ultrasound.

The test is done by placing a scope, like the one used in laparoscopy, through the abdomen. The procedure is similar to amniocentesis, but the fetoscope is larger than the needle used for amniocentesis.

If your healthcare provider suggests fetoscopy, ask about possible risks, advantages and disadvantages of the procedure. The test should be done only by someone experienced in the technique. Risk of miscarriage is 3 to 4% with this procedure. It is not available everywhere. If you have fetoscopy and are Rh-negative, you should receive RhoGAM after the procedure.

Chorionic Villus Sampling

Chorionic villus sampling (CVS) is a highly accurate diagnostic test used to detect genetic abnormalities. Sampling is done early in pregnancy, usually between the 9th and 11th weeks. The test offers an advantage over amniocentesis because it is done much earlier, and results are available in about 1 week. If a pregnancy will be terminated, it can be done earlier and may carry fewer risks to the woman.

Chorionic villus sampling involves placing an instrument through the cervix or abdomen to remove fetal tissue from the placenta, which can be tested for abnormalities. Over 95% of women who have CVS learn their baby does *not* have the disorder for which the test was done.

If your healthcare provider recommends CVS, ask about its risks. The test should be performed only by someone experienced in the technique. The risk of miscarriage is small—between 1 and 2%—and the test is considered as safe as amniocentesis. If you have CVS and are Rh-negative, you should receive RhoGAM after the procedure.

Find Out Baby's Sex This Week?

You may have seen gender tests advertised that use your blood or a urine sample to determine baby's sex. They are often offered on the Internet. But experts agree tests available today may not offer accurate results.

One over-the-counter test claims it can predict your baby's sex as early as this week. Called the *IntelliGender's Gender Prediction Test,* it uses a simple urine test to provide immediate results that indicate baby's gender, based on a color match. Green indicates boy, and orange indicates girl.

However, before you rush off to buy the test, you should realize test results are actually only about 80% accurate. They only indicate the *possibility* of determining whether baby is a girl or a boy.

To do the test, you use your first morning urine. You need to avoid sexual relations for at least 48 hours before taking the test, and you can't be taking any hormones, such as progesterone.

The *Pink or Blue* test is another at-home test developed to determine baby's gender by examining DNA of the mom-to-be. Research has shown fetal DNA can be found in a mother's bloodstream. A woman sends a small sample of her blood to the lab, and results of the test (boy or girl) are sent to the parents-to-be. The makers of the product claim the test is 95% accurate and can predict a baby's sex as early as 6 weeks after conception.

Some medical authorities are concerned some couples may consider ending a pregnancy because of baby's sex, based on the result of these tests. If you have questions or concerns, discuss them with your healthcare provider.

Dad Tip

Are you concerned about sex during pregnancy? You both may have questions, so talk about them together and with your partner's healthcare provider. Occasionally during a pregnancy you'll need to avoid intercourse. However, pregnancy is an opportunity for increased closeness and intimacy for you as a couple. Sex can be a positive part of this experience.

Exercise for Week 10

Kneel on your hands and knees, with your hands directly below your shoulders and knees directly under your hips. Inhale as you raise your head and gaze forward. Then exhale as you slowly bring your head down, round your back and shoulders and tuck in your tummy. Do 4 times. *Stretches back and tummy muscles, and increases flexibility.*

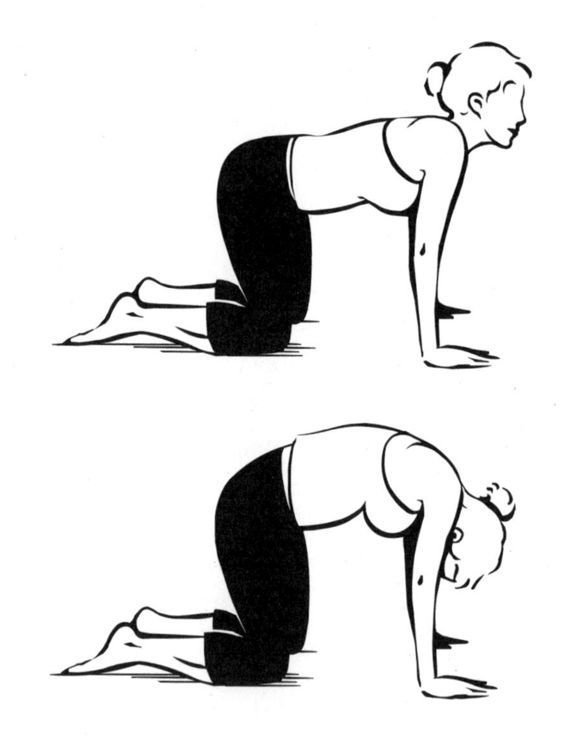

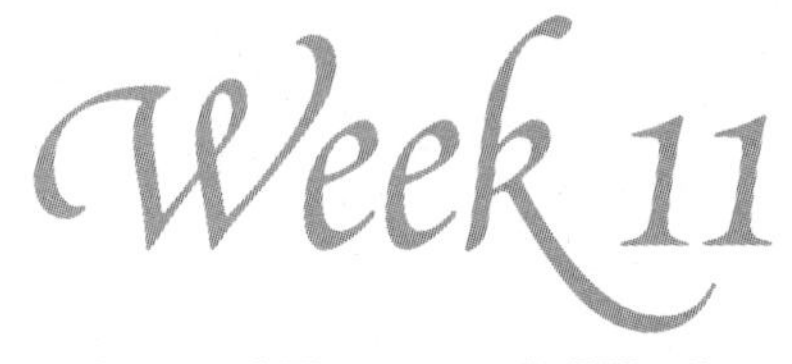

Age of Fetus—9 Weeks

How Big Is Your Baby?

Crown-to-rump length of your baby is 1½ to 2½ inches (4.4 to 6cm). Fetal weight is about 0.3 ounce (8g). Your baby is about the size of a large lime.

How Big Are You?

You're near the end of the first trimester! Your uterus is almost big enough to fill your pelvis and may be felt in your lower abdomen, above the middle of your pubic bone.

How Your Baby Is Growing and Developing

Fetal growth is rapid now. As you can see in the illustration on page 159, the head is almost half the baby's entire length. As the head moves backward toward the spine, the chin rises from the chest, and the neck develops and lengthens. Fingernails appear.

External genitalia are beginning to show distinguishing features. Development into a male or female is complete in another 3 weeks. All embryos begin life looking the same, as far as outward appearances go. Whether the embryo develops into a boy or girl is determined by the genetic information contained within the embryo.

By this time, the small intestine begins to contract and relax, which pushes substances through it. The small intestine is capable of passing sugar from inside itself into the baby's body.

Changes in You

Some women notice changes in their hair, fingernails or toenails during pregnancy. Some lucky pregnant women see an increase in hair and nail growth. Others find they lose some hair during this time, or their nails break more easily. This doesn't happen to everyone, but if it happens to you, don't worry about it.

Some experts believe these changes happen because of increased circulation in your body. Others credit the hormone changes in you. In any event, these changes are rarely permanent.

Pregnancy May Reveal Future Problems

Your body goes through many changes during pregnancy, which begin almost at the time of conception. They allow your body to accept and to tolerate the genetically "different" fetus. Changes also help your body adapt to nourish and to support the fetus and to prepare you for delivery.

Most healthy women don't have problems with changes; however, in some women, these changes result in pregnancy problems. Pregnancy can reveal a woman's likelihood for getting a disease. It can give a woman a hint of what long-term health problems might lie ahead. It may help you take steps now to help prevent serious problems later.

One example is gestational diabetes. Women who have pregnancy-induced diabetes are more likely to have diabetes later in life. Another example is women who have pre-eclampsia; they are at greater risk for stroke in later life.

Talk to your healthcare provider about any changes you experience during your pregnancy. Discuss steps you can take now and after pregnancy to help reduce your risk of problems in later life.

Dad Tip

Remember that despite morning sickness, headaches and a changing waistline, pregnancy is a miracle! Pregnancy and childbirth happen only a few times in your life. Enjoy this special time together. You'll look back fondly at the challenge of becoming parents and probably even say, "That wasn't so bad." We know that because couples get pregnant again and have more kids!

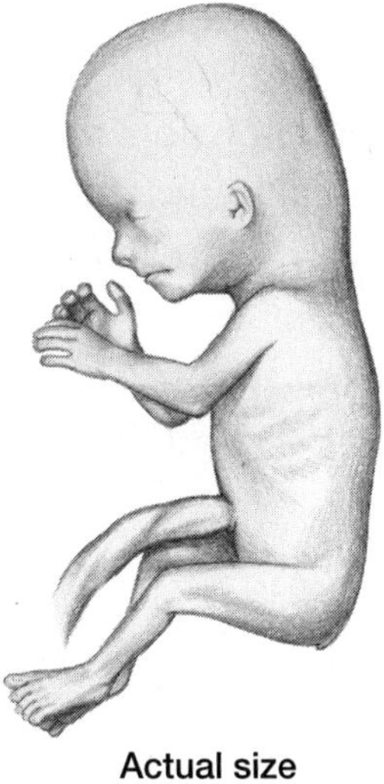

Actual size

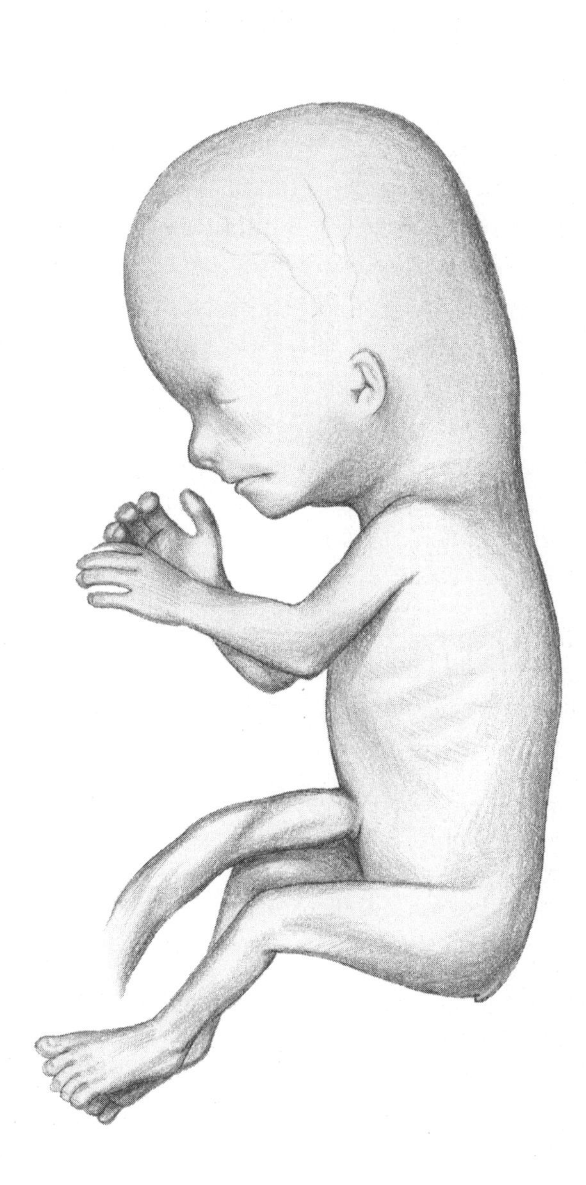

By week 11 of gestation (fetal age—9 weeks),
fingernails are beginning to appear.

How Your Actions Affect Your Baby's Development

Traveling during Pregnancy

Pregnant women frequently ask whether travel can hurt their baby. If your pregnancy is uncomplicated and you aren't at high risk, travel is usually OK. Ask your healthcare provider about any travel you're considering *before* making firm plans or buying tickets.

Whether you travel by car, bus, train, boat or airplane, get up and walk at least every hour. Regular visits to the bathroom may take care of this.

The biggest risk of traveling during pregnancy is developing a problem while you're away from those who know your medical and pregnancy history. If you do decide to take a trip, be sensible in your planning. Don't overdo it. Take it easy! Signs you shouldn't travel include:

- severe swelling of the face, arms, legs, hands or feet
- bleeding
- severe nausea and vomiting
- cramping
- extreme and/or continuing headaches
- fever

Traveling by Air. Air travel is safe for most pregnant women. Most U.S. airlines let women fly up to 36 weeks of pregnancy. For international travel, the cutoff is usually 35 weeks of pregnancy.

Pregnant women who are at high risk should avoid all air travel. You may want to keep the following things in mind if you're considering flying during pregnancy.

- Visit your healthcare provider before you go to be sure your trip is still a "go."
- Avoid high-altitude flights (nonstop overseas or cross-country flights) because they cruise at a higher altitude and oxygen levels can be lower. This increases your heartbeat, as well as your baby's; baby also receives less oxygen.

- If you have problems with swelling, wear loose-fitting shoes and clothes. (This is good advice for every traveler.) Avoid pantyhose, tight clothes, knee socks or stockings, and tight waistlines.
- If you know your flight serves a meal, you can order special meals. If your flight is long and doesn't serve food, bring along nutritious snacks.
- Drink lots of water to keep you hydrated. Take along an empty bottle, and fill it after you go through security.
- Get up and move around when you can during the flight. Try to walk at least 10 minutes every hour. Sometimes just standing up helps your circulation.
- Try to get an aisle seat, close to the bathroom. If you have to go to the bathroom a lot, it's easier if you don't have to crawl over someone to get out.

Auto Safety during Pregnancy

Many women are concerned about driving and using seat belts and shoulder harnesses during pregnancy. There's no reason not to drive while you're pregnant, if your pregnancy is normal and you feel OK (and you know how to drive).

Wearing safety restraints is important during pregnancy; you really lower the chance of getting hurt in an accident. If you don't wear a seat belt, you could cause a serious injury to your baby if you're in an accident.

Seat belts do *not* increase the risk of injury to you or your baby. They actually protect you both from life-threatening injuries. Don't skip wearing seat belts as you get bigger because you're uncomfortable. Studies show pregnant women who weren't wearing seat belts when they were in an accident were twice as likely to have excessive bleeding and were nearly three times more likely to lose their babies.

Below are some common excuses (and our responses) for not using seat belts and shoulder harnesses in pregnancy.

"*Using a safety belt will hurt my baby.*" There's no evidence seat-belt use increases the chance of injury to a baby. Your chance of survival

The Proper Way to Wear a Lap Belt and Shoulder Harness

There is a proper way for you to wear a seat belt during pregnancy. Wear both the shoulder strap and the lap belt. Place the lap-belt portion under your abdomen and across your upper thighs. The shoulder portion of the belt should rest between your breasts and over the middle of your collarbone. Don't slip the belt off your shoulder. Both the shoulder belt and lap belt should be snug but comfortable. Adjust your position so the belt crosses your shoulder without cutting into your neck. You might want to check out a seat-belt extender or a maternity seat belt to help keep the seat belt from riding up on your tummy.

with a seat belt is better than without one. Your survival is important to your unborn baby.

"*I don't want to be trapped in my car if there is a fire.*" Few automobile accidents result in fires. Even if a fire did occur, you could probably undo the restraint and escape if you were conscious. Ejection from a car accounts for about 25% of all deaths in automobile accidents. Seat-belt use prevents this.

"*I'm a good driver.*" Defensive driving doesn't prevent an accident.

"*I don't need to use a safety belt; I'm just going a short distance.*" Most injuries occur within 25 miles of home.

We know the lap/shoulder seat-belt system is safe to wear during pregnancy, so buckle up for you *and* your baby. Move your seat as far away from the air bag as possible—10 inches is a good distance. You might want to consider riding in the back seat when you're not driving. The middle of the back seat is the safest place in the car.

Medication Classification for Pregnancy

Medications a pregnant woman might use have been classified by the Food and Drug Administration (FDA) to show the risk to the baby if a mother-to-be takes it. If you have questions about any medicines you take, ask your healthcare provider about its safety.

We don't know a lot about some medications because we haven't studied their effects on a pregnant woman and/or her baby. That's because we believe these substances may be dangerous and could harm the baby. No one wants to put a growing baby at risk deliberately by exposing it to a harmful substance for the sake of gathering information. So nearly all the information we have comes from accidental exposure.

Category A—Well-controlled studies in pregnant women have not shown any risk to the baby. The possibility of harm appears remote. Few medications have been tested to this level. Prenatal vitamins and folic acid are considered Category-A medications.

Category B—Animal studies indicate risk to a baby is probably low, but human studies have not been done. Examples of Category-B medications include some antibiotics, such as Ceclor (cefaclor).

Category C—Either studies in animals have revealed adverse effects or there are no controlled studies in women. Drugs should be given only if the potential benefits to the pregnant woman justify the potential risks to the fetus. An example of a Category-C medication is codeine.

Category D—Studies using animals have shown a harmful effect on the baby, or studies have not been done in humans or animals. There is evidence of risk to the baby. Benefits from use in a pregnant woman may outweigh risks if the medication is needed for a life-threatening situation or for a serious disease for which safer drugs cannot be used. An example of a Category-D medication is phenobarbital.

Category X—There is evidence the medication causes birth defects in a baby. Risks outweigh any potential benefits for women, and it is not given during pregnancy. Accutane is a Category-X medication.

Your Risk of Food Poisoning Increases

You're at greater risk of food poisoning when you're pregnant. Avoid raw oysters and raw clams. Don't eat smoked or cured seafood unless it's been cooked. Limit your liver consumption. Keep away from refrigerated meat spreads and pâtés.

Your Nutrition

Carbohydrate foods provide the primary source of energy for your growing baby. These foods also help your body use protein efficiently. Foods from this group are almost interchangeable, so it should be easy to get all the servings you need. Some carbohydrate foods you may choose, and their serving sizes, include the following:

- tortilla—1 large
- pasta, cereal or rice, cooked—½ cup
- cereal, ready-to-eat—1 ounce
- bagel—½ small
- bread—1 slice
- roll—1 medium

You Should Also Know

Instant Risk Assessment (IRA)

There is a screening test for Down syndrome called *IRA* (Instant Risk Assessment) that offers women faster results at an earlier stage in pregnancy. It has a 91% accuracy rate. IRA has two parts, a blood test and an ultrasound. Women receive a collection kit from a healthcare provider or the hospital.

The woman pricks her finger and marks a card in the kit with her blood, which is sent to the lab for analysis. It is tested for levels of HCG (human chorionic gonadotropin) and a substance called *pregnancy-associated plasma protein A (PAPP-A)*. Elevated levels have been associated with Down syndrome.

The second part of the test, the ultrasound, is a nuchal translucency exam, in which an ultrasound measures the space on the back of the baby's neck. See Week 13. The larger the space in this area, the higher the chance of the baby having Down syndrome. Your healthcare provider can schedule the ultrasound.

If you're feeling down, take a look at the carbohydrates you eat. Complex carbohydrates that are used slowly by the body result in more-stable blood-sugar levels, which is better for baby. They may also help a bit with mood swings. Complex carbohydrates to choose from include fruits and vegetables as well as beans, lentils and oats.

Fragile-X Syndrome

Fragile-X syndrome is one of the most common inherited causes of mental retardation. The condition can occur in both boys and girls.

Testing for the gene that causes it is done with DNA analysis. Prenatal diagnosis requires DNA from amniotic fluid. Prenatal testing should be offered to known carriers of the fragile-X gene and to families with a history of mental retardation.

Ultrasound in Pregnancy

By this point, you may have discussed ultrasound with your healthcare provider. Or you may already have had an ultrasound test. Ultrasound (also called *sonography* or *sonogram*) is one of our most valuable tools for evaluating a pregnancy. Healthcare providers, hospitals and insurance companies (yes, they get involved in this too) don't agree whether ultrasound should be done or if every pregnant woman needs an ultrasound test during pregnancy. It is a noninvasive test, and there are no known risks associated with it. In the United States, millions of obstetrical ultrasounds are performed each year!

Ultrasound involves the use of high-frequency sound waves made by applying an alternating current to a transducer. A lubricant is rubbed on the skin to improve contact with the transducer. The transducer passes over the tummy, above the uterus. Sound waves are sent from the transducer through the tummy, into the pelvis. As sound waves bounce off tissues, they are directed toward and back to the transducer. The reflection of sound waves can be compared to "radar" used by airplanes or ships.

Different tissues of the body reflect ultrasound signals differently, and we can distinguish among them. Motion can also be seen, so we can detect motion of the baby or parts of the baby, such as the heart. With ultrasound, a fetal heart can be seen beating as early as 5 or 6 weeks into the pregnancy. Your baby's body and limbs can be seen moving as early as 4 weeks of embryonic growth (6th week of pregnancy).

Your healthcare provider uses ultrasound in many ways in relation to your pregnancy, such as:

- helping in the early identification of pregnancy
- showing the size and growth rate of the baby
- identifying the presence of two or more babies
- measuring the fetal head, abdomen or femur to determine the stage of pregnancy
- identifying some fetuses with Down syndrome
- identifying some birth defects
- identifying some internal-organ problems
- measuring the amount of amniotic fluid
- identifying the location, size and maturity of the placenta
- identifying placental abnormalities
- identifying uterine abnormalities or tumors
- determining the position of an IUD
- differentiating between miscarriage, ectopic pregnancy and normal pregnancy
- in connection with various tests, such as amniocentesis, percutaneous umbilical-cord blood sampling (PUBS) and chorionic villus sampling (CVS), to select a safe place to do each test

You may be asked to drink a lot of water before an ultrasound examination. Your bladder is in front of your uterus. When your bladder is empty, your uterus is harder to see because it's farther down inside the pelvic bones. Bones disrupt ultrasound signals and make the picture harder to interpret. With your bladder full, your uterus rises out of the pelvis and can be seen more easily. The bladder acts as a window to look through to see the uterus and the fetus inside.

Other Ultrasound Tests. The *ultrasound vaginal probe,* also called the *transvaginal ultrasound*, can be used in early pregnancy for a better view of the baby and placenta. A probe is placed inside the vagina, and the pregnancy is viewed from this angle.

The *UltraScreen* test identifies babies at increased risk of having certain birth defects. The test combines maternal blood tests and an ultrasound measurement at 11 to 13 weeks. The UltraScreen test is fairly effective in detecting Down syndrome.

Fetal *nasal-bone evaluation* is another type of ultrasound exam that increases Down syndrome detection accuracy to 95%, with a small percentage of false-positives. The benefit of first trimester screening is earlier diagnosis.

Three-dimensional ultrasound is also available in many areas. It is discussed in Week 17.

Can Ultrasound Determine the Baby's Sex? Some couples ask for ultrasound to determine whether they are going to have a boy or girl. If the baby is in a good position and it's old enough for the genitals to have developed and they can be seen clearly, determination may be possible. However, many healthcare providers feel this reason alone is not a good reason to do an ultrasound exam. Discuss it with your healthcare provider. Understand ultrasound is a test, and test results can occasionally be wrong.

Fetal MRI

Ultrasound is the standard test used to diagnose birth defects and other problems. It is often the first test used. However, there are some limitations to ultrasound. If a woman is obese, if there is less amniotic fluid or baby is in an abnormal position, ultrasound may not reveal problems. In addition, midpregnancy is the best time to use ultrasound, so earlier or later use may not be as helpful.

> *Tip for Week 11*
>
> You may be able to get a "picture" of your baby before birth from an ultrasound test. Some facilities can even make a DVD or videotape for you. Ask about it before the test, if you're scheduled to have one.

Relax and Have a Great Pregnancy!

It's natural to feel nervous about being pregnant and what lies ahead—labor and delivery, and going home with baby. It's important to deal with any anxieties you may have, and focus on having a great pregnancy. Below are some guidelines to help you do just that.

- Don't panic if someone bumps you in the tummy. Your baby is well protected.
- It's OK to lift things—just don't lift heavy objects. Sacks from the market and a young child won't hurt you. Stay away from heavy lifting.
- You don't have to worry about using a computer, a cell phone, a microwave oven or going through airport security. None of the machines involved in these procedures produce enough "bad vibes" to hurt you or your baby.
- Coloring or perming your hair is OK. The chemicals used in these preparations won't hurt you. However, if the fumes make you sick, wait until you aren't bothered so much by smells to have a perm or color your hair.
- Ask your partner to take pictures of you as you move through pregnancy. It's fun to look back at them and remember how big you were when.
- Even though you may not feel sexy, wear a beautiful, supportive bra made for expecting moms. It can help you feel pretty and desirable (which you are anyway!). For added comfort for your breasts, check out sleep bras. They can add support to sore breasts while you sleep.
- Pamper your feet. Wear good, comfortable shoes. Get a pedicure or foot massage. Soak your feet when they're sore. Use foot cream to help

Another test healthcare providers use has fewer limitations—fetal MRI. Fetal MRI (magnetic resonance imaging) is most helpful when findings from ultrasound are unclear or cannot be seen clearly.

MRI does not use radiation. Several studies have shown MRI is safe to use during pregnancy. To be cautious, MRI is still not advised during the first trimester. The test is most useful in diagnosing babies with specific birth defects.

It is important to note that ultrasound is more widely available and lower in cost than MRI. Ultrasound is still the first choice for discovering problems. However, MRI can be helpful in special situations, as mentioned above.

Exercise for Week 11

Place your left hand on the back of a chair or against the wall. Lift your right knee up, and put your right hand under your thigh. Round your back, and bring your head and pelvis forward. Hold position for count of 4, straighten up, then lower your leg. Repeat with your left leg. Do 5 or 8 times with each leg. *Reduces back tension, and increases blood flow to the feet.*

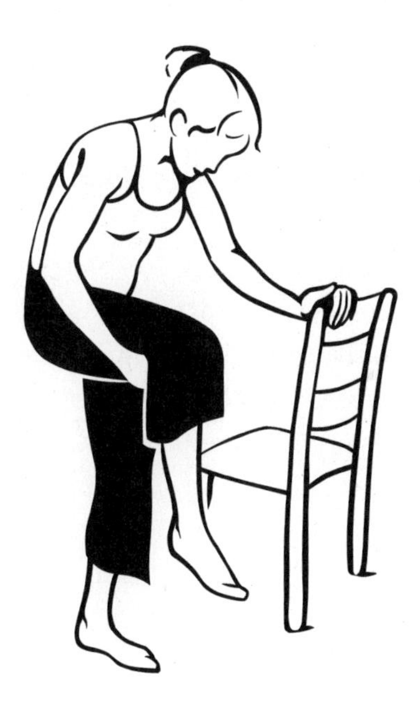

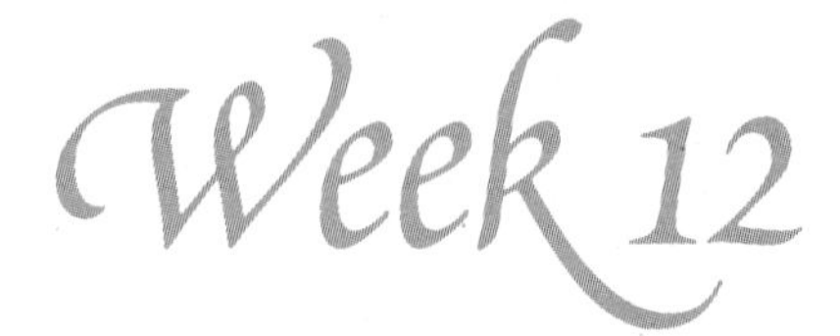

Week 12

Age of Fetus—10 Weeks

How Big Is Your Baby?

Your baby weighs between ⅓ and ½ ounce (8 to 14g), and crown-to-rump length is almost 2½ inches (6.1cm). As you can see on page 172, your baby's size has almost doubled in the past 3 weeks!

How Big Are You?

Around this time, you may be able to feel your uterus above your pubic bone (pubic symphysis). Before pregnancy, your uterus holds ⅓ ounce (10ml) or less. During pregnancy, it becomes a muscular container big enough to hold the baby, placenta and amniotic fluid. The uterus increases its capacity 500 to 1000 times during pregnancy! By the time baby is born, it's grown to the size of a medium-size watermelon. The weight of the uterus also changes. When your baby is born, your uterus weighs almost 40 ounces (1.1kg) compared to 2½ ounces (70g) before pregnancy.

How Your Baby Is Growing and Developing

Few structures in the baby are formed after this week, but the structures already formed continue to grow and to develop. At your 12-week visit (or near then), you'll probably be able to hear your baby's heartbeat! It can be heard with *doppler*, a special listening machine (not a stethoscope), that magnifies the sound of baby's heartbeat so you can hear it.

Bones are forming. Fingers and toes have separated, and nails are growing. Bits of hair begin to appear on the body.

The small intestine is capable of pushing food through the bowels. It is also able to absorb sugar.

Baby's pituitary gland is beginning to work. Its nervous system has developed further. Stimulating baby may cause it to squint, open its mouth and move its fingers or toes.

> **Dad Tip**
>
> At this prenatal visit, it may be possible to hear the baby's heartbeat. If you can't be there, ask your partner to record baby's heartbeat for you to listen to later.

The amount of amniotic fluid is increasing. Total volume is now about 1½ ounces (50ml).

Changes in You

Around this time, morning sickness often begins to improve—that's always a plus. You aren't very big and are probably still quite comfortable.

If it's your first pregnancy, you may still be wearing regular clothes. If you've had other pregnancies, you may start to show earlier and to feel more comfortable in looser clothing, such as maternity clothes.

You may be getting bigger in places besides your tummy. Your breasts are probably growing, and you may notice weight gain in your hips, legs and at your sides.

Changes in Your Skin

During pregnancy, many things can cause changes in your skin, such as hormones and stretching skin. Below we discuss some of the changes you may experience.

Skin-Color Changes. Melanin cells in your skin produce pigment; hormones can cause your body to produce more pigment. These may lead to a variety of skin-color changes. Women of color may be at increased

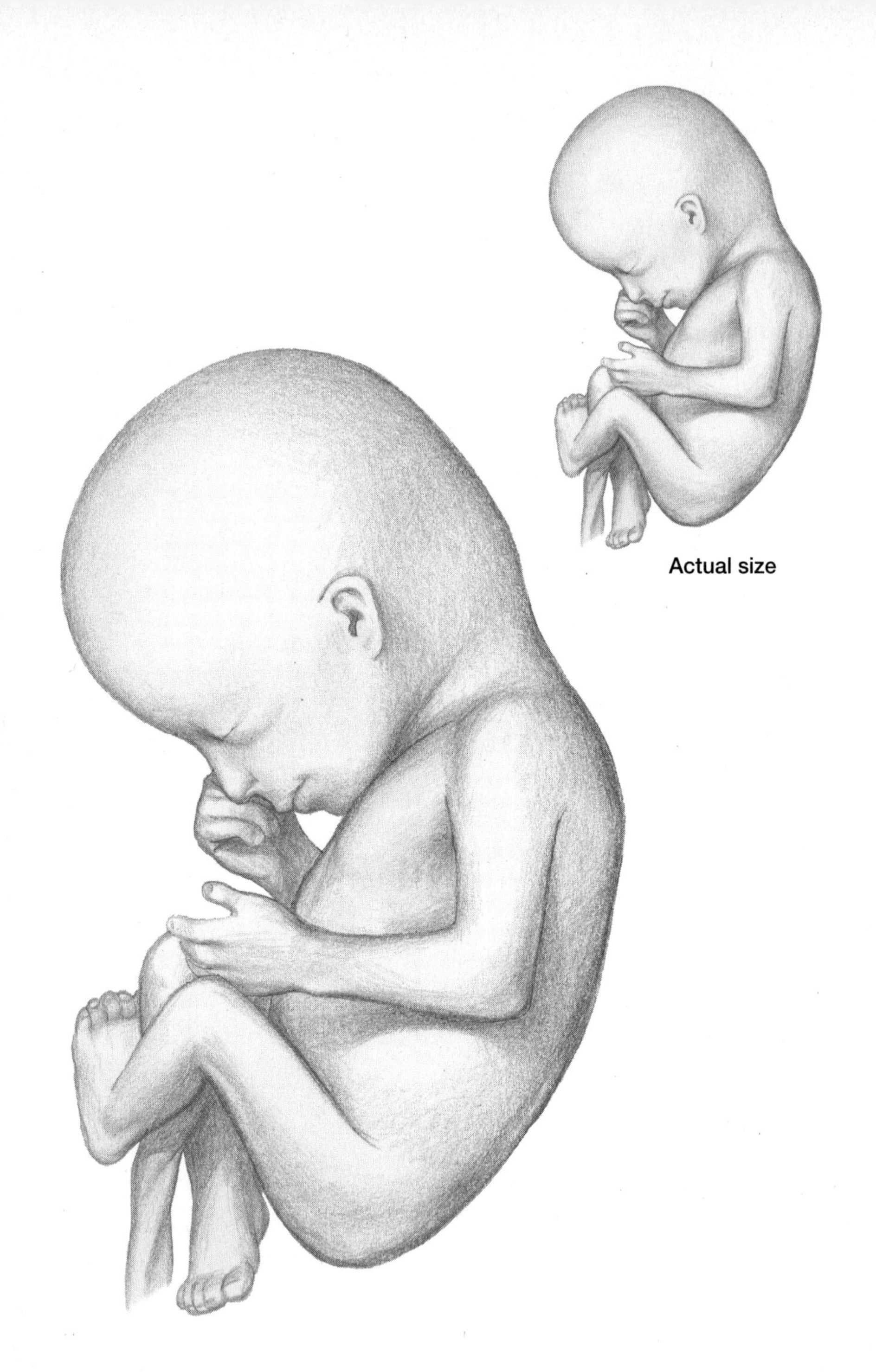

Your baby is growing rapidly. It has doubled
its length in the past 3 weeks.

risk for changes in skin color, which may leave the skin darker or lighter than it was before.

Itchy Skin. Pregnant women often have dry, itchy skin. Moisturizers can help, but you can also help your skin by eating omega-3 fatty acids. They're good for you and baby. Olive oil, almonds and macadamia nuts contain omega-3 fatty acids, so eat these if you do not eat fish.

If you have sensitive skin and experience itchy hives, try rubbing milk of magnesia on the affected area. Rubbing it into the skin helps reduce itching.

Cholestasis of Pregnancy. A sudden attack of itching on the palms and soles may indicate cholestasis of pregnancy. Itching then spreads to the rest of the body. Cholestasis of pregnancy, also called *intrahepatic cholestasis of pregnancy (ICP)* or *prurigo gravidarum,* is a condition in which a woman has severe itching all over the body, but there's no rash.

The condition is rare. We see only about one case in 10,000 pregnancies in the United States.

Intense itching all over begins in the third trimester. Usually it's much worse at night. Other symptoms include jaundice, light-colored stools and dark urine.

Treatment includes anti-itch creams and UVB light treatments. Symptoms generally disappear a few days after baby's birth.

Chloasma. Occasionally irregular brown patches appear on the face and neck, called *chloasma* or *mask of pregnancy.* These disappear or get lighter after delivery. Birth-control pills may cause similar changes. Up to 70% of all pregnant women develop chloasma after exposure to the sun. Women of Asian, Hispanic, North African, Indian and Middle Eastern heritage are more prone to developing chloasma.

The best way to prevent chloasma is to stay out of the sun, especially during the hottest part of the day (between 10am and 3pm). Wear sunscreen and protective clothing (hats, long-sleeved shirts, long pants). Brown patches usually fade in the months after delivery. If they don't, ask your healthcare provider about using Retin-A.

Plaques of Pregnancy (PUPP). Some women have a severe, itchy rash of red bumps that begins on the tummy and spreads to the lower body, then to the arms and legs. This is called *plaques of pregnancy, toxemic rash, polymorphic eruption of pregnancy* or *pruritic urticaria pappules (PUPP)*. With plaques of pregnancy, your healthcare provider may first rule out scabies.

PUPP is the most common skin problem pregnant women experience; it's more common in white women. It may be caused by the skin stretching rapidly, which damages tissue, resulting in bumps and inflammation.

This condition usually appears in first pregnancies during the third trimester. It often affects women who gain a lot of weight or those who are expecting multiples.

The good news is that PUPP won't harm the baby. The bad news is the itching can be so severe that relief may be all you think about, especially at night, which may cause you to lose sleep. PUPP usually resolves within a week of delivery and doesn't usually come back with future pregnancies.

Many treatments have been recommended for relief, including Benadryl, powders, creams, calamine lotion, soaking in cold tubs, oatmeal baths, witch hazel, going without clothes and ultraviolet (UVB) therapy. If you can't find relief, talk to your healthcare provider. He or she may have some recommendations for home remedies that have worked for other women. If all else fails, a prescription for oral antihistamines, topical steroids or cortisone cream may be needed.

Pemphigoid Gestationis (PG; Herpes Gestationis). *Pemphigoid gestationis (PG)* usually begins with blisters around the bellybutton. It may occur in the second or third trimester or immediately after birth. Despite its name, PG has no relationship to the herpes simplex virus. The name came about because the blisters appear similar to herpes infections. It occurs in 1 in 50,000 pregnancies.

The problem begins with sudden onset of intensely itchy blisters on the tummy in about 50% of cases. For the other 50%, blisters can appear anywhere on the body. It often resolves during the last part of pregnancy. It can flare up at delivery or immediately after baby's birth, which happens more than 60% of the time.

The goal of treatment is to relieve itching and to limit blister formation. Oatmeal baths, mild creams and steroids are used. PG usually eases a few weeks after delivery and can recur in your next pregnancies and with oral-contraceptive use. Infants are not at risk.

Other Skin Changes. Vascular spiders (called *telangiectasias* or *angiomas*) are small red elevations on the skin, with branches extending outward. A similar condition is redness of the palms, called *palmar erythema.* Vascular spiders and palmar erythema often occur together. Symptoms are temporary and disappear shortly after delivery.

In many women, skin down the middle of the abdomen becomes markedly darker or pigmented with a brown-black color. It forms a vertical line called the *linea nigra.* It causes no problems and may be permanent.

Atopic eruption of pregnancy (AEP) covers three different pregnancy skin conditions that cause itching—eczema of pregnancy, prurigo of pregnancy and pruritic folliculitis of pregnancy. If you experience *eczema,* you may need prescription skin cream. Research has shown that Elidel and Protopic may have a potential risk for causing cancer. Don't use either to treat diaper rash or any other type of rashes in baby.

Prurigo of pregnancy is a poorly understood pregnancy skin condition. It may look like insect bites, and it itches. Treatment includes anti-itch creams and steroid creams. The condition usually resolves after delivery. There's no risk to you or baby.

Pruritic folliculitis of pregnancy (PFP) occurs in the second and third trimesters. It usually appears as an elevated, red area in hair follicles on the chest and back. Usually some mild itching is involved; the problem resolves 2 to 3 weeks after delivery.

Entering Pregnancy with High Blood Pressure

Blood pressure is the amount of force exerted by blood against arterial walls. If you've had high blood pressure before pregnancy, you have

Tip for Week 12

If you have diarrhea that doesn't go away in 24 hours or it keeps returning, call your healthcare provider. Be sure to drink lots of water and/or hydrating fluids, such as Gatorade. Eat bland foods, such as rice, toast and bananas. Don't use any medicines without your healthcare provider's OK.

chronic hypertension. Your condition will not go away during pregnancy and must be controlled to avoid problems.

If you have chronic high blood pressure, you have a greater chance of having complications during pregnancy. Baby may be low birthweight and/or premature.

If your blood pressure is high when you get pregnant, you may have more ultrasounds to monitor baby's growth. You may want to purchase a blood-pressure monitor to use at home so you can check your pressure any time.

Most blood-pressure medications are safe to use during pregnancy. However, ACE inhibitors should be avoided.

How Your Actions Affect Your Baby's Development

Physical Injury during Pregnancy

Physical injury occurs in 6 to 7% of all pregnancies. Accidents involving motor vehicles account for 65% of these cases; falls and assaults account for the remaining 35%. More than 90% of these are minor injuries.

If you experience any injury, you may be taken care of by emergency-medicine personnel, trauma surgeons, general surgeons and your obstetrician. Most experts recommend observing a pregnant woman for a few hours after an accident to provide adequate time to monitor the baby. Longer monitoring may be necessary in a more serious accident.

It's important to take care during pregnancy so you don't get hurt. There are many ways to do this; it just takes practice and awareness. Use the tips below.

- Keep your eyes open, and pay attention to your surroundings.

If You Have Psoriasis

We know over half of all women with psoriasis find their skin condition improves during pregnancy. This improvement may be due to increased estrogen levels. Treatment for psoriasis during pregnancy may include moisturizers or topical steroids; both are safe to use. Treatment for psoriasis in pregnancy must be very individualized.

- Slow down. Don't be in a rush to get someplace—that's how many accidents occur, whether you're walking, driving or just making your way.
- Don't try to do too much—it can divert your attention from safety.
- Wear clothes and shoes that are comfortable *and* safe. Avoid long skirts that can trip you, carry a smaller purse, put away high heels and opt for comfortable shoes. During pregnancy, comfort and safety can go hand in hand.
- Use handrails when available, such as on stairs, escalators, buses and other places.
- Wear your seat belt *every time* you ride in a car.

Your Nutrition

Some women don't understand the concept of increasing their caloric intake during pregnancy. Don't fall into this trap!

It's unhealthy for you and baby if you gain too much weight, especially early in pregnancy. It makes carrying your baby more uncomfortable, and delivery may be more difficult. It may also be hard to shed the extra pounds after pregnancy.

Chew each mouthful of food for 10 seconds to break down food. It makes it easier for your body to absorb vitamins and minerals.

After baby's birth, most women are anxious to return to "normal" clothes and to look the way they did before pregnancy. Having to deal with extra weight can interfere with reaching this goal.

Junk Food

Is junk food your kind of food? Do you eat it several times a day? Pregnancy is the time to break that habit!

Snack foods account for nearly 20% of the average American's daily calorie intake. Now that you're pregnant, you may need to do away with junk food. What you eat affects someone besides just yourself—your growing baby. If you're used to skipping breakfast, getting something "from a machine" for lunch, then eating dinner at a fast-food restaurant, it doesn't help your pregnancy.

What and when you eat become more important when you realize how your actions affect your baby. Good nutrition takes planning on your part, but you can do it. Avoid foods that contain a lot of sugar and/or fat. Choose healthful alternatives. If you work, take healthy foods with you for lunches and snacks. Stay away from fast food and junk food.

Fats and Sweets

You may need to be cautious with fats and sweets, unless you're underweight and need to gain some weight. Many of these foods are high in calories and low in nutritional value. Eat them sparingly.

Instead of selecting a food with little nutritional value, like potato chips or cookies, choose a piece of fruit, some cheese or a slice of whole-wheat bread with a little peanut butter. You'll satisfy your hunger and your nutritional needs at the same time! Some fats and sweets you may choose, and their serving sizes, include the following:

- sugar or honey—1 tablespoon
- oil—1 tablespoon
- margarine or butter—1 pat
- jam or jelly—1 tablespoon
- salad dressing—1 tablespoon

Watch your intake of peanuts and peanut butter. Research shows eating a lot of peanut products during pregnancy may increase your baby's chances of having asthma.

You Should Also Know

Fifth Disease

Fifth disease, also called *parvo virus B19*, was the fifth disease to be described with a certain kind of rash. (It is *not* related to the parvo virus common in dogs.) It is a mild, moderately contagious airborne infection and spreads easily through groups, such as classrooms or day-care centers. About 60% of pregnant women have previously had fifth disease—that means 40% are at risk. However, you have only a 10% chance of being infected after exposure.

The rash looks like reddened skin caused by a slap. The reddening fades and recurs, and lasts from 2 to 34 days. Joint pains are another symptom. There is no treatment. Fifth disease is most harmful to baby during the first trimester.

If you believe you have been exposed to fifth disease, contact your healthcare provider. A blood test can determine whether you previously had the virus. If you haven't, your healthcare provider can monitor you to detect problems in the baby. Some problems can be dealt with before baby is born.

Cystic Fibrosis

Cystic fibrosis (CF) is a genetic disorder that causes digestive and breathing problems. It causes the body to produce sticky mucus that builds up in the lungs, pancreas and other organs, which can lead to respiratory and digestive problems. Those with the disorder are usually diagnosed early in life.

We are now able to determine whether there is a risk of having a baby with CF. You and your partner can be tested before pregnancy to determine if either of you are carriers. A test can also be done in the first and/or second trimester of pregnancy to see if the baby has cystic fibrosis. Medical experts urge Caucasians to have the CF test. It's the most common birth defect in this group. Screening is also recommended for others at higher risk for CF, such as Ashkenazi Jews. The screening test uses a blood sample or a saliva sample.

For your baby to have cystic fibrosis, *both* parents must be carriers. If only one parent is a carrier, the baby will *not* have CF. A carrier does *not* have CF. You could be a carrier even if no one in your family has CF. You could also be a carrier if you already have children and they do not have CF. Your chance of carrying the gene for cystic fibrosis increases if someone in your family has CF or is a known carrier.

Screening for Cystic Fibrosis. Screening for cystic fibrosis is often offered to couples as part of genetic counseling. One test available is called *Cystic Fibrosis (CF) Complete Test.* It can identify more than 1000 mutations of the CF gene. A panel that screens for 23 CF mutations is the recommended test.

If both of you carry the CF gene, your baby will have a 25% chance of having cystic fibrosis. Your developing baby can be tested during your pregnancy with chorionic villus sampling around the 10th or 11th week of pregnancy. Amniocentesis may also be used to test the baby.

Some CF gene mutations cannot be detected by the current test. This means you could be told you don't carry the gene, when in fact you do. The test cannot detect all CF mutations because researchers don't know all of them at this time. However, unknown CF gene mutations are rare.

Late-night nutritious snacks are beneficial for some women. However, for many women, snacking at night is unnecessary. If you're used to ice cream or other goodies before bed, you may pay for it during pregnancy with excessive weight gain. Food in your stomach late at night may also cause heartburn or indigestion.

If you believe cystic fibrosis is a serious concern or if you have a family history of the disease, talk to your healthcare provider. Testing is a personal decision you and your partner must make.

Many couples choose not to have the test because it would not change what they would do during the pregnancy. In addition, they do not want to expose the mother-to-be or the developing fetus to the risks of CVS or amniocentesis. However, testing is recommended so care can be provided to baby after birth.

Exercise for Week 12

Lie on your left side, with your body in alignment. Support your head with your left hand, and place your right hand on the floor in front of you for balance. Inhale and relax. While exhaling, slowly raise your right leg as high as you can without bending your knee or your body. Keep your foot flexed. Inhale and slowly lower your leg. Repeat on your right side. Do 10 times on each side. *Tones and strengthens hip, buttock and thigh muscles.*

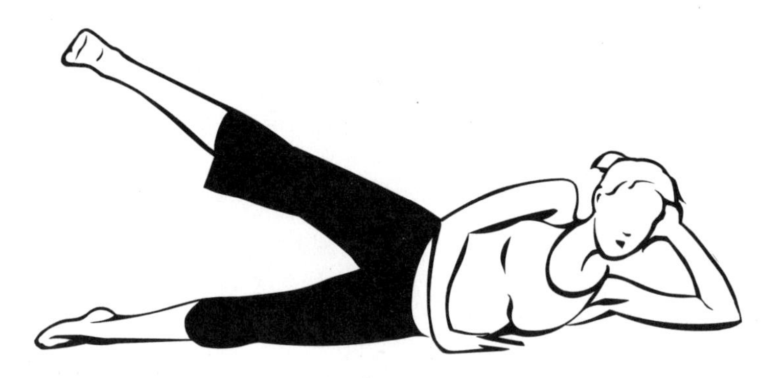

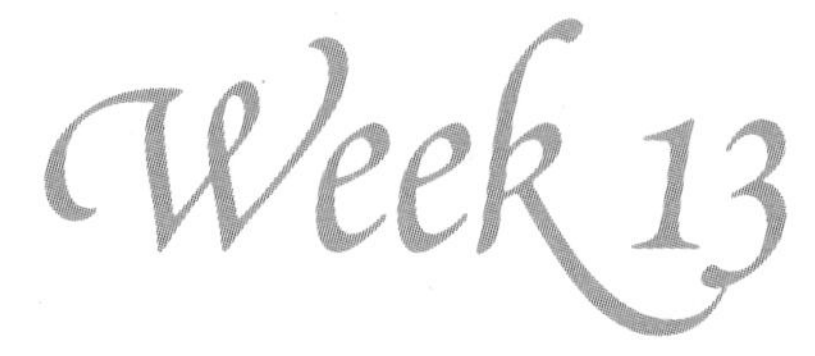

Week 13

Age of Fetus—11 Weeks

How Big Is Your Baby?

Your baby continues to grow rapidly! Its crown-to-rump length is 2½ to 3 inches (6.5 to 7.8cm), and it weighs between ½ and ¾ ounce (13 to 20g). It is about the size of a peach.

How Big Are You?

You can probably feel the upper edge of your uterus about 4 inches (10cm) below your bellybutton. Your uterus fills your pelvis and is growing upward into your abdomen. It feels like a soft, smooth ball.

You have probably gained some weight by now. If morning sickness has been a problem and you've had a hard time eating, you may not have gained much. As you feel better and as your baby rapidly starts to gain weight, you'll also gain weight.

Although this book is designed to take you through pregnancy by examining one week at a time, you may want specific information. Because the book can't include *everything* you need *before* you know you're looking for it, check the index, beginning on page 653, for a particular topic. We may not cover the subject until a later week.

How Your Baby Is Growing and Developing

Fetal growth is particularly striking from now through about 24 weeks of pregnancy. The baby has doubled in length since the 7th week. Changes in fetal weight have also been dramatic.

There is a relative slowdown in the growth of your baby's head compared to the rest of its body. In week 13, the head is about half the crown-to-rump length. By week 21, the head is about ⅓ of baby's body. At birth, your baby's head is only ¼ the size of its body. Body growth speeds up as head growth slows down.

Eyes are moving closer together on the face. The ears move to their normal position on the sides of the head. Sex organs have developed enough so a male can be distinguished from a female, if examined outside the womb.

Intestines begin to develop within a large swelling in the umbilical cord outside the body. About this time, they draw back into the abdominal cavity. If this doesn't occur and the intestines remain outside the abdomen at birth, a condition called an *omphalocele* occurs. It is rare (occurs in 1 of 10,000 births). The condition can usually be repaired with surgery, and babies do well afterward.

Changes in You

Stretch Marks

Many women have stretch marks, called *striae distensae*, during pregnancy. They occur when the elastic fibers and collagen in deeper layers of your skin are pulled apart to make room for baby. When skin tears, collagen breaks down and shows through the top layer of your skin as a pink, red or purple indented streak.

Nearly 9 out of 10 pregnant women develop stretch marks on their breasts, tummy, hips, buttocks and/or arms. They may appear any time during pregnancy. After birth, they may fade to the same color as the rest of your skin, but they won't go away.

You can help yourself by gaining weight *slowly* and *steadily* during pregnancy. Any large increase in weight can cause stretch marks to appear more readily.

Although you'd like to think you can keep stretch marks from happening to you, there really isn't much you can do to prevent them. Creams and lotions you see advertised on TV and in magazines don't really work. You'll get stretch marks if you're going to get them (some lucky women get very few, if any!). They're just a part of being pregnant.

Drink lots of water, and eat healthy foods. Foods high in antioxidants provide nutrients you need to repair and heal tissue. Eating enough protein and smaller amounts of "good" fats, such as flaxseed, flaxseed oil and fish oils, may also help you.

Stay out of the sun! Keep up with your exercise program.

Ask your healthcare provider about using creams with alpha-hydroxy acid, citric acid or lactic acid. Some of these creams and lotions improve the quality of the skin's elastic fibers.

Don't use steroid creams, such as hydrocortisone or topicort, to treat stretch marks during pregnancy without first checking with your healthcare provider. You absorb some of the steroid into your system, and the steroid can pass to baby. And stretch creams really can't penetrate deeply enough to repair damage to your skin.

Treatment after Pregnancy. After pregnancy, you have quite a few treatment options. Some treatments hold promise. If you're left with lots of stretch marks, you may want to ask about prescription creams, such as Retin-A or Renova, or laser treatments.

Retin-A, in combination with glycolic acid, has been shown to be fairly effective. Prescriptions are needed for Retin-A and Renova; you can get glycolic acid from your dermatologist. Cellex-C, with glycolic acid, also helps with stretch marks.

The most effective treatment is laser treatment, but it can be costly. It's often done in combination with the medication methods described above. However, lasers don't work for everyone.

Massage may help—it increases blood flow to the area, which helps gets rid of dead surface cells. Discuss treatment with your healthcare provider if stretch marks bother you after pregnancy.

Changes in Your Breasts

Your breasts are changing. (See the illustration on page 187.) The mammary gland (another name for the breast) got its name from the Latin term for breast—*mamma.*

Before pregnancy, your breasts may weigh about 7 ounces (200g) each. During pregnancy, they increase in size and weight as you add fat in your breast tissue. Near the end of pregnancy, each breast may weigh 14 to 28 ounces (400 to 800g). During nursing, each breast can weigh 28 ounces (800g) or more.

A breast is made up of glands, tissue to provide support and fatty tissue for protection. Each nipple contains nerve endings, muscle fibers, sebaceous glands, sweat glands and about 20 milk ducts. Milk-producing sacs connect with the ducts leading to the nipple.

From the beginning of pregnancy, your body is getting ready to breastfeed. Soon after pregnancy begins, the alveoli begin to increase in number and to grow larger. Milk sinuses, located close to the nipple, begin forming; they hold the milk you will produce. By as early as 20 weeks of pregnancy, your breasts will begin to produce milk. Even if you give birth weeks earlier than your due date, your breast milk will be nutritious enough to nourish a premature baby.

Grandma's Remedy

If you want to avoid using medication, try a folk remedy. If you get a paper cut, apply some lip balm to help heal the cut and reduce skin irritation.

You may notice veins appearing just beneath the skin and a change in nipples. They may get larger and more sensitive. The nipple is surrounded by the areola, a circular, pigmented area. During pregnancy, the areola darkens and grows larger. A darkened areola may act as a visual signal to baby. Bumps on your nipples, called *Montgomery glands,* secrete fluid to lubricate and protect your nipples if you breastfeed.

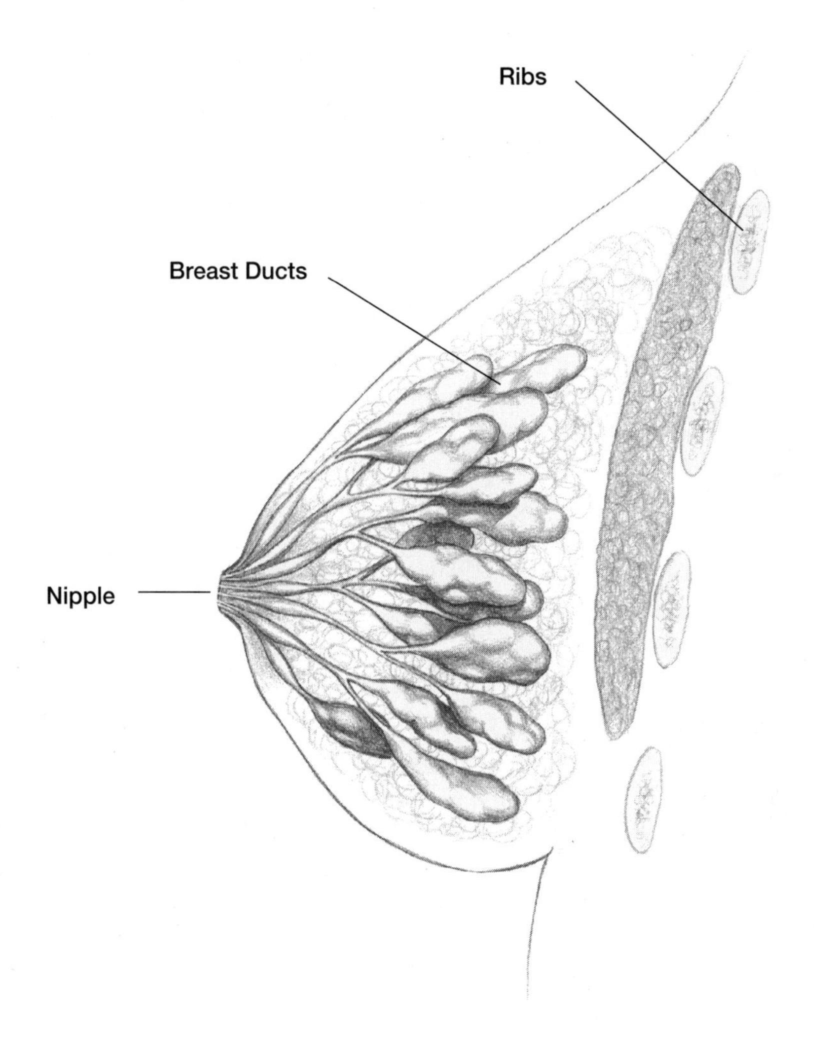

Development of the maternal breast by the end of the first trimester (13 weeks of pregnancy).

During the second trimester, a thin yellow fluid called *colostrum* begins to form. It can sometimes be pressed from the nipple by gentle massage. You may also notice stretch marks on your breasts. During the third trimester, your breasts may itch as skin is stretched. An alcohol-free, perfume-free moisturizer may help. Your breasts will reach their maximum size a few days *after* baby's birth.

How Your Actions Affect Your Baby's Development

Working during Pregnancy

Today, many women work outside the home, and many continue to work during pregnancy. Most pregnant women can work until they deliver, if they choose.

In the United States, millions of babies are born to women who have been employed at some time during pregnancy. These women often have concerns about safety at work. It's common for women and their employers to have questions.

"*Is it safe to work while I'm pregnant?*"

"*Can I work my entire pregnancy?*"

"*Am I in danger of harming my baby if I work?*"

You may feel anxious when you have to tell your boss you're pregnant, but it's something you must do. It's better if he or she hears it from you, not someone else.

Find out your company's maternity leave policy and what benefits it provides to pregnant women and new mothers. Be sure to document everything as you progress through pregnancy.

Legislation That May Affect You. The *U.S. Pregnancy Discrimination Act* prohibits job discrimination on the basis of pregnancy or childbirth. It states pregnancy and related conditions should be treated the same as any other disability or medical condition. A healthcare provider may be asked to certify a pregnant woman can work without endangering herself or her baby.

You may experience a *pregnancy-related disability*. It can come from the pregnancy itself, complications of pregnancy or a job situation, such as standing for a long time or exposure to various substances.

If you have worked for your present employer for at least 1 year, the *Family and Medical Leave Act* (FMLA) may apply to you. The law allows a new parent (mom or dad) to take up to 12 weeks of unpaid leave in any 12-month period for the birth of a baby. If you're covered, you're entitled to the same or equal job after you return to work.

To be eligible, you must work at your job for at least 1250 hours a year (about 60% of a normal 40-hour work week). This act applies only to companies that employ 50 or more people within a 75-mile radius. States may allow an employer to deny job restoration to employees in the top 10% compensation bracket. If *both parents* work for the same employer, only a *total* of 12 weeks off *between them* is allowed.

Any time taken off *before* the birth of a baby is counted toward the 12 weeks a person is entitled to in any given year. (You might have to take time off if you have health or medical problems.) Leave may be taken intermittently or all at the same time.

Dad Tip

Did you know that exercise is important for a pregnant woman? If there are no complications to forbid it, nearly *all* pregnant women are advised to exercise at least 5 times a week. Ask the healthcare provider if there's some exercise you can do together on a regular basis, such as walking, swimming or playing golf or tennis. It can help you get in shape, too.

If you work for a small company, fewer than 15 people, you aren't covered by the FMLA or the Pregnancy Discrimination Act. You'll probably want to find out what your company's policy is regarding pregnancy leave well in advance of your due date. Check out your state laws and any other local laws that apply to you to determine what kind of leave you can take.

The *Health Insurance Portability and Accountability Act* (HIPAA; pronounced hip-ah) may also apply to you. This law protects most women who change health plans or enroll in a new plan after they become pregnant. The law states that if you change jobs and insurance plans during pregnancy, you can't be denied insurance coverage if you had insurance in your former job. And your baby can't be denied coverage if you sign him or her up within 30 days of birth.

State or Provincial Laws and Parental Leave. About half the states in the United States have passed state legislation that deals with parental leave. Some states provide disability insurance if you have to leave work because of pregnancy or birth. If you're self-employed, you aren't qualified to receive state disability payments. You may want to consider a private disability policy to cover you during the time your healthcare provider says you can't work. The glitch here is the policy must be in place *before* you become pregnant.

In Canada, unpaid parental leave is available. The length of time you may take off from work varies from province to province.

State laws about parental leave differ, so check with your state labor office or consult the personnel director in your company's human resources department. A summary of state laws on family leave is also available from:

Women's Bureau
U.S. Department of Labor
200 Constitution Avenue NW
Room S-3311
Washington, DC 20210

In Canada, contact the Human Resources office for information, or call Service Canada at 1-800-206-7218.

You may be wondering about taking some medicine you normally use now that you're pregnant. *Zicam* is an over-the-counter product to help lessen cold symptoms. *Amitiza* is a prescription medication taken for constipation. *Ambien* and *Rozerem* are medications to help you sleep. If you're considering using any of these medications, check first with your healthcare provider, who will determine whether you should use it.

Some Risks If You Work during Pregnancy. It can be hard to know the exact risk of a particular job. In most cases, we don't have enough information to know about everything that can harm a developing baby.

The goal is to minimize the risk to mom and baby while still allowing a woman to work. A normal woman with a normal job should be able to work throughout her pregnancy. However, she may need to change some things about her job. If your job involves lifting, climbing, carrying or standing for a long time, you may need to make some changes. Early in pregnancy, you may feel dizzy, tired or nauseous, which might increase your chance of injury. Extra weight and a large tummy may affect your balance and increase your chance of falling in late pregnancy.

You probably know caffeine is found in lots of foods and beverages. But did you know it's now *added* to some foods? We found it added to some potato chips, candy and cereal. Be sure to read labels because caffeine must be listed as an ingredient; however, the amount may not be listed.

If you're exposed to any hazardous substances, you will want to make changes. You may be exposed to pesticides, harmful chemicals, cleaning solvents or heavy metals, such as lead, if you are employed in a factory, at a dry cleaners, in the printing trade, in an arts-and-crafts business, in the electronics industry or on a farm. Healthcare workers, teachers or child-care providers may be exposed to harmful viruses.

If you have any type of health problem, your healthcare provider may want you to limit activities on and off the job. He or she may also certify you have a pregnancy-related disability. This means you have a health problem caused by your pregnancy that keeps you from doing your normal duties.

Work with your healthcare provider and your employer. If problems arise, such as premature labor or bleeding, listen to your healthcare provider. If bed rest at home is suggested, follow that advice. As your pregnancy progresses, you may have to work fewer hours or do lighter work. Be flexible. It doesn't help you or your baby if you wear yourself out and make things worse.

Take Care of Yourself. If you work, be smart! Don't participate in anything that is dangerous for you or baby. Don't stand for long periods. Don't wear clothes that are tight around the waist, especially if you sit most of the day.

Sit up straight at your desk. Place a low footstool on the floor to rest your feet on. Rest at breaks and during lunch. Get up and walk a little every 30 minutes. Going to the bathroom may be a good reason to get up and move around.

Drink lots of water. Bring a healthy lunch and snack foods to help you keep tabs on your calorie intake. Fast foods can be loaded with empty calories.

Try to keep stress to a minimum. Don't take on new projects or those that take a lot of time and attention.

Your Nutrition

Caffeine is a stimulant found in many beverages and foods, including coffee, tea, various soft drinks and chocolate. It may also be found in some medicine, such as headache remedies.

You may be more sensitive to caffeine during pregnancy. For over 20 years, the Food and Drug Administration (FDA) has recommended pregnant women avoid caffeine. It isn't good for you or baby. If you drink as little as two 8-ounce cups of coffee a day, you may be doubling your risk of early miscarriage.

A Caffeine Warning

If a woman takes a lot of caffeine, it may affect her baby's respiratory system. One study showed exposure before birth might be linked to sudden infant death syndrome (SIDS).

Cut down on caffeine, or eliminate it from your diet. Caffeine crosses the placenta to the baby—if you're jittery, your baby may suffer from the same effects. And caffeine passes into breast milk, which can cause irritability and sleeplessness if you breastfeed baby.

The list below details the amounts of caffeine from various sources:

- coffee, 5 ounces—from 60 to 140mg and higher
- tea, 5 ounces—from 30 to 65mg
- cocoa, 8 ounces—5mg
- 1½ ounce chocolate bar—10 to 30mg
- baking chocolate, 1 ounce—25mg
- soft drinks, 12 ounces—from 35 to 55mg
- pain-relief tablets, standard dose—40mg
- allergy and cold remedies, standard dose—25mg

Tip for Week 13

When cutting down on caffeine during pregnancy, read labels. More than 200 foods, beverages and over-the-counter medicines contain caffeine!

You Should Also Know

Lyme Disease

Lyme disease is transmitted to humans by ticks. About 80% of those bitten have a bite with a distinctive look, called a *bull's eye.* There may also be flulike symptoms. After 4 to 6 weeks, symptoms may become more serious.

Early on, blood tests may not diagnose Lyme disease. A blood test done later can establish the diagnosis.

We know Lyme disease can cross the placenta. However, at this time we don't know if it is dangerous to the baby.

Treatment for Lyme disease requires long-term antibiotic therapy. Many medications used to treat Lyme disease are safe to use during pregnancy.

Avoid exposure if you can. Stay out of areas with ticks, especially heavily wooded areas. If you can't, wear long-sleeved shirts, long pants, a hat or scarf, socks and boots or closed shoes. Be sure to check your hair when you come in; ticks often attach themselves there. Check your clothing to make sure no ticks remain in folds, cuffs or pockets.

Some Information May Scare You

In an effort to give you as much information as possible about pregnancy, we do include serious discussions throughout the book that some might find "scary." The information is not included to frighten you; it's there to provide facts about particular medical situations that may occur during pregnancy.

If a woman experiences a serious problem, she and her partner will probably want to know as much about it as possible. If a woman has a friend or knows someone who has problems during pregnancy, reading about it might relieve her fears. We also hope our discussions can help you start a dialogue with your doctor, if you have questions.

Nearly all pregnancies are uneventful, and serious situations don't arise. However, please know we have tried to cover as many aspects of pregnancy as we possibly can so you'll have all the information at hand that you might need and want. Knowledge is power, so having various facts available can help you feel more in control of your own pregnancy. We hope reading information helps you relax and have a great pregnancy experience.

If you find serious discussions frighten you, don't read them! Or if the information doesn't apply to your pregnancy, just skip over it. But realize information is there if you want to know more about a particular situation.

Gas (Flatulence)

Are you experiencing more gas (flatulence) than normal? It's not uncommon. What you eat definitely has an impact on gas production. And foods that trigger gas may change each trimester.

Eating slowly may help reduce the amount of air you take in, which in turn helps reduce gas. Keep exercising—it can help break up gas pockets. Stay away from certain foods, including sugar, some dairy and bread products. Sorbitol, a sugar substitute found in many "lite" foods, can also cause gas.

Nuchal Translucency Screening

Nuchal translucency screening is a test to help healthcare providers and pregnant women find answers about whether a baby has Down syndrome. An advantage of this test is results are available in the first trimester. Because results are available early, a couple may make earlier decisions regarding the pregnancy, if they choose to do so.

A detailed ultrasound allows the healthcare provider to measure the space behind baby's neck. When combined with the blood tests, the results of these *two* tests (ultrasound and blood test) can be used to predict a woman's risk of having a baby with Down syndrome.

Be careful with bottled waters—some contain caffeine.

Exercise for Week 13

Stand with your feet apart and your knees relaxed. Holding a light weight in your right hand (a 16-ounce can will do fine), extend your right arm straight over your head. Contract your tummy muscles, bend slightly at the waist, then swing your arm down and over your left foot. Complete the exercise by making a complete circle and returning your arm to the original position, above your right shoulder. Repeat 8 times on each side. *Strengthens back and shoulder muscles.*

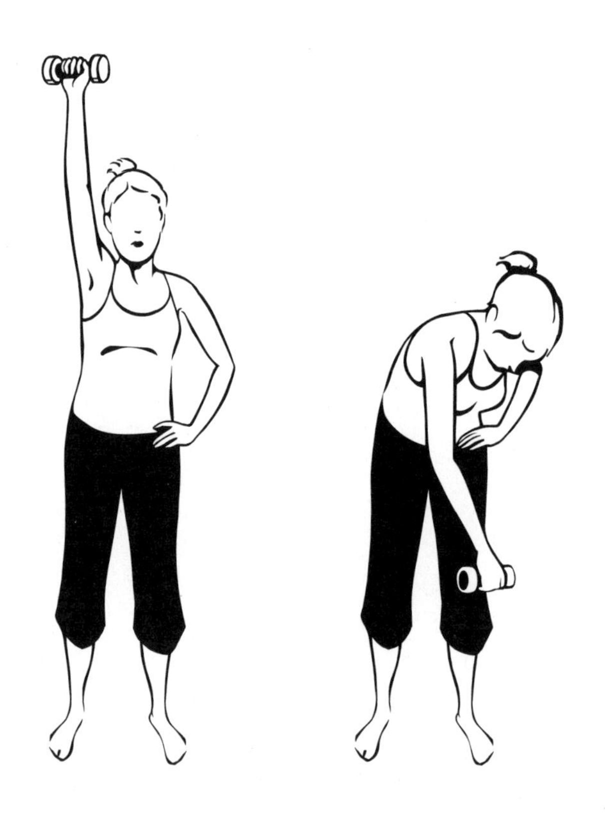

Week 14

Age of Fetus—12 Weeks

How Big Is Your Baby?

The crown-to-rump length is 3¼ to 4 inches (8 to 9.3cm). Your baby is about the size of your fist and weighs almost 1 ounce (25g).

How Big Are You?

Maternity clothes may be a "must" by now. Some women try to get by for a while by not buttoning or zipping their pants all the way or by using rubber bands or safety pins to increase the size of their waistbands. Others wear their partner's clothing, but that usually works for only a short time. You'll enjoy your pregnancy more and feel better with clothing that fits comfortably and provides you room to grow.

How Your Baby Is Growing and Developing

As you can see in the illustration on page 198, baby's ears have moved to the sides of its head. The neck continues to grow, and the chin no longer rests on the chest.

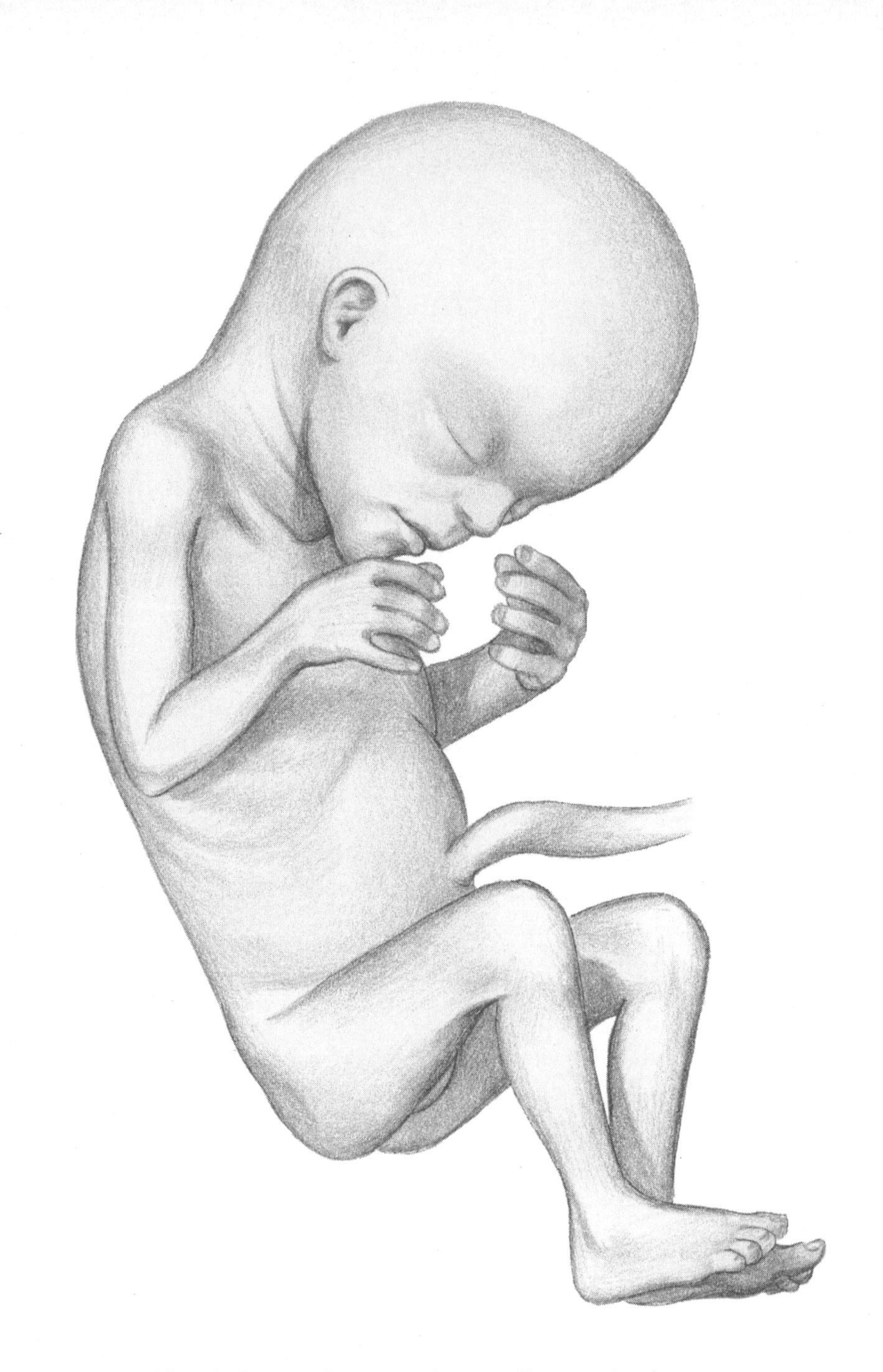

Your baby continues to change. Ears and eyes move to a more normal position by this week.

Changes in You

Skin Tags and Moles

Pregnancy can make skin tags and moles change and grow. *Skin tags* are small tags of skin that may appear for the first time or may grow larger during pregnancy. *Moles* may appear for the first time during pregnancy, or existing moles may grow larger and darken. If you notice any changes in a mole, show it to your healthcare provider!

Do You Have Hemorrhoids?

Hemorrhoids (dilated blood vessels around or inside the anus) are a common problem during or after pregnancy. Pregnant women often develop hemorrhoids during the second and third trimesters. Hormone changes and the growing baby are contributing factors. Hemorrhoids may worsen toward the end of pregnancy. They may also get worse with each succeeding pregnancy.

> Don't take flax oil (it's not the same as flaxseed oil). Flax oil is often recommended as an herbal treatment for constipation. If taken during the second and third trimesters, it may increase your risk of premature birth.

Eat lots of fiber, and drink lots of fluid. Stool softeners and bulk fiber products may also help. Fiber tablets, wafers or fiber products you can add to any food or drink without adding texture may also be good remedies.

If hemorrhoids cause a lot of discomfort, discuss it with your healthcare provider. He or she will know what treatment method is best for you. Try the following for relief.

- Rest at least 1 hour every day with your feet and hips elevated.
- Lie with your legs elevated and knees slightly bent when you sleep at night.
- Eat lots of fiber, and drink lots of fluid.
- Take warm (not hot) baths for relief.
- Suppository medications, available without a prescription, may help.
- Over-the-counter products that contain hydrocortisone may help relieve itching and swelling. Ask your healthcare provider about them.

- Apply ice packs, cold compresses or cotton balls soaked in witch hazel to the affected area.
- Don't sit or stand for long periods.
- Get up and walk often to relieve pressure on the anus.
- If you experience pain, acetaminophen may help relieve it.

After pregnancy, hemorrhoids usually improve, but they may not go away completely. Use the above treatment methods when pregnancy is over.

How Your Actions Affect Your Baby's Development

X-Rays, CT Scans and MRIs during Pregnancy

Some women are concerned about tests that use radiation during pregnancy. Can these tests hurt the baby? Can you have them at any time in pregnancy? Unfortunately, we do not know of any "safe" amount for a developing baby.

Problems, such as pneumonia or appendicitis, can and do occur in pregnant women and may require an X-ray for diagnosis and treatment. Discuss the need for X-rays with your healthcare provider. It's your responsibility to let your healthcare provider and others know you're pregnant or may be pregnant before you have any medical test. It's easier to deal with the questions of safety and risk *before* a test is performed.

If you have an X-ray or a series of X-rays, then discover you're pregnant, ask your healthcare provider about the possible risk to your baby. He or she will be able to advise you.

If you enjoy listening to your baby's heartbeat, devices are available so you can listen at home! Some people believe doing this helps a couple bond with baby. If you're interested in a use-at-home doppler device, check with your healthcare provider at an office visit. Or check out these devices on the Internet.

Computerized tomographic scans, also called *CT* or *CAT scans,* are a form of specialized

X-ray. This technique combines X-ray with computer analysis. Many researchers believe the amount of radiation received by a fetus from a CT scan is much lower than that received from a regular X-ray. However, use caution when having these tests until we know more about the effects of even this small amount of radiation on a baby.

Magnetic resonance imaging, also called *MRI,* is another test widely used today. At this time, no harmful effects in pregnancy have been reported from the use of MRI. However, it may be best to avoid MRI during the first trimester.

Dental Care

See your dentist at least once during pregnancy. Tell your dentist you're pregnant. If you need dental work, postpone it until after the first 13 weeks, if possible. You may not be able to wait if you have an infection; an untreated infection could be harmful to you and your baby.

Antibiotics or pain medicine may be necessary. If you need medication, consult your pregnancy healthcare provider before taking anything. Many antibiotics and pain medications are OK to take during pregnancy.

If brushing your teeth makes you nauseous, try a different toothpaste or plain baking soda. Avoid mouthwashes that contain alcohol.

Be careful about anesthesia for dental work during pregnancy. Local anesthesia is OK. Avoid gas and general anesthesia when possible. If general anesthesia is necessary, make sure an experienced anesthesiologist who knows you're pregnant administers it.

Gum Disease. During pregnancy, hormones can make gum problems worse. Increased blood volume can cause gums to swell and make them more disposed to infection.

If you have a condition during pregnancy that causes severe pain, such as a root canal or a severe sprain, and acetaminophen doesn't take care of it, ask your healthcare provider about using analgesic codeine. It's considered safe during the first and second trimesters.

Tip for Week 14

If you must have dental work or diagnostic tests, tell your dentist or your healthcare provider you're pregnant so they can take extra care with you. It may be helpful for your dentist and healthcare provider to talk before any decisions are made.

Gingivitis is the first stage of periodontal disease. It appears as swollen, bleeding, reddened gums. It's caused by bacteria growing down into the spaces between the gums and teeth. Experts believe these bacteria can enter the bloodstream, travel to other parts of the body and cause infections in you.

Regular flossing and brushing help prevent gingivitis. Brushing with a power toothbrush, especially one with a 2-minute timer, may help clean teeth more thoroughly and may help toughen gums.

Dental Emergencies. Dental emergencies do occur. Emergencies you might face include root canal, pulling a tooth, a large cavity, an abscessed tooth or problems resulting from an accident or injury. A serious dental problem must be treated. Problems that could result from not treating it are more serious than the risks you might be exposed to with treatment.

Eating raisins can inhibit the growth of bacteria that cause gum disease and tooth decay.

Dental X-rays are sometimes necessary and can be done during pregnancy. Your abdomen must be shielded with a lead apron before X-rays are taken.

Your Nutrition

Being overweight when pregnancy begins may present special problems for you. Your healthcare provider may advise you to gain less weight than the average 25 to 35 pounds recommended for a normal-weight woman. You will probably have to choose lower-calorie, lower-fat foods to eat. A visit with a nutritionist may be necessary to help you develop a healthful food plan. You will be advised *not* to diet during pregnancy. See the discussion below dealing with obesity during pregnancy.

You Should Also Know

Overweight/Obesity Bring Special Precautions

If you are overweight when you get pregnant, you're not alone. Statistics show up to 38% of all pregnant women are overweight. About 20% of women are obese when they get pregnant.

A new category has been added to pregnancy weight-gain guidelines. The category is for obese women, and the recommendation is a weight gain of between 11 and 20 pounds for an entire pregnancy. Some experts also cite morbid obesity as a subcategory of obesity; experts suggest weight gain should be determined on an individual basis for women in this category.

You're considered *overweight* if your body mass index (BMI) is between 25 and 29; over 30, you are considered *obese*. If you have a BMI of 40 or over, you are considered *morbidly obese.*

Ask your healthcare provider to help you figure out your BMI at a prenatal appointment, or do it yourself using the formula on page 204. When figuring your BMI, use your *prepregnancy weight.* For example, a woman who is 5'4" tall who weighs 158 pounds has a BMI of 27 and is considered overweight. A woman who is 5'4" tall who weighs 184 pounds has a BMI of 32 and is considered obese. A woman who is 5'4" tall who weighs 239 pounds has a BMI of 41 and is considered morbidly obese.

If you're overweight, it can contribute to a variety of problems. Research shows over 65% of all overweight women gain more weight than their healthcare provider recommends during pregnancy. Gaining too much weight (above the amount advised by your healthcare provider) may increase your chances of a Cesarean delivery. It can also make carrying baby more uncomfortable, and delivery may be more difficult. And it's harder to lose any weight you gain during pregnancy after baby is born.

Calculation of BMI (Body Mass Index)

BMI is determined from the measurement of height and weight. Be sure you use your *prepregnancy weight* for this calculation. It is calculated as shown below:

$$\text{BMI} = \frac{\text{weight (pounds)} \times 703}{\text{height squared (inches)}}$$

For example, the BMI of a woman who is 5'4" tall who weighs 152 pounds would be calculated as follows:

$$\frac{152 \times 703}{64 \times 64} = \text{BMI of 26}$$

Women who are overweight may need to see their healthcare provider more often. Ultrasound may be needed to pinpoint a due date. You may also need other tests.

Take Care of Yourself. Try to gain your total-pregnancy weight *slowly*. Weigh yourself weekly, and watch your food intake. Eat nutritious, healthful foods, and eliminate those with empty calories. A visit with a nutritionist may help you develop a healthful food plan.

Do *not* diet during pregnancy. To get the nutrients you need, choose nonfat or lowfat products, meats, grain products, fruits and vegetables. Many supply a variety of nutrients. Take your prenatal vitamin every day throughout your entire pregnancy.

Talk to your healthcare provider about exercising. Discuss swimming and walking, which are good exercises for *any* pregnant woman.

Eat regular meals—5 to 6 *small* meals a day is a good goal. Your total calorie intake should be between 1800 and 2400 calories a day. Keeping a daily food diary can help you track how much you're eating and when you're eating. It can help you identify where to make changes, if necessary.

Pregnancy in the Military

Are you pregnant and currently on active duty in the military? If you are, you have made the decision to stay in the Armed Forces. Before 1972, if you were on active duty and became pregnant, you were automatically separated from the military, whether you wanted to be or not!

Today, if you want to stay in the service, you can. Each branch of the service has particular policies regarding pregnancy. Below is a summary of those policies for the Army, Navy, Air Force, Marines and Coast Guard.

Army Policies. During pregnancy, you are exempt from body composition and fitness testing. You cannot be deployed overseas. At 20 weeks, you're required to stand at parade rest or attention for no longer than 15 minutes. At 28 weeks, your work week is limited to 40 hours a week, 8 hours a day.

Navy Policies. During pregnancy, you are exempt from body composition and fitness testing. You are not allowed to serve on a ship after 20 weeks of pregnancy. You're limited to serving duty in places within 6 hours of medical care. Your work week is limited to 40 hours, and you're required to stand at parade rest or attention for no longer than 20 minutes.

Air Force Policies. During pregnancy, you are exempt from body composition and fitness testing. Restrictions are based on your work environment. If you are assigned to an area without obstetrical care, your assignment will be curtailed by week 24.

Marine Corps Policies. You will be on full-duty status until a medical doctor certifies full duty is not medically advised. You may not participate in contingency operations nor may you be deployed aboard a Navy vessel. Flight personnel are grounded, unless cleared by a medical waiver. If a medical doctor deems you are unfit for physical training or you cannot stand in formation, you will be excused from these activities. However, you will remain available for worldwide assignments.

Pregnant Marines will not be detached from Hawaii aboard a ship after their 26th week. If serving aboard a ship, a pregnant woman will be reassigned at the first opportunity but no later than by 20 weeks.

U.S. Coast Guard. During pregnancy, you are exempt from body composition and fitness testing. After 28 weeks of pregnancy, your work week will be limited to 40 hours. You will not be assigned overseas. Other duty restrictions are based on your job; however, you will not be assigned to any rescue-swimmer duties during your pregnancy.

You may not be deployed from the 20th week of your pregnancy through 6 months postpartum. You will not be assigned to any flight duties after your second trimester (26 weeks), and you are limited to serving duty in places within 3 hours of medical care.

Dad Tip

Be thoughtful about staying in touch. If you have to go out of town, call your partner at least once a day. Let her know you're thinking about her and the baby. You can also ask friends and family members to check on her and to be available to help out.

Some General Cautions. We know women who get pregnant while they're on active duty face many challenges. The pressure to meet military body-weight standards can have an effect on your health; that's the reason these requirements are relaxed during pregnancy.

Work hard to eat healthy foods so you have adequate levels of iron and folic acid. Examine your job for any hazards you may be exposed to, such as standing for long periods, heavy lifting and exposure to toxic chemicals. Before receiving any vaccinations or inoculations, discuss them with your healthcare provider. Any of these factors can impact your pregnancy.

If you are concerned about any of the above, discuss it with a superior. Changes beyond those described above may have to be made.

Taking Others to Prenatal Visits

Take your partner with you to as many prenatal appointments as possible. It's nice for your partner and healthcare provider to meet before labor begins. Maybe your mother or the other grandmother-to-be would like to go with you to hear the baby's heartbeat. Or you may want to

Bed Bugs

There's a lot of information in the news about bed bugs. Many pregnant women want to know if bed-bug bites or the chemicals used to kill them are dangerous for a woman and her baby, before and after it is born.

Bed bugs are round, wingless insects that hide in the cracks of beds, mattresses, baseboards and couches. It doesn't hurt when they bite you, but you awake the next morning with bites similar to those of a mosquito or other insect. A bed-bug bite can't be identified just by looking at it. If you're bitten, look in folds, creases and under mattresses for the insects–they're pretty tiny, so it may be hard to spot them.

Bed-bug bites can be more of a nuisance than a health hazard. Bites can cause itching and even secondary infections from scratching. Bed bugs aren't known to transmit infectious diseases to humans, so you don't have to worry about who was bitten before you if you get a bite.

If you get bed-bug bites, don't panic—they won't hurt your baby. But try not to scratch. Anti-itch creams and antibiotic creams to use on your skin should be OK. Call your healthcare provider and ask what he or she recommends.

Don't go overboard with insecticides trying to get rid of them—exposure to the chemicals could be worse than the bugs themselves. If you find bed bugs and are sure you have a problem, get help from an expert. Treatments to get rid of them include insecticides and heat treatments. Whatever you do, be careful and know what you're being exposed to.

record the heartbeat for others to hear. Things have changed since your mother carried you; many grandmothers-to-be enjoy this type of visit.

It's a good idea to wait until you have heard baby's heartbeat before bringing other people. You don't always hear it the first time, and this can be frustrating and disappointing.

Some women bring their children with them to a prenatal appointment. Most office personnel don't mind if you bring your children occasionally. They understand it isn't always possible to find someone to watch them. However, if you have problems or have a lot to discuss with your healthcare provider, don't bring your child or children.

If a child is sick, has just gotten over chicken pox or is getting a cold, leave him or her at home. Don't expose everyone else in the waiting room.

Some women like to bring one child at a time to a visit if they have more than one. That makes it special for mom and for the child. Crying or complaining children can create a difficult situation, however, so ask your healthcare provider when it's good to bring family members with you before you come in with them.

Exercise for Week 14

The Kegel exercise strengthens pelvic muscles; practicing it helps relax your muscles for delivery. This exercise can also be helpful in getting vaginal muscles back in shape after delivery of your baby. You can do it anywhere, anytime, without anyone knowing that you're doing it!

While sitting, contract the lowest muscles of your pelvis as tightly as you can. Tighten the muscles higher in the pelvis in stages until you reach the muscles at the top. Count to 10 slowly as you move up the pelvis. Hold briefly, then release slowly in stages, counting to 10 again. Repeat 2 or 3 times a day.

You can also do a Kegel exercise by tightening the pelvic muscles first, then tightening the anal muscle. Hold for a few seconds, then release slowly, in reverse order. To see if you're doing the exercise correctly, stop the flow of urine while you're going to the bathroom.

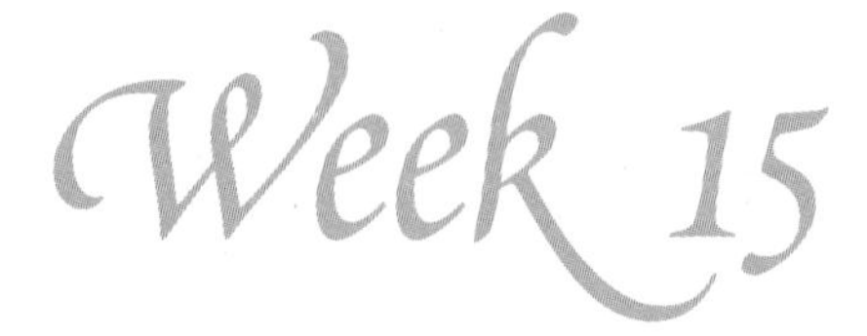

Week 15

Age of Fetus—13 Weeks

How Big Is Your Baby?

The fetal crown-to-rump length by this week of pregnancy is 4 to 4½ inches (9.3 to 10.3cm). The fetus weighs about 1¾ ounces (50g). It's close to the size of a softball.

How Big Are You?

Changes in your lower abdomen change the way your clothes fit. Your pregnancy may not be obvious to other people when you wear regular clothes. But it may become obvious if you start wearing maternity clothes or put on a swimming suit. You may be able to feel your uterus about 3 or 4 inches (7.6 to 10cm) below your belly button.

How Your Baby Is Growing and Developing

It's still a little early to feel movement, although you should feel your baby move in the next few weeks! Your baby's skin is thin, and you can see blood vessels through the skin.

Your baby may be sucking its thumb. This has been seen with ultrasound examination.

As you can see in the illustration on page 212, ears now look more normal. In fact, your baby looks more human every day. Bones that have already formed are getting harder. If an X-ray were done at this time, the baby's skeleton would be visible.

Alpha-Fetoprotein (AFP) Testing

As baby grows, it produces *alpha-fetoprotein* (AFP) in its liver and passes some of it into your bloodstream. It's possible to measure AFP by drawing your blood; too much or not enough of the protein in your blood can be a sign of problems.

An AFP test is usually done between 16 and 18 weeks of gestation. Timing is important and must be tied to the gestational age of your pregnancy and to your weight. An important use of the test is to help a woman decide whether to have amniocentesis.

An elevated AFP level can indicate problems in the baby. A connection has been found between a low level of AFP and Down syndrome. If your AFP level is abnormal, your healthcare provider may choose to do other tests to look for problems.

The AFP test is not done on all pregnant women, although it is required in some states. It is not used routinely in Canada. AFP is often used with other tests. If the test isn't offered to you, ask about it. There's little risk, and it helps your healthcare provider determine how baby is growing and developing.

> *Tip for Week 15*
>
> **Start now to learn to sleep on your side; it will pay off later as you get bigger. Sometimes it helps to use a few extra pillows. Put one behind you so if you roll onto your back, you won't lie flat. Put another pillow between your legs, or rest your top leg on a pillow. Consider using a "pregnancy pillow" that supports your entire body.**

Changes in You

During your first prenatal visit, you probably had a Pap smear; one is usually done at the beginning of pregnancy. By now, the result is back, and you've discussed it with your healthcare provider, particularly if it was abnormal.

A Pap smear identifies cancerous or precancerous cells coming from the cervix. This test has helped decrease the number of deaths from cervical cancer because of early detection and treatment.

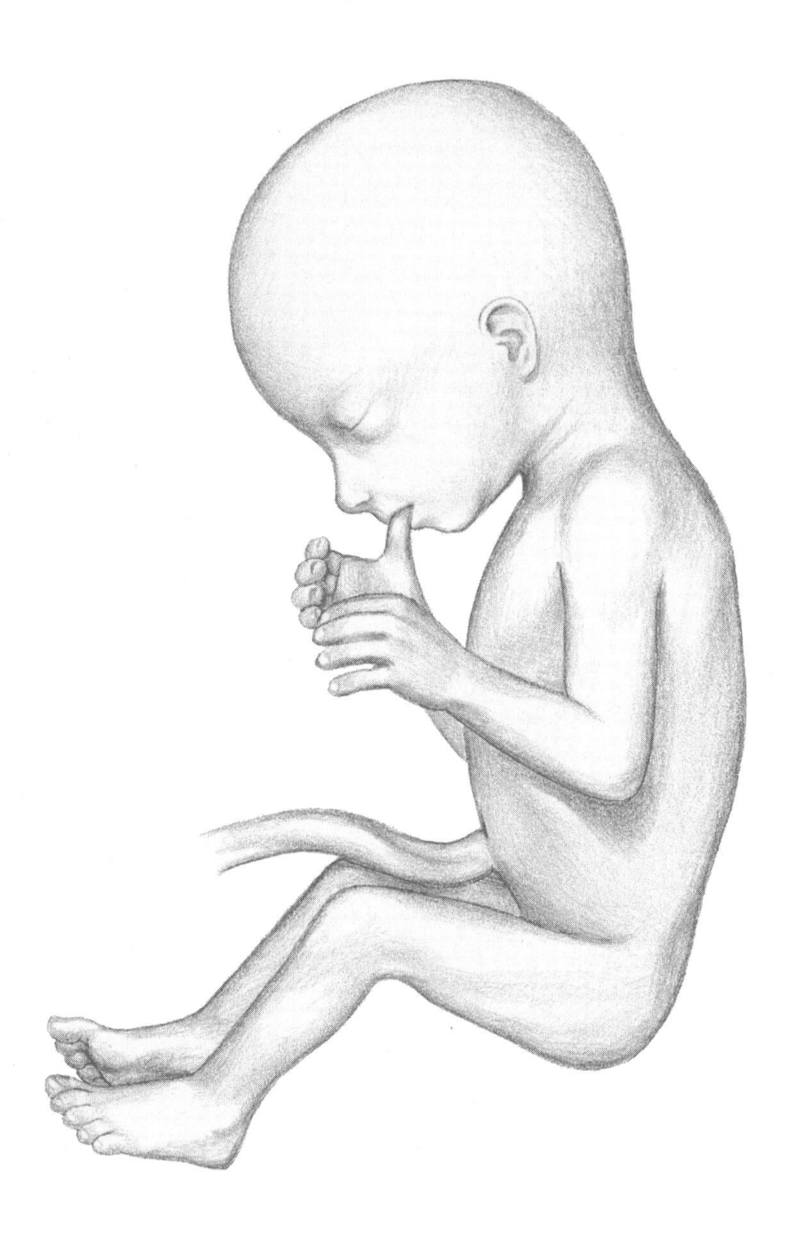

By week 15 of pregnancy (fetal age—13 weeks), your baby may suck its thumb. Eyes are at the front of the face but are still widely separated.

An abnormal Pap smear during pregnancy must be handled individually. When abnormal cells are "not too bad" (premalignant or not as serious), it may be possible to watch them during pregnancy.

If your healthcare provider is concerned, he or she may do a *colposcopy,* a procedure to examine the cervix. Abnormal areas can be seen so biopsies can be taken after pregnancy. Most obstetricians/gynecologists can do this procedure in the office.

There are several ways to treat abnormal cells on the cervix, but most treatment methods aren't done during pregnancy. After pregnancy, the problem will be revisited.

Women who deliver vaginally may see a change in abnormal Pap smears. One study showed over half of the women who had problems before giving birth had normal Pap smears after their baby was born.

How Your Actions Affect Your Baby's Development

Ultrasound during the Second Trimester

Ultrasound can be used during the second trimester for several reasons. These include diagnosis of multiple fetuses, with amniocentesis, with bleeding related to placenta previa or placental abruption, intrauterine-growth restriction (IUGR) and evaluation of baby's well-being. Ultrasound at around 20 weeks may be done to determine if the placenta has attached normally and is healthy.

Change Sleeping Positions Now

Some women have questions about their sleeping positions and sleep habits while they're pregnant. Some want to know if they can sleep on their stomachs. Lying on your stomach puts extra pressure on your growing uterus. Others want to know if they should stop sleeping on their waterbed. (It's OK to continue to sleep on a waterbed.)

As you get bigger, finding comfortable sleeping positions will get harder. Don't lie on your back when you sleep. As your uterus gets larger, lying on your back can place the uterus on top of the aorta and the inferior vena cava that run down the back of your abdomen. This can decrease circulation to your baby and parts of your body. Some pregnant women also find it harder to breathe when lying on their backs.

It's important to learn to sleep on your side. For some women, their favorite thing after delivery is to be able to sleep on their stomach again!

Communicating with Your Healthcare Provider

Communication between you and your healthcare provider is critical for a successful relationship; poor communication may affect your ability to get the best medical care possible. Being able to communicate effectively will help you deal more easily with personal issues relating to pregnancy, sexuality and intimacy. It's worth the effort to find a provider with whom you can establish this type of relationship.

For a successful healthcare provider–patient relationship, you both must be willing to try to understand and to respect each other. Sometimes communication is hard because everyone is so busy.

To get the best care possible, find someone you're comfortable with and with whom you can communicate easily and effectively. Miscommunication between healthcare provider and patient is often the source of many conflicts.

If language is a barrier, try to find a healthcare provider who speaks your language fluently. If this isn't possible, find out if anyone on the staff speaks your language or if there are other resources available to you. If language is still a barrier, find someone (a friend or even a professional interpreter) to attend every office visit with you so you can ask questions and receive accurate information. You'll be better able to understand advice and instructions, treatment plans or directions.

To receive the best care possible, *you* have to be the best patient you can be. Follow your healthcare provider's instructions; if you have questions or disagree with something, don't ignore the advice. Instead, discuss it. Speak up when you're confused or dissatisfied. When a test or procedure is ordered, ask why it is being done. And be sure you get test results later.

Don't withhold information, even if you feel it's embarrassing. Tell your healthcare provider everything he or she needs to know about you.

In this way, your healthcare team will have all the information they need to provide you and your baby the best care possible.

Go to visits prepared with your questions and concerns written down. Then write down answers you receive or have someone come with you to help you remember important instructions or suggestions. Be an active participant in your health care for your good health and the good health of your baby.

Dad Tip

Having a baby can mean a lot of financial changes in your life. You need to examine your wills and update them, if necessary. You also need to name a guardian for your child, in case something happens to both of you. Other important tasks include checking your life insurance and medical-health insurance to be sure coverage is enough for your family. You also need to consider child-care costs, if one of you is not going to be a stay-at-home parent.

Changing Healthcare Providers. If all these suggestions don't work, it's OK to change healthcare providers—it happens all the time. If you think you need to find someone new, start as soon as possible. You might consider calling the labor-and-delivery department of the hospital where you plan to deliver. Ask nurses whom they would recommend.

When you select a new healthcare provider, be sure he or she is accepting new patients. Also check whether your insurance plan covers this healthcare provider. Tell your current healthcare provider you're leaving, and explain why. Writing a letter may be a good way to do this.

Ask for your records. It's better to take them with you instead of having them sent, which can take some time. Be sure also to request copies of all tests and test results.

Take your records to your first office visit. Bring a list of all prescription and over-the-counter medications, including any herbs, supplements or other substances, you take. Be prepared to cover your health and pregnancy history in detail to provide your new healthcare provider a complete picture of your health care to date.

Your Nutrition

About this time, you'll probably need to start adding an extra 300 calories to your meal plan to meet the needs of your growing baby and your changing body. Below are some choices of extra food for one day to get those 300 calories. Be careful—300 calories is *not* a lot of food.

- Choice 1—2 thin slices pork, ½ cup cabbage, 1 carrot
- Choice 2—½ cup cooked brown rice, ¾ cup strawberries, 1 cup orange juice, 1 slice fresh pineapple
- Choice 3—4½ ounces salmon steak, 1 cup asparagus, 2 cups Romaine lettuce
- Choice 4—1 cup cooked pasta, 1 slice fresh tomato, 1 cup 1% milk, ½ cup cooked green beans, ¼ cantaloupe
- Choice 5—1 container of yogurt, 1 medium apple

You Should Also Know

Getting a Good Night's Sleep

Sleeping soundly may be difficult for you now or later in pregnancy. The discomforts of pregnancy may impact on your sleep.

Research shows if a woman experiences sleep disruption during pregnancy, she may be at higher risk of some pregnancy problems. Less sleep may also increase your risk of postpartum depression. And if you're exhausted when you begin labor, you may be at a higher risk for a Cesarean delivery.

Lack of sleep can impact you in other ways. Studies show if you get less than 6 hours of sleep a night during the last few weeks of pregnancy, your labor may be longer. If you get less than 7 hours of sleep a night, you're at higher risk of getting a cold when exposed to the virus.

Sleep disturbances are common in pregnancy—between 65 and 95% of all pregnant women experience some sleep changes. Try some of the following suggestions to help you get a good night's sleep.

- Develop a nighttime ritual. Go to bed and wake up at the same time each day.
- Don't drink too much after 4pm so you don't have to get up to go to the bathroom all night long.
- Avoid caffeine after late afternoon.
- Slowly drink a glass of milk before bed.
- Get regular exercise.
- Keep your bedroom dark and cool.
- The scent of jasmine may help you fall asleep faster, sleep better and wake up feeling more refreshed.
- Record favorite late-night TV shows, and watch them the next day.
- Even if you feel exhausted, don't nap close to your bedtime.
- If you get heartburn at night, sleep propped up or sitting in a comfortable chair.

Studies show listening to soothing sounds before bedtime can train your brain to fall asleep faster and sleep as long as if you took a sleep medication. It takes about 10 days of consistent listening to train your brain to this calming effect.

Stretching for 15 to 30 minutes during the day may also help you sleep better. Stretching eases muscle tension so you're more relaxed when you go to bed. Try sitting on the edge of a chair and leaning forward far enough to touch your knees with your chest. Let your arms hang by your sides, and gently stretch your fingertips to the floor.

Research shows if you eat a lot of high-fat food during the day, you may pay for it at night by tossing and turning more. Pastas and other complex carbohydrates may help relax you.

If you still have trouble sleeping after trying the above suggestions, talk to your healthcare provider. He or she may prescribe a medication for you. You may also want to ask your healthcare provider to check your iron levels, which can impact on sleep.

You may experience shortness of breath due to your bigger tummy, which can interfere with sleep. Lie on your left side. Prop up your head and shoulders with extra pillows. If this doesn't help, a warm shower or a soak in a warm (not hot) tub might help. If you just can't get comfortable in bed, try sleeping partially sitting up in a recliner.

Domestic Violence

Domestic violence is an epidemic problem in the United States; every year almost 5 million women experience a serious assault by someone who says they love them. The term *domestic violence* refers to violence against adolescent and adult females within a family or intimate relationship. It can take the form of physical, sexual, emotional, economic or psychological abuse. Actions or threats of action are intended to frighten, intimidate, humiliate, wound or injure a person. Abuse affects all income levels and all ethnic groups.

Unfortunately, abuse does not usually stop during pregnancy. Research shows most women who experience violence during pregnancy may have experienced it before.

Research shows one in six women is abused during pregnancy; abuse occurs in 4 to 8% of all pregnancies. Domestic violence kills more pregnant women than any single medical complication of pregnancy. In fact, it accounts for 20% of all pregnancy-related deaths. Some studies indicate abuse may *begin* during pregnancy; still other studies show abuse escalates during pregnancy. A startling fact to be aware of—up to 60% of men who abuse their partners also abuse their children.

Abuse can be an obstacle to prenatal care. Some abused pregnant women do not seek prenatal care until later in pregnancy. They may miss more prenatal appointments. Women at risk may not gain enough weight, or they may suffer from more injuries during pregnancy. Other risks include trauma to the mother, miscarriage, preterm delivery, vaginal bleeding, low-birthweight infants, fetal injury and a greater number of Cesarean deliveries.

If you're unsure if you are in an abusive relationship, ask yourself the following questions.

- Does my partner threaten me or throw things when he's angry?
- Does he make jokes at my expense and put me down?
- Has he physically hurt me in the past year?

- Has he forced me to perform a sexual act?
- Does he say it's my fault when he hits me?
- Does he promise me it won't happen again, but it does?
- Does he keep me away from family and friends?

If you answered "yes" to any of these questions, your relationship may be unhealthy, and it may be abusive.

Many victims of abuse blame themselves; *you are not to blame.* It isn't your fault, no matter what a boyfriend or spouse may say. If you're being abused, we encourage you to seek help immediately. Intervention can be lifesaving for you and your unborn child.

Talk to someone—a friend, relative, someone at your church or your healthcare provider are good resources. There are many domestic violence programs, crisis hotlines, shelters and legal-aid services available to help you. Call the 24-hour National Domestic Violence Hotline at 800-799-7233 for help and advice.

Plan for your safety. This may include a "fast exit." A recommended safety plan includes the following.

- Pack a suitcase.
- Arrange for a safe place to stay, regardless of the time of day or night.
- Hide some cash.
- Know where to go for help if you are hurt.
- Keep needed items in a safe place, such as prescription medicines, health insurance cards, credit cards, checkbook, driver's license and medical records.
- Be prepared to call the police.

If you're hurt before you can leave permanently, go to the nearest emergency room. Tell personnel at the emergency room how you were hurt. Ask for a copy of your medical records, and give them to your own healthcare provider.

These steps may seem drastic, but remember—domestic violence is a serious problem with serious consequences. Protect yourself and your unborn baby!

Old Wives' Tales

Now that you're pregnant, you may receive all sorts of information—whether or not you welcome it. Some may be useful, some may be frightening and some may be laughable. Should you believe everything you hear? Probably not.

Below is a list of old wives' tales that you can definitely ignore. When you hear one of them, smile and nod. You'll know the truth and *not* worry this will happen to you!

- You need calcium if you crave ice cream.
- Cold feet indicate a boy.
- Refusing to eat the heel on a loaf of bread means you're going to have a girl.
- Dangling a wedding ring over your tummy indicates the sex of your baby.
- Your baby will be born with a hairy birthmark if you see a mouse.
- If you carry out in front, it's a boy—carrying around your middle means it's a girl.
- Eating berries causes red splotches on your baby's skin.
- If you perspire a lot, it's a girl.
- Taking a bath can hurt, or even drown, a fetus. (But do be careful of soaking for a long time in hot water, like in a spa—that could harm the fetus.)
- It's a girl if you crave orange juice.
- Stretching your arms over your head can cause the umbilical cord to wrap around baby's neck.
- If you carry high, it's a boy—carrying low means it's a girl.
- Dry hands means you're going to have a boy.
- Craving greasy foods means your labor will be short.
- Craving spinach signifies you need iron.
- Your baby will be cross-eyed if you wear high heels.
- Your moods during pregnancy affect your baby's personality.
- Using various techniques or substances will start labor. Do not try to induce labor by walking, exercising, drinking castor oil, going on a bumpy ride (not a good idea during pregnancy anyway) or using laxatives.

There are some old wives' tales that are true. If you've heard that if you suffer from heartburn, baby will have a full head of hair, this is true! Studies show over 80% of women who experienced moderate to severe heartburn during pregnancy had babies with lots of hair! Hormones that cause heartburn also control hair growth. Who knew?

Another tale to believe is that if you have sex during late pregnancy, it may cause labor to start. If you have sex after 36 weeks of pregnancy, you're more likely to deliver sooner than women who don't have sex. Semen contains prostaglandin, and when combined with your hormones, it may cause contractions to begin.

Tay-Sachs Disease

Tay-Sachs disease is an inherited disease of the central nervous system. The most common form of the disease affects babies, who appear healthy at birth and seem to develop normally for the first few months of life. Then development slows, and symptoms begin to appear. Unfortunately, there is no treatment and no cure for Tay-Sachs disease at this time, and death usually occurs before age 5.

The disease occurs most frequently in descendants of Ashkenazi Jews from Central and Eastern Europe. About one out of every 30 American Jews carries the Tay-Sachs gene. Some non-Jewish people of French-Canadian ancestry (from the East St. Lawrence River Valley of Quebec) and members of the Cajun population in Louisiana are also at increased risk. These groups have about 100 times the rate of occurrence of other ethnic groups. The juvenile form of Tay-Sachs, however, may not be increased in these groups. See the discussion below.

Babies born with Tay-Sachs disease lack a protein called *hexosaminidase A* or *hex-A*. This protein is necessary to break down certain fatty substances in brain and nerve cells. When hex-A isn't available, substances build up and gradually destroy brain and nerve cells, until the central nervous system stops working.

Tay-Sachs disease can be diagnosed before birth. Amniocentesis and chorionic villus sampling (CVS) can diagnose it during a pregnancy. If prenatal testing shows hex-A is present, the baby will *not* have Tay-Sachs.

The disease is hereditary; a Tay-Sachs carrier has one normal gene for hex-A and one Tay-Sachs gene. A person can be tested to measure the amount of the hex-A enzyme in the blood. Tay-Sachs carriers have about half as much of the enzyme as noncarriers, which is enough for their own needs. A carrier does not have the illness and leads a normal, healthy life.

When two carriers become parents, there is a one-in-four chance that any child they have will inherit a Tay-Sachs gene from each parent and have the disease. There is a two-in-four chance the child will inherit one of each kind of gene and be a carrier like the parents. There is a one-in-four chance the child will inherit the normal gene from each parent and be completely free of the disease. If only one parent is a carrier, none of the children can have the disease, but each child has a 50–50 chance of inheriting the Tay-Sachs gene and being a carrier.

There are various types of Tay-Sachs disease. The classic type, which affects babies, is the most common. Other rare deficiencies of the hex-A enzyme are sometimes included under the umbrella of Tay-Sachs disease. These often are referred to as *juvenile*, *chronic* and *adult-onset* forms of hex-A deficiency.

Affected individuals have low levels of the hex-A enzyme (it is completely missing in the type that babies have). Symptoms begin later in life and are generally milder. Children with juvenile hex-A deficiency develop symptoms between the ages of 2 and 5 similar to those of the classical, infantile form. The course of the disease is slower; however, death usually occurs by age 15.

Were You Hard to Live with When You Had Morning Sickness?

If you suffered with morning sickness and you're starting to feel better, you may want to take stock of your relationship with your partner. Were you hard to get along with when you weren't feeling good? Your partner needs your support as pregnancy progresses, just as you need his support. You may need to make an effort to work very hard at treating each other well—you're both in this together!

Symptoms of chronic hex-A deficiency may also begin by age 5, but they are more often milder than those with infantile and juvenile forms. Vision and hearing remain intact, but slurred speech, muscle weakness, muscle cramps, tremors, unsteady gait and, sometimes, mental illness may appear. Individuals with adult-onset hex-A deficiency experience many of the same symptoms as individuals with the chronic form, but symptoms begin later in life.

Exercise for Week 15

Place a chair in the corner so it won't slide when you push against it. Place your right foot on the chair seat; support yourself against the wall with your hand, if necessary. Stretch your left leg behind you, lift your chest and arch your back. Turn your shoulders and lean your torso to the right. Hold 25 to 30 seconds. Do 3 stretches for each side. Do this stretch before beginning tummy exercises. *Tones back muscles.*

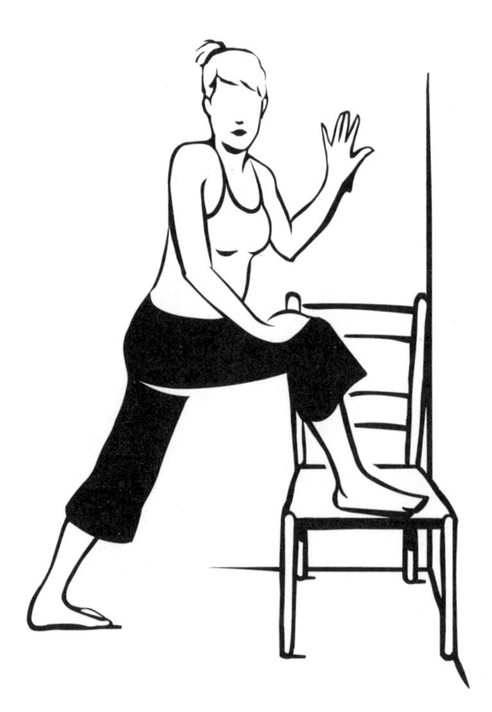

Week 16

Age of Fetus—14 Weeks

How Big Is Your Baby?

The crown-to-rump length of your baby by this week is 4⅓ to 4⅔ inches (10.8 to 11.6cm). Weight is about 2¾ ounces (80g).

How Big Are You?

Six weeks ago, your uterus weighed about 5 ounces (140g). Today, it weighs about 8¾ ounces (250g). The amount of amniotic fluid around the baby is increasing. There is now about 7½ ounces (250ml) of fluid. You can easily feel your uterus about 3 inches (7.6cm) below your bellybutton.

How Your Baby Is Growing and Developing

Fine hair covers your baby's head. The illustration on page 226 shows soft hair, called *lanugo*. The umbilical cord is attached to the abdomen; this attachment has moved lower on the body of the fetus. Fingernails are well formed.

At this stage, arms and legs are moving. You can see movement during an ultrasound examination. You may also be able to feel baby move; many women describe feelings of movement as a "gas bubble" or "fluttering." Often, it's something you may have noticed for a few days, but you didn't realize what you were feeling. Then you realize you're feeling baby moving inside you!

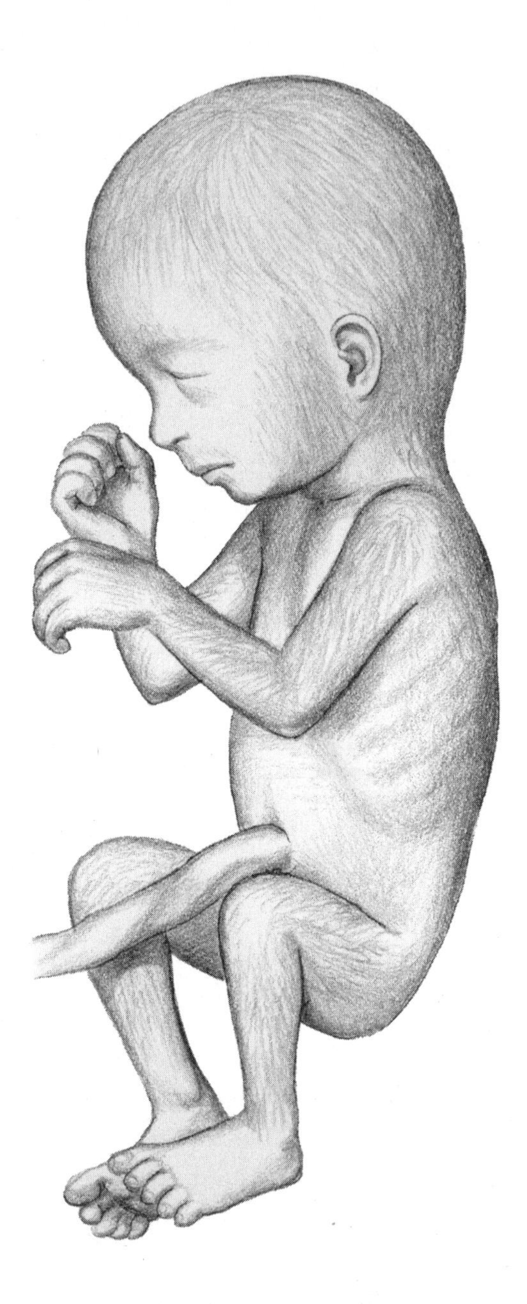

By this week, soft lanugo hair covers
the baby's body and head.

Changes in You

If you haven't felt your baby move yet, don't worry. Fetal movement, also called *quickening*, is usually felt between 16 and 20 weeks of pregnancy. The time is different for every woman and can be different from one pregnancy to another. One baby may be more active than another. The size of the baby or the number of fetuses can also affect what you feel.

Multiple-Marker Tests

Multiple-marker tests, such as the triple-screen and quad-screen tests, are usually done 15 to 18 weeks after your last menstrual period. These tests measure levels of certain substances in your blood and are based on your age, weight, race and whether you smoke or have diabetes requiring insulin. The triple-screen test is discussed below. The quad-screen test is discussed in Week 17.

> **Dad Tip**
>
> Do you have concerns you haven't shared with anyone? Are you concerned about your partner's health or the baby's? Do you wonder about your role in labor and delivery? Are you worried about being a good father? Share your thoughts with your partner. You won't burden her. In fact, she'll probably be relieved to know she's not alone in feeling a little overwhelmed by this monumental life change.

Triple-Screen Test. The *triple-screen test* can go beyond alpha-fetoprotein testing in helping your healthcare provider determine if you might be carrying a child with Down syndrome. The triple-screen checks your alpha-fetoprotein level, along with the amounts of human chorionic gonadotropin (HCG) and unconjugated estriol (a form of estrogen produced by the placenta). Abnormal levels can indicate baby has a problem.

This test has a higher level of false-positives, which means the test says there's a problem when there really isn't. One reason for this is a wrong due date. If you believe you're 16 weeks pregnant, but are actually 18 weeks pregnant, hormone levels will be off, which could make test results incorrect. If you're carrying more than one baby it can also cause inaccurate tests results. If you have an abnormal result, ultrasound and amniocentesis may be recommended.

This blood test is used to find *possible* problems. It is a *screening* test. A *diagnostic* test will usually be done to confirm any diagnosis.

How Your Actions Affect Your Baby's Development

Amniocentesis

If necessary, amniocentesis is often performed around 16 to 18 weeks of pregnancy. By this point, your uterus is large enough and there is enough fluid surrounding the baby to make the test possible.

Fetal cells that float in amniotic fluid can be grown in cultures and can be used to identify some birth defects. We know of more than 400 abnormalities a child can be born with—amniocentesis identifies about 40 (10%) of them, including the following:

- chromosomal problems, particularly Down syndrome
- fetal sex, if sex-specific problems, such as hemophilia or Duchenne muscular dystrophy, must be identified
- skeletal diseases
- fetal infections
- central-nervous-system diseases
- blood diseases
- chemical problems or enzyme deficiencies

Ultrasound is used to locate a pocket of fluid where the baby and placenta are out of the way. The abdomen above the uterus is cleaned. Skin is numbed, and a needle is passed through the abdominal wall into the uterus. About 1 ounce of fluid is withdrawn from the amniotic cavity (area around the baby) with a syringe; if you are carrying twins, fluid may be taken from each sac.

Risks from amniocentesis include injury to the baby, placenta or umbilical cord, infection, miscarriage or premature labor. The use of ultrasound to guide the needle helps avoid problems but doesn't eliminate all risk.

Bleeding from the baby to the mother can occur, which can be a problem because fetal and maternal blood are separate and may be different types. This is a particular risk to an Rh-negative mother carrying an Rh-positive baby (see the discussion that begins on page 234) and may cause isoimmunization. An Rh-negative woman should receive RhoGAM at the time of amniocentesis to prevent isoimmunization.

Over 95% of women who have amniocentesis learn their baby does *not* have the disorder the test was done for. Fetal loss from amniocentesis is estimated to be less than 3%. The procedure should be done only by someone who has experience doing it.

Are You an Older Mother-to-Be?

More women are getting pregnant in their 30s or 40s. If you waited to start a family, you're not alone. Close to 15% of the mothers of newborns are now 35 or older.

When you're older, your partner may also be older. You may have waited to get married, or you may be in a second marriage and starting a new family. Some couples have experienced infertility and do not achieve a pregnancy until they have gone through testing or surgery. Or you may be a single mother who has chosen donor insemination to achieve pregnancy.

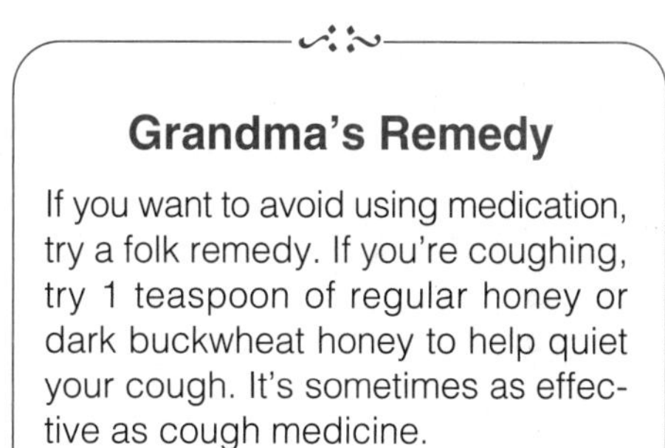

Grandma's Remedy

If you want to avoid using medication, try a folk remedy. If you're coughing, try 1 teaspoon of regular honey or dark buckwheat honey to help quiet your cough. It's sometimes as effective as cough medicine.

Today, many healthcare professionals gauge pregnancy risk by the pregnant woman's health status, not her age. Pre-existing medical conditions have the greatest impact on a woman's well-being during pregnancy. For example, a healthy 39-year-old is less likely to develop problems than a diabetic woman in her 20s. A woman's fitness can also have a greater effect on her pregnancy than her age.

Most older women who become pregnant are in good health. A woman in good physical condition who has exercised regularly may go through pregnancy as easily as a woman 15 to 20 years younger. An exception—women in a first pregnancy who are over 40 may have more problems than women the same age who have previously had children. But most healthy women will have a safe delivery.

Some health problems can be age related, and the risk of developing a condition increases with age. You may not know you have a problem unless you see your healthcare provider regularly.

Genetic Counseling May Be a Wise Choice. If either you or your partner is over 35, genetic counseling may be recommended; this can raise many questions for you. The risk of chromosome problems exceeds 5% for the over-35 age group.

Genetic counseling brings together a couple and professionals who are trained to deal with the questions about the occurrence, or risk of occurrence, of a genetic problem. With genetic counseling, information about human genetics is applied to a particular couple's situation. Information is interpreted so the couple can make informed decisions.

When a mother is older, the father is often older; the father's age can affect a pregnancy. It can be difficult to determine whether the mother's age or the father's age matters more. More research is needed before we definitely know the effects of a father's age on pregnancy.

Will Your Pregnancy Be Different If You're Older? If you're older, your healthcare provider may see you more often or you may have more tests. You may be advised to have amniocentesis or CVS to find out whether your child has Down syndrome. Even if you would never terminate a pregnancy, this information helps you and your healthcare team prepare for the birth of your baby.

If you're over 35, you have a greater chance of having problems. You may be watched more closely during pregnancy for signs of those problems. Some can be troublesome, but with good medical care, they can usually be handled fairly well.

Pregnancy when you're older can take its toll. You may gain more weight, see stretch marks where there were none before, notice your breasts sag lower and feel a lack of tone in your muscles. Attention to nutrition, exercise and rest can help a great deal.

Because of demands on your time and energy, fatigue may be one of your greatest problems. It's a common complaint. Rest is essential to your health and to your baby's. Rest and nap when possible. Don't take on more tasks or new roles. Don't volunteer for any big projects. Learn to say "No." You'll feel better!

Moderate exercise can help boost energy levels and may ease some discomforts. However, check first with your healthcare provider before starting any exercise program.

Stress can also be a problem. Exercise, eating healthfully and getting as much rest as possible may help relieve stress. Take time for yourself.

Some women find a pregnancy support group is an excellent way to deal with difficulties they may experience. Ask your healthcare provider for further information.

Through research, we know labor and delivery for an older woman may be different. Labor may last longer. Older women also have a higher rate of Cesarean deliveries. After baby's birth, your uterus may not contract as quickly; postpartum bleeding may last longer and be heavier.

For an in-depth look at pregnancy for women over age 35, we suggest your read our book *Your Pregnancy after 35.*

Your Nutrition

Good news—pregnant women should snack often, particularly during the second half of pregnancy! You should have three or four snacks a day, in addition to your regular meals. There are a couple of catches, though. First, snacks must be nutritious. Second, meals may need to be smaller so you can eat those snacks. One nutritional goal in pregnancy is to eat enough food so nutrients are always available for your body's use and for use by the growing fetus.

Usually you want a snack to be quick and easy. It may take some planning and effort on your part to make sure nutritious foods are available for snacking. Prepare things in advance. Cut up fresh vegetables for later use in salads and for munching with low-cal dip. Keep some hard-boiled eggs on hand. Lowfat cheese and cottage cheese provide calcium. Peanut butter (reduced-fat or regular), pretzels and plain popcorn are good choices. Replace soda with fruit juice. If juice has more sugar than you need, cut it with water.

You Should Also Know

No More Lying on Your Back

Week 16 is the turning point—no more lying flat on your back while resting or sleeping, or lying flat on the floor while exercising or relaxing. Reclining in a chair or propped against pillows is OK. Just don't lie flat on your back!

Lying on your back puts extra pressure on the aorta and vena cava, which can reduce blood flow to your baby. Baby won't get all the nutrients it needs to develop and to grow. Don't endanger baby's well-being by forgetting this important action.

Have a Green Pregnancy

Today, many people are looking for ways to become "greener." They want to do what they can to help protect the environment for themselves, their children and the rest of the world. One way to begin is to have a *green pregnancy.*

Having a green pregnancy can range from being selective about the products you use to how you treat your body. We've gathered together some ideas about ways to have a green pregnancy and list them below.

- Check cosmetics and other personal products you use to see if any contain harmful chemicals. Choose ones that are good for the environment.
- Eat organic foods some of the time to cut down on your exposure to pesticides and other harmful substances.
- Ask friends to give you a green shower. Register for eco-friendly products.
- Buy secondhand baby clothes.
- Make recycling a part of your life every day.
- Donate or sell items you don't need anymore to make room for baby and all the stuff you'll need for him or her.
- Try to avoid outdoor pollutants, such as car exhaust and smog.
- Walk when you can instead of driving.
- Grow your own vegetables when possible. A garden can be a wonderful addition to your lifestyle.

- Use energy-efficient light bulbs in your lamps and fixtures.
- Use green cleaning products, laundry detergents and other household products. Check to be sure they're safe to use during pregnancy–not all green products are.
- Buy a water bottle for your personal use, and use it every day.

Take 1200mg of calcium every day while you breastfeed to help reduce the amount of lead in your milk. If you don't have enough calcium in your bones, your body will pull lead out of them.

If you have an older home, run cold water for 30 seconds to 2 minutes before you drink it or use it for cooking. Running cold water helps flush out any lead in the pipes—hot water tends to leach lead from pipes. A good water filter can also help.

When fixing up baby's room, choose no- or low-VOC paint, which has fewer pollutants. (*VOC* means volatile organic compounds.) If you're going to install carpet, select natural fibers when possible, such as wool, jute or sisal. Or look for carpets with the *Green Label Plus* logo—they contain lower amounts of VOC chemicals. You might also ask the salesperson to air out carpet for 24 hours before installation to help reduce harmful chemicals. After carpet is installed, close the door to the room, and open windows and leave them open for 72 hours.

You might also want to keep baby's bed and bedding natural. Many products are available that are free of dioxins, synthetic petrochemicals and formaldehyde, including crib mattresses and crib bedding.

Watch your energy consumption, and try to live light. The lower your CO_2 footprint, the better it is for the environment. For example, drinking tap water releases almost no CO_2 into the atmosphere. However, if you drink bottled water, *every* bottle of water accounts for the release of 1 pound of CO_2! If you take a hot shower for 5 minutes, 3.5 pounds of CO_2 are released into the atmosphere. If

Tip for Week 16

Some of the foods you normally love may make you sick to your stomach during pregnancy. You may need to substitute other nutritious foods you tolerate better.

your shower lasts 10 minutes, 7 pounds of CO_2 are released. If you take the bus, 0.2 pounds of CO_2 are released per mile, compared with 0.9 pounds if you drive a car that gets 23 miles per gallon.

Remember—if it's not good for you, it's not good for baby!

Rh Disease and Sensitivity

It's important during pregnancy to know your blood type (O, A, B, AB) and your Rh-factor. The Rh-factor is a protein in your blood, determined by a genetic trait.

Everyone has either Rh-positive blood or Rh-negative blood. If you have the Rh factor in your blood, you are Rh-positive—most people are Rh-positive. If you do not have the Rh-factor, you are Rh-negative. Rh-negativity affects about 15% of the white population and 8% of the Black/African-American population in the United States.

An Rh-negative woman who carries an Rh-positive child could face problems, which could result in a very sick baby. If you are Rh-positive, you don't have to worry about any of this. If you are Rh-negative, you *do* need to know about it.

Rh Disease. *Rh disease* is a condition caused by incompatibility between a mother's blood and her baby's blood. If you are Rh-negative, you can become sensitized if your growing baby is Rh-positive. Your baby may be Rh-positive *only* if your partner is Rh-positive. If you are Rh-positive and your partner is Rh-negative, you won't have a problem.

Over 4000 babies develop Rh disease before birth every year. If you're Rh-negative and your baby isn't or if you have had a blood transfusion or received blood products of some kind, you might have a problem. There's a risk you could become Rh-sensitized or isoimmunized. *Isoimmunized* means you make antibodies that circulate inside your system. The antibodies don't harm you but they can attack the Rh-positive blood of your growing baby. (If your baby is Rh-negative, there is no problem.)

Cause of Problems. You and your fetus do not share blood systems during pregnancy. However, in some situations, blood passes from the baby to the mother. Occasionally when this happens, the mother's body reacts as if she were allergic to the fetus's blood. She becomes sensitized and makes antibodies. These antibodies can cross the placenta and attack the fetus's blood. Antibodies can break down the baby's red blood cells, which results in anemia in the baby and can be very serious.

With a first baby, if fetal blood enters the mother's bloodstream, the baby may be born before the woman's body can become sensitized. She probably won't produce enough antibodies to harm the baby. However, antibodies stay in the woman's circulation forever. In the next pregnancy, anemia can occur in the fetus because antibodies in the mom are already formed. If these antibodies cross the placenta, they can attack the baby's red blood cells, resulting in anemia.

Preventing Problems. If you're Rh-negative, you'll be checked for antibodies at the beginning of pregnancy. If you have antibodies, you are already sensitized. If you don't have antibodies, you're unsensitized (this is good).

Rh-positive blood can mix with an Rh-negative woman's blood, causing sensitization, in many ways. These include miscarriage, abortion, ectopic pregnancy, amniocentesis, chorionic villus sampling, PUBS or cordocentesis, blood transfusion, bleeding during pregnancy, such as with placental abruption, or in an accident or injury, such as blunt-force trauma to the uterus in an auto accident.

If you're Rh-negative and are *not* sensitized, a treatment is available to prevent you from becoming sensitized. It is called *RhoGAM* and *Rh immune globulin* (RhIg)–they're the same thing. RhoGAM is a product extracted from human blood. (If you have religious, ethical or personal reasons for not using blood or blood products, consult your physician or minister.) If your blood mixes with baby's blood, RhoGAM keeps you from becoming sensitized. If you're already sensitized, RhoGAM doesn't help.

Your healthcare provider will probably suggest you receive RhoGAM around the 28th week of pregnancy to prevent sensitization in the last part of your pregnancy. You're more likely to be exposed to baby's blood during the last 3 months of pregnancy and at delivery. If you go beyond your due date, your healthcare provider may suggest another dose of RhoGAM.

RhoGAM is given within 72 hours after delivery, if your baby is Rh-positive. If your baby is Rh-negative, you don't need RhoGAM after delivery and you didn't need the shot during pregnancy. But it's better not to take that risk and to have the RhoGAM injection during pregnancy.

After delivery, if blood tests show a larger than normal number of Rh-positive blood cells (from baby) have entered your bloodstream, you may be given RhoGAM. The RhoGAM treatment is necessary for every pregnancy.

At the beginning of your pregnancy, a blood test is done to determine if you are Rh-positive or Rh-negative, and if you have antibodies. If you're Rh-positive, like most people, you don't need to worry about any of this. If you are Rh-negative, you may:

- be *sensitized* (already have antibodies)—your pregnancy will be monitored closely for fetal anemia and other problems
- be *unsensitized* (do not have antibodies)—you will receive a RhoGAM injection at 28 weeks
- receive a RhoGAM injection at 40 weeks, if you are still pregnant

Your baby is checked at delivery with a blood test to see if it is Rh-positive or Rh-negative.

- If baby is Rh-negative, nothing further will be done.
- If baby is Rh-positive, a test is done on your blood to determine how much RhoGAM you should receive.

Rh Disease and Your Growing Baby. When Rh disease destroys a fetus's blood cells, it can cause blood disease of the fetus or newborn. If your healthcare provider suspects fetal problems from Rh disease, amniocentesis and cordocentesis can help determine whether baby is developing anemia and how severe it is. These tests may need to be repeated every 2 to 4 weeks. Amniocentesis can also determine whether the fetus is Rh-negative or Rh-positive.

Ultrasound may be used to measure the speed of blood flowing through an artery in the baby's head. This can help detect moderate to severe anemia but not mild anemia.

A blood test on you is done to help provide your medical team with information on the fetus. The test determines Rh status in the fetus, which may mean you won't need amniocentesis in the future to determine this factor.

If your baby has a problem, there are actions that can be taken before birth. Babies have been treated with blood transfusions as early as 18 weeks of pregnancy.

Exercise for Week 16

You now know why you shouldn't lie on your back to exercise after the 16th week, so no more abdominal crunches. However, you can do a modified, pregnancy-friendly crunch. Sit on the floor in a crossed-leg position. Brace your back against the wall. Use pillows for added comfort. Exhaling through your nose, pull your bellybutton in toward your spine. Hold for 5 seconds, then inhale through your nose. Begin with 5 repetitions and work up to 10. *Strengthens stomach muscles, and keeps lower back and spine strong.*

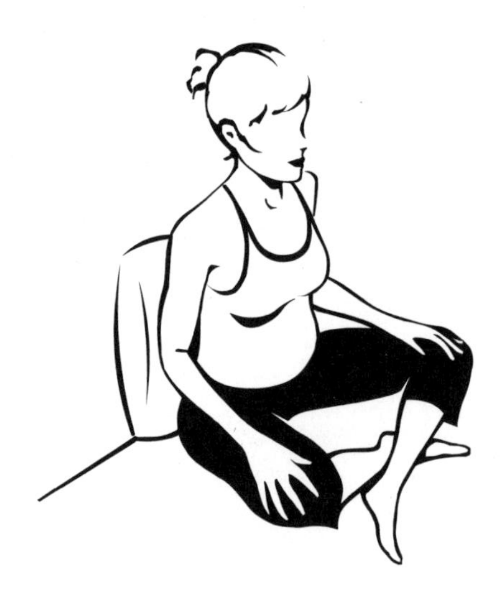

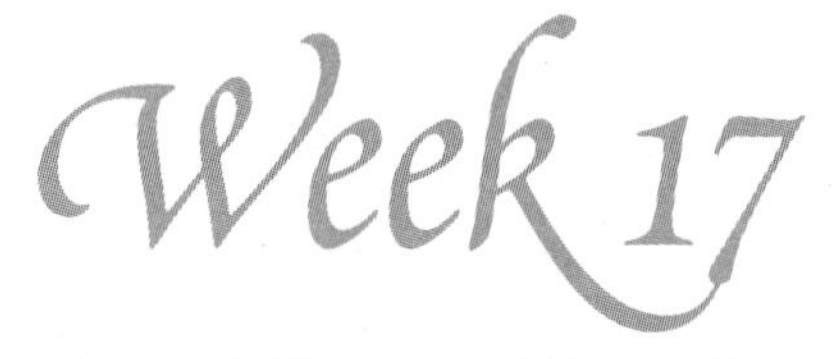

Age of Fetus—15 Weeks

How Big Is Your Baby?

The crown-to-rump length of your baby is 4½ to 4¾ inches (11 to 12cm). Fetal weight has doubled in 2 weeks and is now about 3½ ounces (100g). By this week, your baby is about the size of your hand spread open wide.

How Big Are You?

Your uterus is 1½ to 2 inches (3.8 to 5cm) below your bellybutton. You now have an obvious swelling in your lower abdomen. Expanding or maternity clothing is a must for comfort's sake. When your partner gives you a hug, he may feel the difference in your lower abdomen. A total 5- to 10-pound (2.25 to 4.5kg) total weight gain by this point in your pregnancy is normal.

How Your Baby Is Growing and Developing

If you look at the illustration on page 240, then look at earlier weeks, you'll see the incredible changes occurring in your baby. Fat, also called *adipose tissue,* begins to form this week. It's important to baby's heat production and metabolism. At birth, fat makes up about 5¼ pounds (2.4kg) of the total average weight of 7¾ pounds (3.5kg).

You have felt your baby move, or you will soon. You may not feel it every day. As pregnancy progresses, movements become stronger and more frequent.

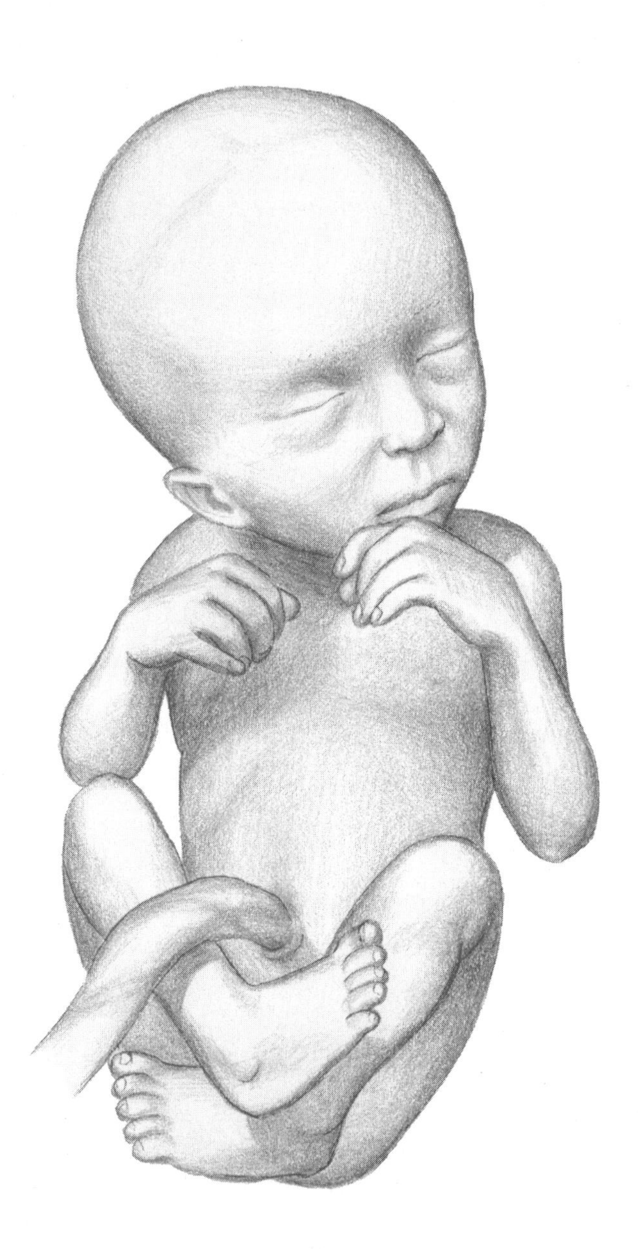

Your baby's fingernails are well formed.
The baby is beginning to accumulate a little fat.

Changes in You

Feeling your baby move can reassure you things are going well with your pregnancy. This is especially true if you've had problems.

As pregnancy advances, the uterus becomes more oval than round as it fills the pelvis and starts to grow into the abdomen. Your intestines are pushed upward and to the sides. Your uterus eventually reaches almost to your liver.

When you stand, your uterus touches your abdominal wall in the front. You may feel it most easily in this position. When you lie on your back, it can fall backward onto your spine and blood vessels (vena cava and aorta).

Round-Ligament Pain

Round ligaments are attached to each side of the upper uterus and to the pelvic side wall. With the growth of the uterus, these ligaments stretch and pull, and become longer and thicker. Moving may cause pain or discomfort called *round-ligament pain*. Pain may occur on one side only or both sides, or it may be worse on one side than another. This pain does not harm you or your baby.

If you have this pain, you may feel better if you lie down and rest. Talk to your healthcare provider if pain is severe or if other symptoms arise. Warning signs of serious problems include bleeding from the vagina, loss of fluid from the vagina or severe pain.

Tip for Week 17

If you experience leg cramps during pregnancy, there are some things to try. Don't stand for long periods. Rest on your side as often as possible. Do stretching exercises. You may also use a heating pad on the cramped area, but don't use it for longer than 15 minutes at a time. Eat raisins and bananas—they're great sources of potassium. Inadequate calcium intake can also affect leg cramps. Be sure you take in 1200mg of calcium every day. Drinking lots of water may also help. Also try Grandma's Remedy for leg cramps; see the box in Week 25.

How Your Actions Affect Your Baby's Development

Ultrasound at This Time

Ultrasound is performed at different times for different reasons. During the second trimester, it can be used with amniocentesis, with bleeding related to placenta previa or abruption, when there is concern about intrauterine-growth restriction (IUGR), to evaluate fetal well-being and to diagnose multiple fetuses.

Ultrasound has proved very effective for diagnosing problems and giving reassurance. It is often combined with other tests.

3-Dimensional Ultrasound. A 3-dimensional ultrasound available in many areas provides detailed, clear pictures of the baby inside you. Images almost look like photos. For the pregnant woman, the test is almost the same as a 2-dimensional ultrasound. The difference is that computer software "translates" the picture into a 3-D image.

A 3-D ultrasound may be used when there is suspicion of problems with the baby and the healthcare provider wants to take a closer look. Three-dimensional ultrasound can furnish information that helps with diagnosis and treatment. It helps medical personnel understand the severity of the problem so a treatment program can be planned that can be started immediately after birth.

This ultrasound is most helpful in assessing babies with facial problems, hand and foot problems, spine problems and neural-tube defects. Some studies show 3-D images can be a valuable teaching aid for parents, who may have trouble visualizing the defects. Medical personnel have found many uses for 3-D ultrasound, including:

- measurement of volume, such as when measuring the amount of amniotic fluid
- more-accurate measurements of nuchal translucency
- better pictures of baby's skull
- evaluation of the spine
- seeing subtle differences with cleft-lip and cleft-palate problems

- seeing defects in the abdominal wall
- better evaluation of the placenta, which can be very helpful when you are carrying more than one baby
- helping the healthcare provider see some abnormalities of the umbilical cord
- helping to rule out some birth defects

Increased Vaginal Discharge

During pregnancy, it's normal to have an increase in vaginal discharge, called *leukorrhea*. This discharge is usually white or yellow and fairly thick. It's not an infection. We believe it's caused by increased blood flow to the skin and muscles around the vagina; this also causes a violet or blue coloration of the vagina. This appearance, visible to your healthcare provider early in pregnancy, is called *Chadwick's sign*.

You may have to wear sanitary pads if you have a heavy discharge. Avoid wearing pantyhose and nylon underwear. Choose underwear with a cotton crotch to allow more air circulation.

> **Dad Tip**
>
> **Massage can work wonders to help relieve your partner's discomforts and tiredness. It can also help ease any anxiousness she may be having. Massage can be very relaxing for her and you! Offer your partner tension-relieving, muscle-relaxing head, back and foot massages. It may make you both feel great.**

Vaginal infections can and do occur during pregnancy. The discharge with these infections is often foul-smelling. It is yellow or green and causes irritation or itching around or inside the vagina. If you have any of these symptoms, call your healthcare provider. Many creams and antibiotics are safe to use during pregnancy.

Douching during Pregnancy

Most healthcare providers agree you should not douche during pregnancy. Bulb-syringe douches are definitely out! Douching may cause you to bleed or may cause more serious problems. Avoid this practice.

Your Nutrition

Are You a Vegetarian?

Some women choose to eat a vegetarian diet because of personal or religious preferences. Other women are nauseated by meat during pregnancy. Is it safe to eat a vegetarian diet while you're pregnant? It can be, if you pay close attention to the types and combinations of foods you eat.

Research shows most women who eat a vegetarian diet eat a more nutrient-rich variety of foods than those who eat meat. Vegetarians may make an extra effort to include more fruits and vegetables in their food plans when they eliminate meat products. If you're a vegetarian by choice, and have been for a while, you may know how to get many of the nutrients you need. If you have questions, talk to your healthcare provider. He or she may want you to see a nutritionist if you have any pregnancy risk factors.

During pregnancy, you need to eat between 2200 and 2700 calories a day. And you must eat the *right* kind of calories. Choose fresh foods to supply you a variety of vitamins and minerals. Eat enough different sources of protein to provide energy for you and baby. Discuss your diet with your healthcare provider at your first prenatal visit.

There are different vegetarian nutrition plans, each with unique characteristics.

- If you are an *ovo-lacto vegetarian,* you eat milk products and eggs.
- If you are a *lacto vegetarian,* your diet includes milk products.
- A *vegan* diet includes only foods of plant origin, such as nuts, seeds, vegetables, fruits, grains and legumes.
- A *macrobiotic* diet limits foods to whole grains, beans, vegetables and moderate amounts of fish and fruits.
- A *fruitarian* diet is the most restrictive; it allows only fruits, nuts, olive oil and honey.

Macrobiotic and fruitarian diets are too restrictive for a pregnant woman. They do not provide enough vitamins, minerals, protein and calories needed for baby's development.

Your goal is to eat enough calories to gain weight during pregnancy. You don't want your body to use protein for energy because you need it for your growth and your baby's growth.

By eating a wide variety of whole grains, legumes, dried fruit, lima beans and wheat germ, you should be able to get enough iron, zinc and other trace minerals. If you don't drink milk or include milk products in your diet, you must find other sources of vitamins D, B_2, B_{12} and calcium.

Getting enough folic acid is usually not a problem for vegetarians. Folate is found in many fruits, legumes and vegetables (especially dark leafy ones).

Women who eat little or no meat are at greater risk of iron deficiency during pregnancy. To get enough iron, eat an assortment of grains, vegetables, seeds and nuts, legumes and fortified cereal every day. Spinach, prunes and sauerkraut are excellent sources of iron, as are dried fruit and dark leafy vegetables. Tofu is also a good source. Cook in cast-iron pans because traces of iron will attach to whatever you're cooking.

If you're not eating meat because it makes you ill, ask for a referral to a nutritionist. You may need help developing a good eating plan.

If you are a lacto or ovo-lacto vegetarian, do not drink milk with foods that are iron rich; calcium reduces iron absorption. Don't drink tea or coffee with meals because tannins present in those beverages inhibit iron absorption by 75%. Many breakfast foods and breads are now iron-fortified. Read labels.

To get omega-3 fatty acids, add canola oil, tofu, flaxseed, soybeans, walnuts and wheat germ to your food plan. These foods contain linolenic oil, a type of omega-3 fatty acid. You can also eat flaxseed flour and flaxseed oil—both are available in markets and health-food stores. But avoid plain flax.

Vegetarians and pregnant women who can't eat meat may have a harder time getting enough vitamin E. Vitamin E is important during pregnancy because it helps metabolize polyunsaturated fats and contributes to building muscles and red blood cells. Foods rich in the vitamin include olive oil, wheat germ, spinach and dried fruit.

Vegetarians are more likely to have a zinc deficiency, so pay close attention to getting enough zinc every day. Lima beans, whole-grain products, nuts, dried beans, dried peas, wheat germ and dark leafy vegetables are good sources of zinc. If you're an ovo-lacto vegetarian, it may be harder for you to get enough iron and zinc.

Almonds contain high levels of magnesium, vitamin E, protein and fiber.

If you're a vegan, eating no animal products may make your task more difficult. You may need to ask your healthcare provider about supplements for vitamin B_{12}, vitamin D, zinc, iron and calcium. Eat turnip greens, spinach, beet greens, broccoli, soy-based milk products and cheeses, and fruit juices fortified with calcium.

You Should Also Know

Quad-Screen Test

The quad-screen test is another test that can help find out if you might be carrying a baby with Down syndrome. This blood test can also help rule out other problems, such as neural-tube defects.

The quad-screen test is the same as the triple-screen test, with the addition of a fourth measurement—your inhibin-A level. Measuring the level of inhibin-A, along with the three factors tested for in the triple-screen test, increases the detection rate of Down syndrome and lowers the false-positive rate.

The quad-screen test is able to identify 79% of those fetuses with Down syndrome. It has a false-positive result of 5%.

Complementary and Alternative Medical Techniques

There are many complementary and alternative medicine techniques that may help a woman during pregnancy. *Complementary medicine* refers to treatments and products that are not considered part of traditional medicine. Healthcare providers don't learn about them during training, and they are not usually practiced by healthcare providers. When used with traditional medicine, they are called *complementary medical techniques.* When used in place of traditional medicine, they are called *alternative medicine.*

Many complementary and alternative treatments are untested scientifically. There is no definite way to determine if a treatment is safe or effective, so it's important to talk to your healthcare provider about any of these treatments *before* you have one.

The exception to the rule stated above is *osteopathy.* It uses manipulation and physical therapies to restore structural balance and improve the function of the body. Doctors of osteopathic medicine have graduated from an accredited osteopathic school of medicine and have fulfilled the requirements for a medical license. Treatments by an osteopathic physician are learned in osteopathic schools of medicine and are safe.

Homeopathy uses small, highly diluted substances to alleviate symptoms. In high doses, these same substances *cause* these symptoms. *Chiropractic* involves manipulating the spine to relieve pain and to assist the body's ability to heal itself.

The *Alexander technique* is a gentle approach to movement that can help you rebalance faulty posture through awareness, movement and touch. *Electromagnetic fields,* also called *energy healing,* uses magnets to relieve nerve and joint pain. Low-frequency thermal waves, electrical nerve stimulation and electromagnetic waves provide energy to heal the body.

Acupuncture is the practice of placing tiny needles along pathways believed to connect energy points in your body with specific organs. It is performed by trained practitioners. Research shows acupuncture has many benefits, including changes in blood flow to the brain, as well as helping the body produce its own pain-killing substances. *Acupressure* is similar to acupuncture, except it uses pressure instead of needles on key acu-points on the body.

Biofeedback employs various devices to give you visual or audio feedback about your effort to control automatic body functions, such as blood pressure, heart rate, temperature and brain-wave activity. *Guided imagery* uses imaginary mental pictures, combined with your senses of sight, smell and hearing, to focus on imagining yourself being well. It is particularly useful for managing common stress-related problems, such as headaches or high blood pressure.

Therapeutic touch involves having a therapist pass his or her hands over a person's body to bring energy into balance. *Reflexology* applies pressure to specific points on the hands and feet, especially tender points, believed to be linked to specific organs in the body.

Mind-body therapies involve the mind and body to treat a problem. Some common therapies include massage, meditation, yoga and various relaxation methods. *Massage therapy* employs the ancient healing art of rubbing and manipulating body tissue to help make your body, mind and spirit relax. You can massage your own head and neck, forehead, temple, hands and feet, or go to a trained professional for a complete body massage that may help many common ailments.

Meditation relaxes your mind and helps you get in touch with deeper thoughts. There are different kinds of meditation; some involve focusing on breathing, visualizing different objects or repeating a word or mantra. Other types, such as mindfulness meditation, allow the body to become less reactive to stress. *Yoga,* which comes from the word "union," uses postures designed to align every aspect of a person—spiritual, mental, emotional and physical.

Aromatherapy uses scented plant oils that are added to products to be smelled or applied to the skin. *Dietary supplements* include vitamins, minerals, herbs and supplements to help prevent illness. Herbs and herbal preparations are used as medicine. *Chinese medicine* is based on the belief that balanced energy (qi) flows through the body of a healthy person, and disease causes the flow to be interrupted.

Are You Thinking about Using a Doula?

You may be wondering if you want a doula to help you during baby's birth. A *doula* is a woman who is trained to provide support and assistance during labor and delivery. The doula remains with you from the onset of labor until baby is born.

Doula is the Greek term for *female helper.* Doulas don't deliver babies, replace a doctor or midwife, or play the role of a nurse. They are there to comfort the mom-to-be, to soothe her fears and to help her

Questions to Ask a Prospective Doula

If you are considering a doula, interview more than one before you choose someone. Some questions you may want to ask and some perceptions you might want to analyze after your interview are listed below.

- What are your qualifications and training? Are you certified? By which organization?
- Have you had a baby yourself? What childbirth method did you use?
- What is your childbirth philosophy?
- Are you familiar with the childbirth method we have chosen (if you have a particular method you want to use)?
- What kind of plan would you use to help us through our labor?
- How available are you to answer our questions before the birth?
- How often will we meet before the birth?
- How do we contact you when labor begins?
- What happens if you aren't available when we go into labor? Do you work with other doulas? May we meet some of them?
- Are you experienced in helping a new mom with breastfeeding? How available are you after the birth to help with this and other postpartum issues?
- What is your fee?

Perceptions include how easy the doula is to talk to and to communicate with. Did she listen well and answer your questions? Did you feel comfortable with her? If you don't hit it off with one doula, try another!

through labor. They can provide continuous care through labor. They provide pain relief through massage, breathing techniques and water therapy. In some cases a doula can guide partners in helping during labor and delivery. A doula may even be able to help you begin breastfeeding your baby.

Another strength of a doula is to provide support to a woman who has chosen to have a drug-free labor and delivery. If you've decided you want anesthesia, no matter what, a doula may not be a good choice for you.

Although a doula's primary function is to provide support to the mom during labor, she often assists the labor coach. She does not displace a labor coach; she works with him or her. In some situations, a doula may serve as the labor coach.

The services of a doula may be expensive and can range from $250 to $1500. This usually covers meetings before birth, attendance at labor and delivery, and one or more postpartum visits.

If you and your partner choose to have a doula present during labor and the birth, talk to your healthcare provider about your decision. He or she may find her presence intrusive and veto the idea. Or the healthcare provider may be able to give you the name of someone he or she often works with.

If you decide to use a doula, begin early to search for someone. Start looking as early as your 4th month of pregnancy—certainly no later than your 6th month. If you wait any longer, you may still be able to find someone, but choices may be limited. Starting early allows you to relax and to evaluate more critically any women you interview. Look in your local phone book for the names of doulas, or visit DoulaNetwork.com to find a doula in your area.

Postpartum Doulas. In addition to doulas who help during labor and delivery, there are also *postpartum doulas.* These women help ease the transition into parenthood. A postpartum doula will help a new mother and her family learn to enjoy and to care for the new baby through education and hands-on experience.

A postpartum doula provides emotional and breastfeeding support, and makes sure a new mother is fed, hydrated and comfortable. She may go with mom and baby to pediatric appointments. A postpartum doula may also take care of grocery shopping, preparing meals and other household tasks. She may even help tend older children.

A postpartum doula's services are most often used in the first 2 to 4 weeks after birth, but support can last anywhere from one or two visits to visits for 3 months or longer. Some doulas work all day; others work 3- to 5-hour shifts during the day or after-school shifts until Dad gets home. Some doulas work evenings and/or overnight.

Doulas don't treat postpartum depression but can offer support to a woman who experiences it. Some postpartum doulas are trained to help women screen themselves for depression and will make referrals to healthcare providers and support groups.

Tips for Choosing Maternity Clothes

Wearing maternity clothes may be the first public sign you're pregnant. Luckily, today's maternity clothes are more stylish than in the past. Below are some suggestions to help you choose fashionable, comfortable clothes to grow with you.

- Be sure maternity clothes provide you room to grow in your pregnancy.
- A waistband shouldn't be too tight. You have a long way to go before baby arrives. Clothing that fits tightly at the waist can put pressure on veins in the tummy, which can cut off circulation to the legs. Adjustable-waist pants, skirts and shorts help avoid this problem.
- Select a pregnancy bra with wide straps to help avoid putting pressure on the trapezius muscle in your back. If this muscle becomes tight and knotted, you may experience neck pain, a headache or tingling and/or numbness in your arms. A sports bra with a racer back evenly distributes the weight of the breasts.
- Choose clothes you can use for work (if you work outside your home) and for leisure. Pants and comfortable tops can often do double duty.
- You may want to buy one nice dress to have on hand for special occasions.
- Don't forget about shoes—low-heeled styles can work with pants and dresses.

If you think you may want a postpartum doula, make arrangements a few months before your due date. Even though you don't know exactly when your baby will arrive (unless you're having a scheduled Cesarean delivery), contract with a postpartum doula in advance to be sure of her availability. Costs range between $15 and $30 an hour for this service, depending on the postpartum doula's additional training and experience.

Exercise for Week 17

Sit on the floor with your legs out straight in front of you. Lift your arms straight out in front of you, to shoulder height. "Walk" forward on your buttocks for 6 paces, then return to the starting position by "walking" backward. Repeat 7 times forward and backward. *Strengthens abdominal muscles and lower-back muscles.*

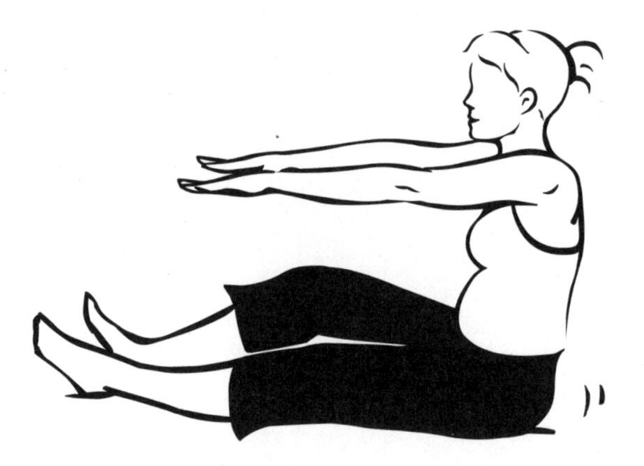

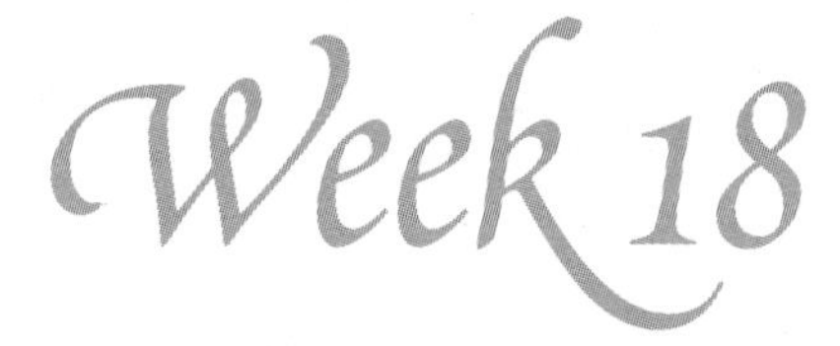

Age of Fetus—16 Weeks

How Big Is Your Baby?

The crown-to-rump length of your growing baby is 5 to 5½ inches (12.5 to 14cm) by this week. Weight of the fetus is about 5¼ ounces (150g).

How Big Are You?

If you put your fingers sideways and measure, your uterus is about two finger-widths (1 inch) below your bellybutton. It's the size of a cantaloupe or a little larger.

Total weight gain to this point should be 10 to 13 pounds (4.5 to 5.8kg), but this can vary. If you've gained more weight than this, talk to your healthcare provider. You may need to see a nutritionist. You still have more than half of your pregnancy ahead of you, and you'll definitely gain more weight.

How Your Baby Is Growing and Developing

Baby continues to develop, but the rapid growth rate slows. As you can see in the illustration on page 254, your baby has a human appearance now.

Ultrasound can detect some fetal problems. If one is suspected, further ultrasound exams may be ordered to follow baby's development as pregnancy progresses.

Blood from your baby flows to the placenta through the umbilical cord. In the placenta, oxygen and nutrients are carried from your blood

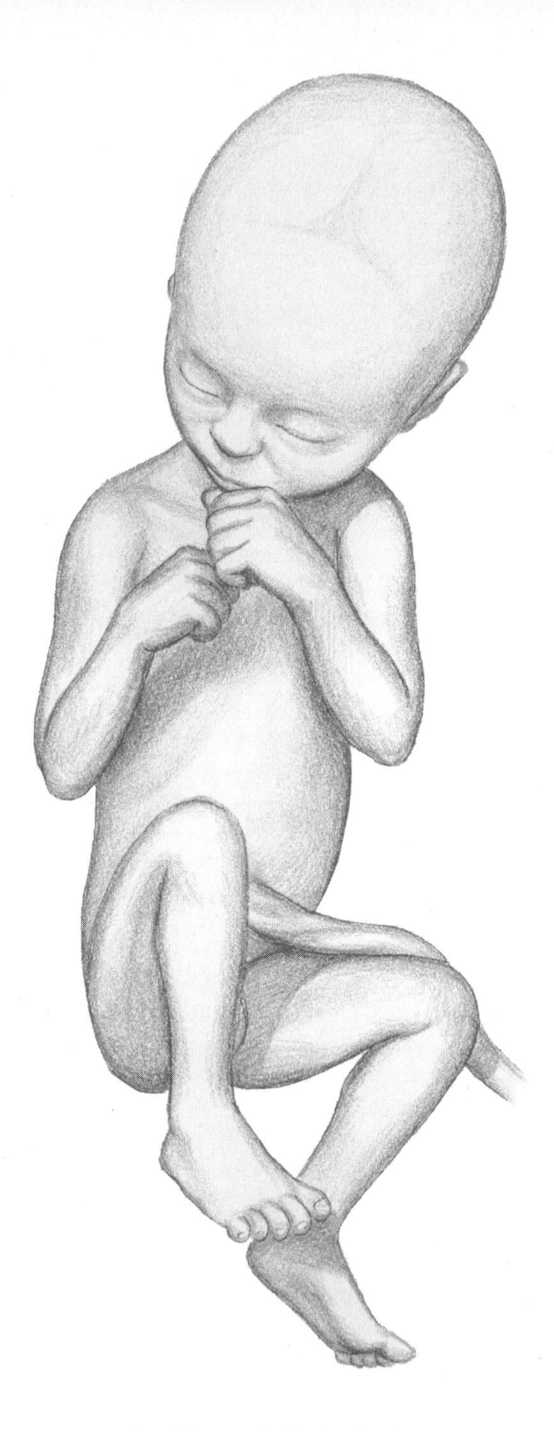

By this week, baby is about
5 inches (12.5cm) from crown to rump.
It looks much more human now.

to the fetal blood. At birth, baby must go rapidly from depending on you for oxygen to depending on its own heart and lungs. The foramen ovale closes at birth, and blood goes to the right ventricle, the right atrium and the lungs for oxygenation. It is truly a miraculous conversion.

Changes in You

Does Your Back Ache?

Between 50 and 80% of all pregnant women have back and hip pain at some time. Pain usually occurs during the third trimester as your tummy grows larger. However, pain may begin early in pregnancy and last until well after delivery (up to 5 or 6 months).

It's more common to have mild backache than severe problems. Some women have severe back pain after excessive exercise, walking, bending, lifting or standing. Some women need to be careful getting out of bed or getting up from a sitting position. In extreme cases, some women find it difficult to walk.

The hormone relaxin may be part of the problem. It's responsible for relaxing joints that allow your pelvis to expand to deliver your baby. However, when joints relax, it can lead to pain in the lower back and legs. Other factors include your weight gain (another good reason to control your weight), larger breasts and your bigger tummy, which can cause a shift in posture.

Lumbar-spine pain (LSP) is an aching feeling that spreads throughout the center lower back. It often begins in the first or second trimester. If you've had lower-back pain before pregnancy, you may experience this discomfort during pregnancy. A prenatal yoga class may offer relief. Staying off your feet is also a good remedy.

A change in joint mobility may cause a change in your posture and may cause discomfort in the lower back, especially during the last part of pregnancy. The growth of the uterus moves your center of gravity forward, over your legs, which can affect the joints around the pelvis. All your joints are looser. Hormone increases are likely causes. Check with your healthcare provider if back pain is a problem for you.

Actions You Can Take to Relieve Back Pain. What can you do to prevent or lessen your pain? Try some or all of the following tips as early in pregnancy as possible. They'll pay off later in pregnancy.

- Watch your weight gain; avoid gaining too much weight or gaining weight too fast.
- Stay active; continue exercising during pregnancy.
- Lie on your side when you sleep.
- Get off your feet and lie down for 30 minutes on your side.
- Practice good posture.
- If you have other children, take a nap when they take theirs.
- It's OK to take acetaminophen for back pain.
- Use heat on the painful area.
- If pain becomes constant or more severe, talk to your healthcare provider about it.

When you have lower-back pain, use an ice pack for up to 30 minutes three or four times a day. If pain lasts, switch to a heating pad, sticking with the same regimen. Stretching gently may also help.

Prenatal massage may help relieve pain—ask your healthcare provider about it. He or she may be able to suggest some qualified massage therapists. Or he or she may suggest a lower-back brace or pregnancy support garment.

Exercise may help relieve back pain. Swimming, walking and nonimpact aerobics may be beneficial. See the discussion of exercise that begins on page 259.

Discomfort may also indicate more serious problems. Bring up any concerns you have with your healthcare provider.

Although this book is designed to take you through pregnancy by examining one week at a time, you may want specific information. Because the book can't include *everything* you need *before* you know you're looking for it, check the index, beginning on page 655, for a particular topic. We may not cover the subject until a later week.

Inflammatory Bowel Disease (IBD)

Inflammatory bowel disease (IBD) describes two common problems—ulcerative colitis and Crohn's disease. (Crohn's disease is discussed in Week 24.) IBD affects about 2 million Americans. (IBD is not the same as IBS—irritable bowel syndrome. See Week 30 for a discussion of IBS.)

With ulcerative colitis, the inner lining of the intestine gets red and swollen, and develops ulcers. It may be most severe in the rectal area, which can cause frequent diarrhea. Mucus and blood often appear in the stool if the colon lining is damaged

IBD can be caused by many things, including environment and diet. Lifestyle choices may affect IBD. Not smoking and taking omega-3 fatty acids seem to help. A defective immune system may also be a cause.

The problem seems to run in families. This has led researchers to believe a gene variant may affect how the immune system works.

The most common symptoms of IBD are diarrhea and stomach pain. Diarrhea can range from mild to severe. At times, IBD may also cause constipation. People with the problem may lose fluid and nutrients from diarrhea, which can lead to fever, fatigue, weight loss and malnutrition. Stomach pain is caused by irritation of the nerves and muscles that control intestinal contractions.

Some people with IBD may experience inflammation in other parts of the body, including the joints, eyes, skin and liver. Skin tags may also develop around the anus.

> **Dad Tip**
>
> **You may be surprised how tired your pregnant partner seems. Doing anything may take a lot of effort on her part, especially if she works outside your home. You can help out by offering to run errands. Take her dry cleaning in, and pick it up when it's ready. Stop by the bank for her. Take her car to a car wash. Return her library books or rented DVDs.**

Diagnosing and Treating IBD. Diagnosing the problem can be difficult because IBD symptoms often resemble those of other conditions. If you lose weight, have repeated bouts of diarrhea or abdominal cramping, IBD may be suspected.

Your healthcare provider may order blood tests to look for inflammation, to check for anemia and to look for other causes of symptoms. A stool test might also be done to check for blood, or a barium study of the intestines may be ordered.

Drug treatment is most often used to treat IBD symptoms. You may be prescribed anti-inflammatory drugs and/or immunosuppressive agents. If symptoms don't respond to either medication, surgery may be necessary. If needed during pregnancy, it should be performed during the second trimester.

Gaining more than the recommended weight can make pregnancy and delivery harder on you. And extra pounds may be hard to lose afterward, so keep watching what you eat. Choose food for the nutrition it provides you and your growing baby.

You may need more tests during pregnancy. Experts believe it's safe to have a colonoscopy, sigmoidoscopy, upper endoscopy, rectal biopsy or abdominal ultrasound during pregnancy. Avoid X-rays and CT scans. Ask your OB/GYN about an MRI if one is recommended. It's important to involve your gastroenterologist. Ask your pregnancy healthcare provider how to go about this.

IBD and Pregnancy. Most women who have IBD can have a normal pregnancy and give birth to a healthy baby. If you didn't talk to your healthcare provider before you got pregnant, contact your healthcare provider before you stop taking any medication.

If your IBD is in remission when you get pregnant, it may stay in remission during pregnancy. This happens with about 65% of all pregnant women. If your disease is active, it will probably remain active throughout pregnancy.

A third of all women with ulcerative colitis relapse during pregnancy, usually during the first trimester. Flare-ups occur most often during the first trimester and immediately after birth.

Women who have severe IBD have a higher risk of problems. You may be seen more often during your pregnancy, and you may have more tests.

How Your Actions Affect Your Baby's Development

Exercise in the Second Trimester

Everyone has heard stories of women who continued with strenuous exercise or arduous activities until the day of delivery without problems. Stories are told of Olympic athletes who were pregnant at the time they won medals. This kind of training and physical stress isn't a good idea for most pregnant women.

As you grow, your sense of balance may be affected. You may feel clumsy. This isn't the time for contact sports or sports where you might fall easily, injure yourself or be struck in the tummy.

Pregnant women can usually participate safely in many sports and exercise activities throughout pregnancy. This is a different attitude from 30 and 40 years ago; decreased activity was common then. Exercise and activity can benefit you and your growing baby.

Discuss your activities at a prenatal visit. If your pregnancy is high risk or if you have had several miscarriages, it's particularly important to discuss exercise with your healthcare provider *before* starting any activity. Now is not the time to train to increase activity. In fact, this may be a good time to decrease the amount or intensity of exercise you do. Listen to your body. It will tell you when it's time to slow down.

What about activities you're already involved in or would like to begin? Below is a discussion of various activities and how they will affect you in your second and third trimesters.

> **Tip for Week 18**
>
> **During exercise, your oxygen demands increase. Your body is heavier, and your balance may change. You may also tire more easily. Keep these points in mind as you adjust your fitness program.**

Activities You May Enjoy. *Swimming* can be good for you. The support and buoyancy of the water can be relaxing. If you swim, swim throughout pregnancy. If you can't swim and have done water exercises (exercising in the shallow end of a swimming pool), you can continue during your pregnancy. This is an exercise you can begin at any time during pregnancy, if you don't overdo it.

Walking is great during pregnancy. It can be a good time for you and your partner to talk. Even when the weather is bad, you can walk in many places, such as an enclosed shopping mall, to get a good workout. Two miles of walking at a good pace is adequate. As pregnancy progresses, you may need to decrease your speed and distance. Walking is an exercise you can begin at any time during pregnancy, if you don't overdo it.

If you're comfortable riding and have safe places to ride, you can enjoy *bicycling* with your partner or family. But now is not the time to learn to ride a bike. Your balance changes as your body changes. This can make getting on and off a bicycle difficult. A fall from a bicycle could injure you or your baby.

A *stationary bicycle* is good for bad weather and for later in pregnancy. Many experts suggest you ride a stationary bike in the last 2 to 3 months of pregnancy to avoid the danger of a fall. Spinning—a high-intensity stationary cycling workout—may not be recommended during pregnancy because it may cause dehydration and a rapid heart rate.

Jogging may be permitted during pregnancy, but check with your healthcare provider first. Some women continue to jog during pregnancy. If your pregnancy is high risk, jogging may not be a good idea. Pregnancy is not the time to increase mileage or to train for a race. Wear comfortable clothing and supportive athletic shoes with good cushioning. Allow plenty of time to stretch and to cool down.

During your pregnancy, you'll probably need to slow down and to decrease the number of miles you run. You may even change to walking. If you have pain, bleeding, contractions or other symptoms during or after jogging, call your healthcare provider immediately.

We are often asked about other sports activities. Below is a discussion of various sports you may want information about.

- Tennis and golf are safe to continue in the second and third trimesters but may provide little actual exercise.
- Horseback riding is not advisable during pregnancy.
- Avoid water skiing.

- Bowling is OK, although the amount of exercise you get varies. Be careful in late pregnancy; you could fall or strain your back. As balance changes, bowling could be more difficult for you.
- Talk to your healthcare provider about skiing before you hit the slopes or the trails. Both may be OK during pregnancy. Also discuss snowboarding, if this is a sport you enjoy. Your balance changes significantly during pregnancy; a fall could be harmful to you and your baby. Some healthcare providers may allow skiing or boarding in early pregnancy, but many agree these activities in the second half of pregnancy are not a good idea.
- Riding snowmobiles, jet skis or motorcycles is not advised. Some experts feel it's OK to ride if it isn't strenuous. However, most believe the risk is too great, especially if you have had problems during this or a previous pregnancy.

Your Nutrition

You need about 30mg of iron a day to meet the increased needs of pregnancy. Baby draws on your iron stores to create its own stores for its first few months of life. This helps protect baby from iron deficiency if you breastfeed.

Your prenatal vitamin contains about 60mg of iron, which should be enough for you. If you must take iron supplements, take your iron pill with a glass of orange juice or grapefruit juice to increase its absorption. Avoid drinking milk, coffee or tea when taking iron supplements; they prevent the body from absorbing the mineral.

If you feel tired, have trouble concentrating, suffer from headaches, dizziness or indigestion, or if you get sick easily, you may have iron deficiency. An easy way to check is to examine the inside of your lower eyelid. If you're getting enough iron, it should be dark pink. Your nail beds should also be pink.

Only 10 to 15% of the iron you consume is absorbed by the body. You need to eat iron-rich foods on a regular basis to maintain those stores. Foods rich in iron include chicken, red meat, organ meats (liver, heart, kidneys), egg yolks, dark chocolate, dried fruit, spinach, kale and tofu. Combining a vitamin-C food and an iron-rich food ensures better iron absorption. A spinach salad with orange sections is a good example.

If you eat a well-balanced diet and take your prenatal vitamin every day, you may not need additional iron. Discuss it with your healthcare provider if you're concerned.

You Should Also Know

Chronic Fatigue Syndrome (CFS)

Chronic fatigue syndrome (CFS) is a condition in which a person experiences long periods of severe fatigue not directly caused by another condition. Resting doesn't help relieve symptoms. We don't know a lot about CFS and pregnancy. CFS affects about 1 million Americans; 80% are women.

Other problems may also be present. Research suggests about 65% of all people diagnosed with the problem also have symptoms of fibromyalgia. (For more on fibromyalgia, see Week 21.)

CFS often affects women during childbearing years. Many women with chronic fatigue syndrome have had successful pregnancies and healthy babies. Symptoms improve in some pregnant women. Improvement usually occurs after the first trimester and may be due to pregnancy hormones. Some pregnant women experience no change, and some worsen. A woman may also feel worse during subsequent pregnancies.

If you have CFS and are pregnant, you will probably need extra rest during pregnancy. Some women may need bed rest.

Within weeks of delivery, about 50% of all new mothers relapse or feel worse than before pregnancy. This may be caused by the demands on a woman taking care of a newborn, along with the loss of pregnancy hormones. We don't know if women with CFS pass the condition to their babies during pregnancy or breastfeeding.

Talk to your healthcare provider about any over-the-counter or prescription medicine you take. Some medicine may need to be stopped or dosages reduced. Folic acid has been shown to be beneficial before and during pregnancy.

Avodart and Propecia

You may have heard on TV or read in magazines that pregnant women shouldn't handle certain medications, especially *Avodart* and *Propecia.* Should you take these warnings seriously? Can you harm your growing baby by just touching them?

You shouldn't handle either of these pills during pregnancy because of possible problems if pills are crushed or broken, then handled. Medication could be absorbed into your body. If contact is accidentally made, wash the area immediately with soap and water. Let's examine each medication more closely.

Avodart (dutasteride) is used to treat benign enlargement of the male prostate. This potent hormone can pass through the skin, so don't handle it, even if it's not broken. Handling it may cause a birth defect in a baby boy. Men shouldn't donate blood while taking Avodart because blood could be given to a pregnant woman and cause a birth defect.

> If UTIs are a problem, try eating less poultry and pork. These foods may contain an antibiotic-resistant form of *E. coli*.

Research also found dutasteride is present in the semen of a man taking Avodart, so don't have unprotected sex during the first trimester, when baby is forming. Use a condom during sex.

Propecia (finasteride) is used to treat male-pattern baldness. Propecia tablets are coated, but it's probably a good idea not to handle them at all. It could cause problems for a baby boy. No birth defects have been found in baby girls if a mother-to-be accidentally comes in contact with finasteride.

Bladder Infections

A urinary-tract infection (UTI) is the most common problem involving your bladder or kidneys during pregnancy. As the uterus grows, it sits

> ### *Keep Your Urinary Tract Healthy*
>
> - Don't hold your urine—go when you feel the urge.
> - Drink at least 100 ounces of fluid every day to flush bacteria from the urinary tract; include cranberry juice.
> - Urinate immediately after sexual intercourse.
> - Don't wear tight underwear or slacks.
> - Wipe from the front of the vagina to the back after a bowel movement.

directly on top of your bladder and the tubes leading from the kidneys to the bladder. This can block the flow of urine. Other names for urinary-tract infections are *bladder infections* and *cystitis.*

Symptoms include the feeling of urgency to urinate, frequent urination and painful urination, particularly at the end of urinating. A severe UTI may cause blood in the urine.

Your healthcare provider may do a urinalysis and urine culture at your first prenatal visit. He or she may check your urine for infection at other times during pregnancy and when bothersome symptoms arise.

You can help avoid infection by not holding your urine. Empty your bladder as soon as you feel the need. It also helps to empty the bladder after having intercourse.

Drink plenty of fluid. Cranberry juice may help. Don't take cranberry supplements without first asking your healthcare provider.

If you have a UTI during pregnancy, call your healthcare provider. Bacteria could pass through the placenta and affect baby. If left untreated, UTIs may cause other pregnancy problems.

There are many safe antibiotics available to treat a UTI infection, but some antibiotics may not be safe during pregnancy. Your healthcare provider can advise you.

Take the full course of any antibiotic prescribed for you. It may be harmful to baby if you don't treat the problem!

Other Kidney Problems. A more serious problem resulting from a bladder infection is *pyelonephritis.* This type of infection occurs in 1 to 2% of all pregnant women. Symptoms include frequent urination, a burning sensation during urination, the feeling you need to urinate and nothing will come out, high fever, chills and back pain.

Pyelonephritis may require hospitalization and treatment with intravenous antibiotics. If you have pyelonephritis or recurrent bladder infections during pregnancy, you may have to take antibiotics throughout pregnancy to prevent reinfection.

Another problem involving the kidneys and bladder is *kidney stones* (*renal calculi; nephrolithiasis*). They occur about once in every 1500 pregnancies. Kidney stones cause severe pain in the back or lower abdomen and may cause blood in the urine.

Pain with kidney stones may be severe enough to require hospitalization. A kidney stone can usually be treated with pain medication and by drinking lots of fluids. In this way, the stone may be passed without surgical removal or lithotripsy (an ultrasound procedure).

Some women have *chronic kidney disease*, which raises risks during pregnancy. Research has shown a greater risk of various problems in women with chronic kidney disease.

Some Information May Scare You

In an effort to give you as much information as possible about pregnancy, we do include serious discussions throughout the book that some might find "scary." The information is not included to frighten you; it's there to provide facts about particular medical situations that may occur during pregnancy.

If a woman experiences a serious problem, she and her partner will probably want to know as much about it as possible. If a woman has a friend or knows someone who has problems during pregnancy, reading about it might relieve her fears. We also hope our discussions can help you start a dialogue with your doctor, if you have questions.

Nearly all pregnancies are uneventful, and serious situations don't arise. However, please know we have tried to cover as many aspects of pregnancy as we possibly can so you'll have all the information at hand that you might need and want. Knowledge is power, so having various facts available can help you feel more in control of your own pregnancy. We hope reading information helps you relax and have a great pregnancy experience.

If you find serious discussions frighten you, don't read them! Or if the information doesn't apply to your pregnancy, just skip over it. But realize information is there if you want to know more about a particular situation.

Exercise for Week 18

Stand with your feet flat on the floor and your arms by your sides. As you lift your arms straight in front of you and over your head, lunge forward with your right leg. Step back into the starting position as you lower your arms to your sides. Repeat 7 times, then lunge with your left leg. *Tones and strengthens arms, upper back, back of legs and buttocks muscles.*

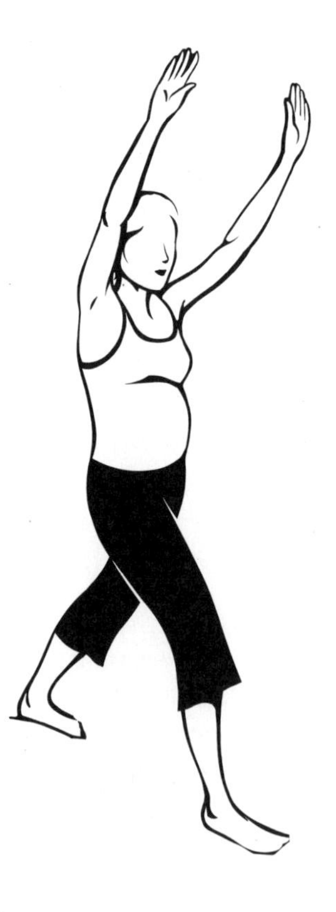

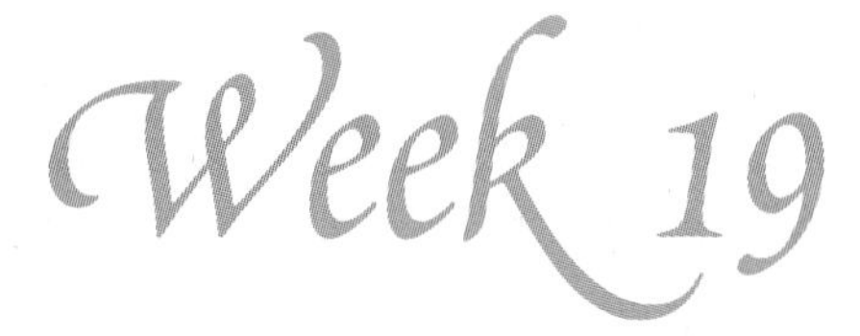

Age of Fetus—17 Weeks

How Big Is Your Baby?

Crown-to-rump length of the growing fetus is 5¼ to 6 inches (13 to 15cm) by this week. Your baby weighs about 7 ounces (200g). It's incredible to think your baby will increase its weight more than 15 times between now and delivery!

How Big Are You?

You can feel your uterus about ½ inch (1.3cm) below your bellybutton. The illustration on page 269 gives you an idea of the relative size of you, your uterus and your growing baby. A side view really shows the changes in you!

Your total weight gain at this point should be between 8 and 14 pounds (3.6 and 6.3kg). Only about 7 ounces (200g) is baby. The placenta weighs about 6 ounces (170g); the amniotic fluid weighs another 11 ounces (320g). The uterus weighs 11 ounces (320g). Your breasts have each increased in weight by about 6½ ounces (180g). The rest of the weight you have gained is due to increased blood volume and other maternal stores.

How Your Baby Is Growing and Developing

Around this time, your baby begins hearing sounds from you—your beating heart, lungs filling with air, swishing blood and digesting food.

Eat More Meals Every Day!

Eating frequent, small meals during the day may provide better nutrition to baby than if you eat three large meals. Though you're eating the same amount of calories, there is a difference. Studies show keeping your blood level of nutrients constant (by eating frequent, small meals) is better for baby than if you eat a large meal, then don't eat again for quite a while. Three larger meals means nutrient levels rise and fall during the day, which isn't as good for the growing baby. Eating small meals frequently can also help ease or avoid some pregnancy problems.

"Hearing" in a fetus is really a matter of feeling vibrations in the skull that are then transmitted to baby's inner ear. Baby "hears" your voice as it vibrates through your bones. Research shows lower-pitched sounds are heard more clearly in utero than high-pitched ones.

Hydrocephalus

Hydrocephalus causes enlargement of baby's head. Occurring in about 1 in 2000 babies, it is responsible for about 12% of all severe birth defects. Hydrocephalus is often associated with spina bifida, meningomyelocele and omphalocele.

Between 15 and 45 ounces of fluid (500 to 1500ml) can accumulate in the skull, but more has been found. Brain tissue is compressed by all this fluid, which is a major concern.

Ultrasound is the best way to diagnose the problem. Hydrocephalus can usually be seen on ultrasound by 19 weeks of pregnancy. Occasionally it is found by routine exams and by "feeling" or measuring your uterus.

In the past, nothing could be done until after delivery. Today, treatment while the fetus is still in the uterus can be done in some cases. There are two methods of treating hydrocephalus inside the uterus. In one method, a needle passes through the mother's abdomen into the area of the baby's brain where fluid is collecting. Some fluid is removed

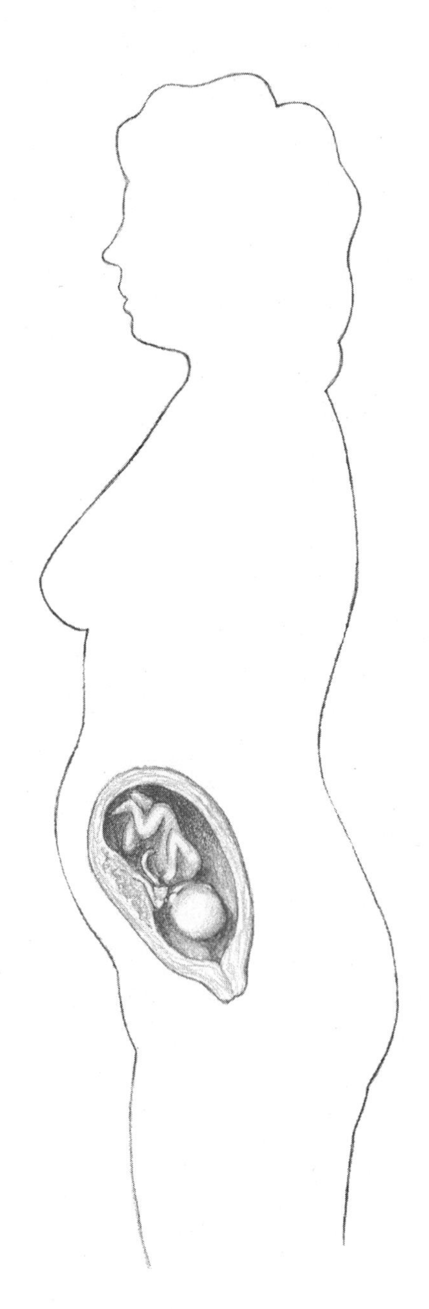

Comparative size of the uterus at 19 weeks of pregnancy
(fetal age—17 weeks). The uterus can be felt
just under the umbilicus (bellybutton).

to relieve pressure on the baby's brain. In another method, a small plastic tube is placed into the area where fluid collects in the baby's brain. This tube is left in place to drain fluid continuously.

Hydrocephalus is a high-risk problem. These procedures are highly specialized and should be performed only by someone experienced in the latest techniques. It requires consultation with a perinatologist specializing in high-risk pregnancies.

Changes in You

Feeling Dizzy

Feeling dizzy during pregnancy is a fairly common symptom, often caused by low blood pressure (hypotension). It usually doesn't appear until the second trimester but may occur earlier.

There are two common reasons for hypotension during pregnancy. It can be caused by the enlarging uterus putting pressure on your aorta and vena cava. This is called *supine hypotension* and occurs when you lie down. You can help ease it or prevent it by not sleeping or lying on your back. The second cause is rising rapidly from a sitting, kneeling or squatting position. This is called *postural hypotension*. Blood pressure drops when you rise rapidly; the problem is cured by rising slowly.

If you're anemic, you may feel dizzy, faint or tired, or you may tire easily. Your blood is checked routinely during pregnancy. Your healthcare provider can tell you if you have anemia.

Pregnancy also affects blood-sugar level. High blood sugar (hyperglycemia) or low blood sugar (hypoglycemia) can make you feel dizzy or faint. Many healthcare providers routinely test pregnant women for blood-sugar problems during pregnancy, especially if they have problems with dizziness or a family history of diabetes.

Most women can avoid or improve the problem by eating a balanced diet, not skipping meals and not going a long time without eating. Carry a piece of fruit or several crackers with you for a quick boost in blood sugar when you need it. You might also try crossing your ankles and squeezing your thighs together, or squeeze a rubber ball in your hand.

Both actions tense muscles, which improves blood flow to your head, which can help you stop feeling faint.

Snoring

More than 35% of all pregnant women snore. When you snore, your upper airway relaxes and partially closes. It may prevent you from inhaling adequate amounts of oxygen and exhaling adequate amounts of carbon dioxide.

In the past, experts believed if you snored during pregnancy, you had a greater chance of having problems, such as high blood pressure and giving birth to a low-birthweight baby. Recent studies show snoring has no damaging effect on baby's growth and development. If you have questions, talk to your healthcare provider.

Thrombophilia

Some women experience blood clots during pregnancy; the term *thrombophilia* describes the condition. Thrombophilia encompasses a broad range of blood-clotting disorders.

Inherited thrombophilias occur in up to 10% of women and can lead to problems during pregnancy in both mother and baby. The condition has been associated with an increased risk of blood clots and other problems during pregnancy.

Many healthcare providers don't screen women for this problem. Ask for a test if you have a family history of the disorder. Some researchers have found inherited thrombophilias are tied to second- or third-trimester fetal loss, not first-trimester loss.

Tests can be done to see if you are at risk. If a blood test shows you have a problem, your healthcare provider may advise aspirin and low-molecular-weight heparin during pregnancy. This treatment has been shown to be effective for some women.

Bikini Waxes

Bikini waxes are OK during pregnancy. Just be careful around the pubic area, and avoid Brazilian waxes. They involve putting hot wax on the tissue on either side of the vaginal opening (labia), which could be more sensitive when you're pregnant.

> *Tip for Week 19*
> Fish can be a healthful food choice during pregnancy, but don't eat more than 12 ounces total of all fish in any one week.

Complications from thrombophilia can recur in subsequent pregnancies. It's important for a woman who has had thrombophilia to cut down the risks in her next pregnancy. Some treatments include folic-acid supplementation, the use of heparin and a low-dose aspirin regimen.

How Your Actions Affect Your Baby's Development

Warning Signs during Pregnancy

Many women are nervous because they don't think they would know if something important or serious happened during pregnancy. Most women have few, if any, problems during pregnancy. If you're concerned, the list below includes the most important symptoms to watch for. Call your healthcare provider if you experience any of the following:

- vaginal bleeding
- severe swelling of the face or fingers
- severe abdominal pain
- loss of fluid from the vagina, usually a gush of fluid, but sometimes a trickle or continuous wetness
- a big change in the baby's movement or a lack of movement
- high fever (more than 101.6F) or chills
- severe vomiting or an inability to keep food or liquid down
- blurring of vision
- painful urination
- a headache that won't go away or a severe headache
- an injury or accident, such as a fall or automobile accident, that causes you concern about the well-being of your baby

Later in pregnancy, if you can't feel baby moving, sit or lie down in a quiet room after eating a meal. Focus on how often the baby moves. If you don't feel at least 10 fetal movements in 2 hours, call your healthcare provider.

Be sure to talk about any concerns you have. Don't be embarrassed to ask questions about anything; your healthcare provider has probably heard it before. He or she would rather know about problems while they may be easier to deal with.

If necessary, you may be referred to a *perinatologist,* an obstetrician who has spent an additional 2 years or more in specialized obstetrical training. These specialists have experience caring for women with high-risk pregnancies.

You may not have a high-risk pregnancy at the beginning of your pregnancy. But if problems develop with you or baby, you may be referred to a perinatologist for consultation and possible care. You may be able to return to your regular healthcare provider for your delivery.

If you see a perinatologist, you may have to deliver your baby at a hospital other than the one you had chosen. This is usually because the hospital has specialized facilities or can administer specialized tests and/or care to you or your baby.

Dad Tip

You're nearly halfway through your pregnancy. Time may be passing very quickly for you both. Make an effort to spend some couple time with your partner. When you can, take some time off from work or other obligations. Together, focus on the pregnancy and preparing for the birth of your baby. You might even suggest a babymoon to guarantee you have quality couple time together. See the discussion in Week 27.

Your Nutrition

Herbal Use in Pregnancy

If you normally use herbs and botanicals—in the forms of teas, tinctures, pills or powders—to treat various medical and health problems, stop! We advise you *not* to treat yourself with any herbal remedy during pregnancy *without checking first with your healthcare provider!*

You may believe an herbal remedy is OK to use, but it could be dangerous during pregnancy. For example, if you're constipated, you may decide to use senna as a laxative. However, senna may cause a miscarriage. Or you may have used St. John's wort before pregnancy. Avoid it now—St. John's wort can interfere with various medicines. Avoid dong quai, pennyroyal, rosemary (used for digestive problems, not cooking), juniper, thuja, blue cohosh and senna during pregnancy.

> If you have hay fever during early pregnancy, your baby is 6 times more likely also to have hay fever.

Play it safe—be extremely careful with any substance your healthcare provider has not specifically recommended for you. Always check with him or her first before you take anything!

You Should Also Know

Allergies during Pregnancy

Allergies occur when the immune system reacts to a substance as if it's harmful. The body releases chemicals to fight the substance. Common reactions include nasal congestion, sneezing, runny nose, and itchy eyes and inner ears. Allergies can be caused by pollen in grasses, weeds, trees and mold.

Forty million people in the United States suffer from allergies. Nearly 10% of all pregnant women have seasonal allergies. They may get a little worse during pregnancy. Some fortunate women notice they get better during pregnancy, and symptoms improve.

If you use allergy medicine, don't assume it's safe during pregnancy. Some may not be advised, such as sudafed during the first trimester. Many are combinations of several medicines. Ask your healthcare provider about your medicine, whether prescription or nonprescription, including nasal sprays.

Medicines that are OK to use during pregnancy include antihistamines and decongestants. Ask your healthcare provider which brands are safest for you. Under his or her supervision, you can continue taking allergy shots, but don't start them now.

Try to avoid anything that triggers your allergies. If dust bothers you, keep windows closed. Use the air conditioner in your car and home. Don't hang clothes, towels or sheets outside to dry.

Avoid outdoor activities in the morning, when the pollen is usually at its worst. Wear a pollen-filtering mask when you're outside. Take a shower as soon as you come in from outdoors to wash away pollen.

Thoroughly clean the inside of your home. Wear a mask when you vacuum, and use a vacuum cleaner with a HEPA filter. Use a humidifier if you live in a very dry climate. Clean the filter in your home at least once a month.

> If you have a ragweed allergy, don't eat bananas, cucumbers, zucchini, melons or sunflower seeds. Avoid drinking chamomile tea. These are all in the ragweed family and may make symptoms worse.

Nasal Congestion

Congestion during pregnancy is normal in many women. It can be especially bad during allergy season when you're pregnant, so you may feel very stuffed up!

Decongestants reduce nasal swelling by narrowing blood vessels in the nose. Most experts agree you can use Afrin as short-term relief to help reduce swelling. For longer relief, talk to your healthcare provider about using long-term-relief products, such as Nasalcrom, which are considered safe during pregnancy. Discuss it with your healthcare provider.

Will You Be a Single Mother?

In the past years, we have seen an increase in the number of single moms. Today, over 40% of all babies in the United States are born to unmarried women. The largest number of single moms is women in their 20s—the average age is 26½.

Nearly 75% of all unmarried moms-to-be got pregnant by accident. Under 15% of single mothers are divorced. Nearly 45% of single mothers consider themselves truly single. Eight percent of single moms have a same-sex partner.

Many women choose to have a child without a spouse; situations vary. Some women are deeply involved with baby's father but have chosen not to marry. Some women are pregnant without their partner's support. Still other single women have chosen donor (artificial) insemination as a means of getting pregnant.

No matter what the personal situation is, many concerns are shared by all single moms-to-be. This discussion reflects some of the issues they have raised.

In most situations—whether a mother is single, widowed or divorced—a child's overall environment is more important than the presence of a man in the household. Over 85% of single-parent households in the United States are headed by women. Studies show if a woman has other supportive adults to depend on, a child can fare well in a home headed by a single woman. However, both boys and girls benefit from male involvement in their lives from an early age.

If you will be a single mother, seek support from family and friends. Mothers of young children can identify with your experiences—they've had similar ones recently. If you have friends or family members with young children, talk with them.

Raising a child alone can be both challenging and joyful. A single mother must take extra-good care of herself physically and emotionally. You may feel isolated and overwhelmed, so it's important to have a strong support system of family and/or friends. Many single moms find it easier to live and parent when they share expenses and daily activities with family or friends by living together.

Find people you can count on for help during your pregnancy and after your baby arrives. One woman said she thought about whom she would call at 2am if her baby were crying uncontrollably. When she answered that question, she had the name of someone she believed she could count on in any type of emergency—during and after pregnancy!

You may want to choose someone to be with you when you labor and deliver, and who will be there to help afterward. A doula can be a good choice for you, if you're going to have natural childbirth. Your insurance company may even pay for a doula's services.

Childbirth classes are now offered in many places for single moms. Many hospitals and birthing centers have options for single women when they give birth. Ask at your healthcare provider's office for further information.

The only part of the birth experience that might require special planning is your plan to get to the hospital when you go into labor. One woman wanted her friend to drive, but couldn't reach her when the time came. Her next option (all part of her plan) was to call a taxi, which got her to the hospital in plenty of time.

Wondering how much it will cost *you* to raise your child until he or she is 18? The U.S. Department of Agriculture (USDA) has information on its website to help you figure it out. Visit the USDA website and search for *Cost of Raising a Child Calculator* for more information.

After the birth, you'll need support when you go home with baby. Consider asking family members, friends, co-workers and neighbors to help out. You'll probably need the most help the first month home. Some chores and errands people can do include some alone time for you, laundry, cooking, cleaning and shopping.

If you find yourself feeling apart from family and friends, make friends with other single moms for emotional and spiritual support. This can also provide you a support group for social interaction and exchanging child care and other tasks.

You Need a Will. You need a will. If you don't have one, now's the time to make one. If you already have a will, check it before baby's birth for any changes or additions you may want to make.

If something happens to you, someone will have to care for your child. Your will should name a legal guardian for your child. Naming a guardian may be one of the most important things you can address at this time. Without a will that names a guardian, the courts decide who will care for your child.

After you decide on a guardian, *ask* that person before naming him or her as guardian in your will. He or she may have reasons you don't know about for not being able to accept this important role. Choose at least two people who could be the guardian of your child. Ask your first choice, and if he or she accepts, put the name in your will. Choose an alternative guardian (again, be sure to ask the person you select about it first), and tell that person that he or she will be named as the alternative.

If you believe you would prefer to have someone else handle finances for your child, you can name a separate *property guardian.* This person's main responsibility is to take care of any financial assets you leave your child.

Some people will say you don't need an attorney to draw up your will if you don't have a lot of property or many assets. They believe do-it-yourself will kits available in some stores or on various computer programs cover all the bases. Some are fairly thorough; however, if you're not an attorney, you may be saving money now, but it could cost your child or family later. If you're unmarried, an attorney may be helpful in covering all the necessary aspects so your child and/or partner will inherit your assets.

If you do use a do-it-yourself will kit, you may want to ask an attorney to check it over when you're finished, to be sure you have covered everything. It may cost a little extra, but it could be well worth it if it saves your child problems in the future.

Check Your Insurance. Be sure to check your insurance coverage before baby's birth. You must arrange where money will come from to care for your child in case of your death. You also need enough disability insurance to provide for your future and baby's future.

If something happens to you, you want to know your child will be provided for and financially taken care of until he or she is an adult. This is most often provided through a life-insurance policy. When examining your life insurance, look at other types of insurance you have. Examine coverage you have now, and determine what type of coverage you'll need after baby's arrival. It's time to make necessary changes!

When insurance is provided by your employer, check with the human resources (HR) representative for specific information about the insurance and its benefits. Don't overlook this important resource.

It's important to have enough life insurance to cover raising your child through college. The U.S. government estimates it costs between $225,000 and $300,000 to raise a child born today through the age of 18. Add to that what the projected costs of college may be in 18 years. This is the amount of coverage you should have. You need sufficient life-insurance coverage to be sure there will be enough money to care for your child into adulthood.

You should also review your health insurance. If you don't have healthcare coverage, you may find it difficult to get coverage at this time. Many companies have a waiting period of 1 year before they will cover costs associated with childbirth. You might want to check to see if there is any type of coverage that might be available through various community programs. Or check out children's health-insurance programs in your state. Some provide medical coverage for a pregnant woman and her baby (after birth). Some programs are free; others are low-cost. These may be available to you even if you are working.

Check your health-insurance policy to see what the time limit is for adding baby to your health insurance. In some cases, a baby must be added within 30 days following the birth or no coverage will be provided.

If you have an accident that requires you to take time off your job, disability insurance is good coverage to have. It pays you a predetermined amount of money while you're disabled. Most employers provide some disability insurance, but *every working parent* should have enough insurance to cover between 65 and 75% of his or her income.

Your employer may provide disability insurance. The drawback to disability insurance through your employment is coverage stops when you leave the job, and benefits may be fairly low. You may also need to be on the job a certain amount of time before you're covered. If your employer doesn't provide disability insurance, consider purchasing a policy on your own. Consult an insurance specialist for further information.

Protect Your Documents

Once you've made your will, keep the original in a safe place. If an attorney prepares yours, he or she will keep an original at the office. You might consider keeping a copy in a fireproof safety box at home.

If you use a do-it-yourself will kit, keep your original document in a safe-deposit box at the bank and a copy in a fireproof safety box at home. If you choose a relative to be the executor of your estate, you might also consider giving him or her a copy to have at hand.

Legal Questions. Because your situation is unique, various situations may occur that will raise questions. You may be wondering how to fill out baby's birth certificate. You have options. You can fill in the father's name or leave it blank. If you don't want people to know the father's identity, you can leave it off the birth certificate. If baby's father is a donor, you can list the name as *unknown* or *confidential.*

Today, a father is required by law to pay child support, even if he isn't involved in his child's life. Consult an attorney to check the laws in your state. If you put baby's father's name on the birth certificate, it may be easier to ask legally for child support. However, this gives the father some legal rights. In some states, a man must sign a *parental acknowledgment* form before you can list him as baby's father on the birth certificate.

You may also have questions about the last name to give your baby. You need to make a decision as to what it will be. Yours? Dad's? In some states, if you're not married, the father must grant permission for you to use his last name.

You don't have to fill out a birth certificate before leaving the hospital. You may have a few months before this must be turned in. However, you can't get a social-security number for your baby without providing a birth certificate. A social-security number is necessary to open a bank account in baby's name and to claim him or her on tax forms. It may also be needed to add baby to your health insurance.

It's important to have answers to your questions. The following questions have been posed by women who chose to be single mothers. We repeat them here without answers because they are legal questions that should be reviewed with an attorney in your area who specializes in family law. These can help you clarify the kinds of questions you need to consider as a single mother. If you become pregnant through donor insemination, much of the legal issues will be dealt with in your dealings with the organization through which you received your donor sperm.

- A friend who had a baby by herself told me I'd better consider the legal ramifications of this situation. What was she talking about?
- I've heard that in some states, if I'm unmarried, I have to get a special birth certificate. Is that true?
- I'm having my baby alone, and I'm concerned about who can make medical decisions for me and my expected baby. Can I do anything about this concern?
- I'm not married, but I am deeply involved with my baby's father. Can my partner make medical decisions for me if I have problems during labor or after the birth?
- If anything happens to me, can my partner make medical decisions for our baby after it is born?
- What are the legal rights of my baby's father if we are not married?
- Do my partner's parents have legal rights in regard to their grandchild (my child)?
- My baby's father and I went our separate ways before I knew I was pregnant. Do I have to tell him about the baby?
- I chose to have donor (artificial) insemination. If anything happens to me during my labor or delivery, who can make medical decisions for me? Who can make decisions for my baby?
- I got pregnant by donor insemination. What do I put on the birth certificate under "father's name"?
- Is there a way I can find out more about my sperm donor's family medical history?
- Will the sperm bank send me notices if medical problems appear in my sperm donor's family?
- As my child grows up, she may need some sort of medical help (such as a donor kidney) from a sibling. Will the sperm bank supply family information?

- I had donor insemination, and I'm concerned about the rights of the baby's father to be part of my child's life in the future. Should I be concerned?
- Someone joked to me that my child could marry its sister or brother some day and wouldn't know it because I had donor insemination. Is this possible?
- Are there any other things I should consider because of my unique situation?

If the baby's father could claim custody of your child, it's best to work out details with an attorney. Don't assume you will automatically have sole custody if the father wasn't a participant in the pregnancy and/or birth.

Exercise for Week 19

Stand with your right side about 2 feet away from the wall. Put your left foot 12 inches in front of your right foot. Bend both knees slightly. Place your right hand on the wall for support. Lift your left arm up and stretch toward the wall, bending your head. Next, encircling your head with your left arm, touch your right ear. Hold for 5 seconds. Return to standing position. Repeat 5 times, then turn and stretch for the wall with your right arm. *Stretches lower-back and side muscles.*

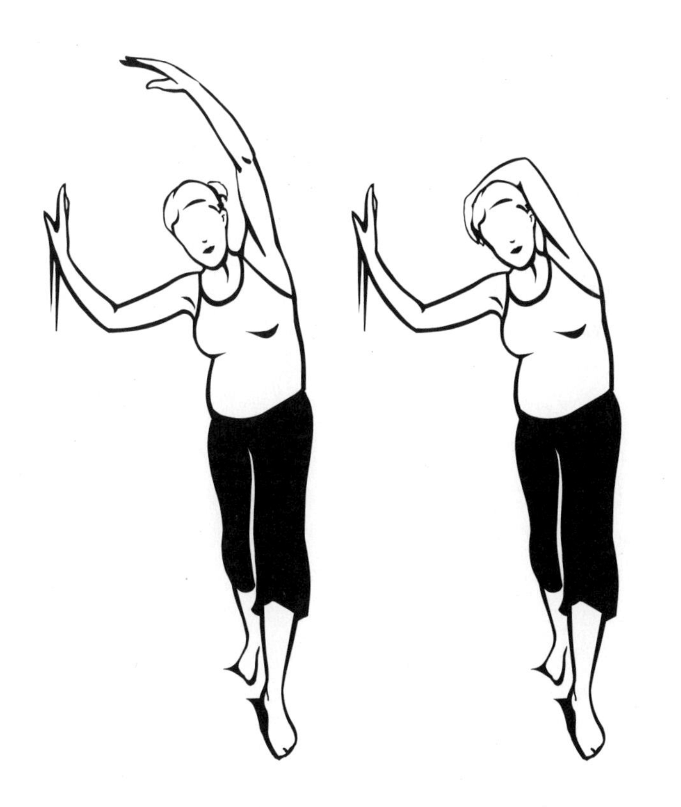

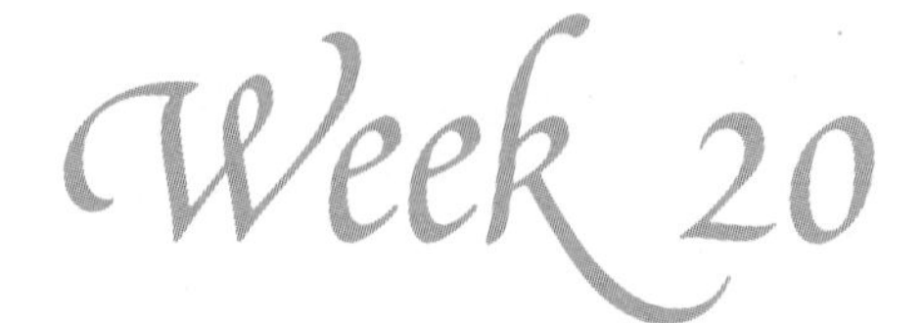

Week 20

Age of Fetus—18 Weeks

How Big Is Your Baby?

At this point in development, the crown-to-rump length is 5⅔ to 6½ inches (14 to 16cm). Your baby weighs about 9 ounces (260g).

How Big Are You?

Congratulations—20 weeks marks the midpoint. You're halfway through your pregnancy!

Your uterus is probably about even with your bellybutton. Your healthcare provider has been watching your growth and the enlargement of your uterus. Growth to this point may have been irregular but usually becomes more regular after the 20th week.

Measuring the Growth of Your Uterus

Your uterus is measured to keep track of your baby's growth. Your healthcare provider may use a measuring tape or his or her fingers and measure by finger breadth. He or she needs a point of reference against which to measure growth. Some healthcare providers measure from your bellybutton. Many measure from the pubic symphysis, the place where the pubic bones meet in the middle-lower part of your abdomen, 6 to 10 inches (15.2 to 25.4cm) below the bellybutton. It may be felt near your pubic hairline.

Not every healthcare provider measures the same way, and not every woman is the same size. And babies vary in size. Measurements differ among women and are often different for a woman from one pregnancy to another.

If you see a healthcare provider you don't normally see or if you see someone new, you may measure differently. This doesn't mean there's a problem or that someone is measuring incorrectly. It's just that everyone measures a little differently.

Measurements are made from the pubic symphysis to the top of the uterus. After this point, you should grow almost ½ inch (1cm) each week. If you're 8 inches (20cm) at 20 weeks, at your next visit (4 weeks later), you should measure about 10 inches (24cm).

If you measure 11¼ inches (28cm) at this point in pregnancy, an ultrasound may be recommended to see if you're carrying twins or to see if your due date is correct. If you only measure 6 inches (15 to 16cm), your due date could be wrong, or there may be a concern about intrauterine-growth restriction (IUGR) or some other problem.

Within limits, changing measurements are a sign of fetal well-being and fetal growth. If they aren't normal, it can be a warning sign. If you're concerned about your size and the growth of your pregnancy, discuss it with your healthcare provider.

How Your Baby Is Growing and Developing

Your Baby's Skin

The skin covering your baby began growing from two layers, the *epidermis,* which is on the surface, and the *dermis,* which is the deeper layer. By this point, there are four layers. One of these layers contains ridges, which are responsible for patterns on fingertips, palms and soles. They are genetically determined.

When a baby is born, its skin is covered by a white substance that looks like paste, called *vernix.* It is

> **Tip for Week 20**
>
> If you have an ultrasound test now, it may be possible to find out the sex of the baby, but baby must cooperate. You have to be able to see the genitals. Even if the sex looks obvious, ultrasound operators have been known to make mistakes!

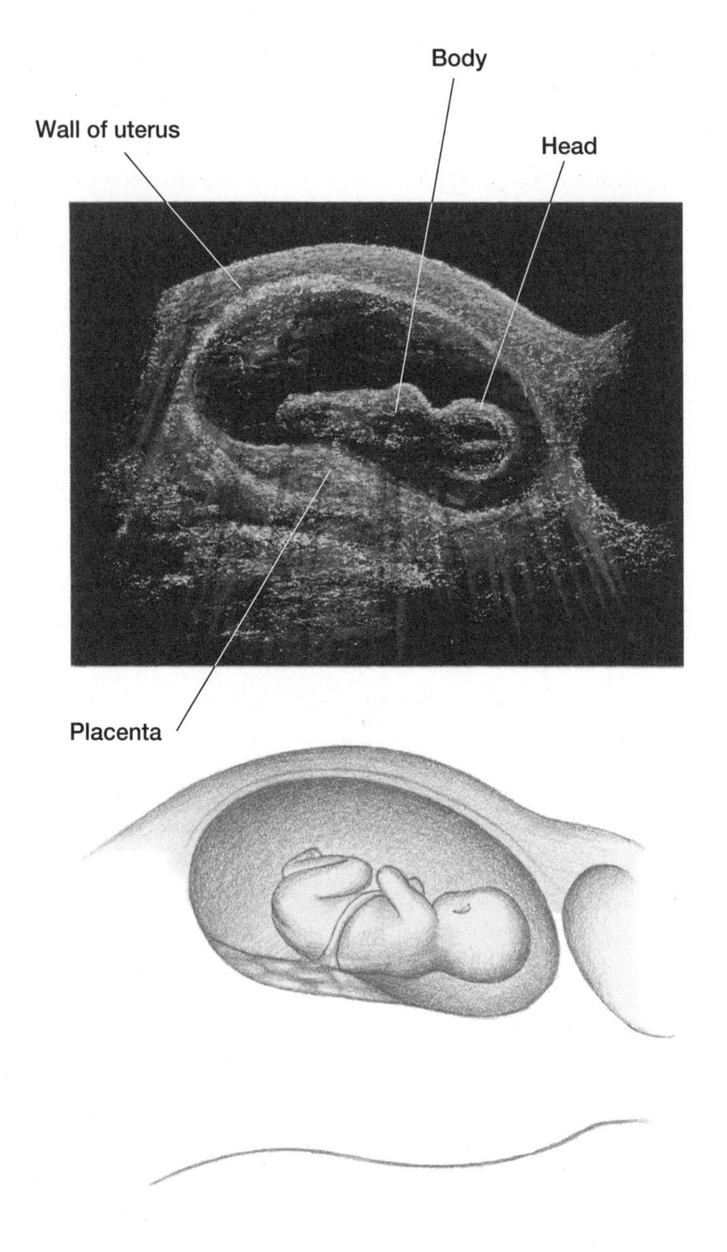

Ultrasound of a baby at 20 weeks gestation (fetal age—18 weeks). The interpretive illustration may help you see more detail.

secreted by the glands in the skin beginning around this week. Vernix protects your growing baby's skin from amniotic fluid.

Hair appears at around 12 to 14 weeks and grows from the epidermis. Hair is first seen on the baby's upper lip and eyebrow. This hair is usually shed around the time of birth and is replaced by thicker hair from new follicles.

Ultrasound Pictures

The illustration on page 286 shows an ultrasound exam (and an interpretive illustration) in a pregnant woman at about 20 weeks. An ultrasound is often easier to understand when it is actually being done. The pictures are more like motion pictures.

If you look closely at the illustration, it may make more sense to you. Read the labels, and try to visualize the baby inside the uterus. An ultrasound picture is like looking at a slice of an object. The picture you see is 2-dimensional.

> Don't have one of those ultrasound "keepsakes" done at your local mall. Ultrasound at the mall can be risky to you and baby because untrained technicians doing the test may not use equipment correctly. In addition, in 2002, the FDA ruled that performing an ultrasound without a prescription is illegal.

Ultrasound done at this point in pregnancy is helpful for confirming or helping to establish your due date. If this test is done very early or very late (first or last 2 months), the accuracy of dating a pregnancy may not be as good. If two or more babies are present, they can usually be seen. Some fetal problems can also be seen at this time.

Percutaneous Umbilical-Cord Blood Sampling (PUBS)

Percutaneous umbilical-cord blood sampling (PUBS), also called *cordocentesis,* is a test done on the fetus inside your uterus. Test results are available in a few days. The test carries a slightly higher risk of miscarriage than amniocentesis.

Guided by ultrasound, a fine needle is inserted through the mother's abdomen into a tiny vein in the umbilical cord. A small sample of the baby's blood is removed for analysis. PUBS detects blood disorders, infections and Rh-incompatibility.

A baby can be checked before birth and a blood transfusion can be given, if necessary. PUBS can help prevent life-threatening anemia that may develop if the mother is Rh-negative and has antibodies that are destroying her baby's blood. If you're Rh-negative, you should receive RhoGAM after this procedure.

Changes in You

Stretching Abdominal Muscles

Your abdominal muscles are being stretched and pushed apart as your baby grows. Muscles attached to the lower portion of your ribs run vertically down to your pelvis. They may separate in the midline. These muscles are called the rectus muscles; when they separate, it is a hernia called a *diastasis recti.*

You may notice the separation when you lie down and you raise your head, tightening your abdominal muscles. It may look like there's a bulge in the middle of your tummy. You might even feel the edge of the muscle on either side of the bulge. It isn't painful and doesn't harm you or baby. What you feel in the gap between the muscles is the uterus. You may feel the baby's movement more easily here.

If this is your first baby, you may not notice the separation. With each pregnancy, separation is often more noticeable. Exercising can strengthen these muscles, but you may still have the bulge or gap.

Following pregnancy, these muscles tighten and close the gap. The separation won't be as noticeable, but it may still be present.

Rheumatoid Arthritis (RA)

Rheumatoid arthritis (RA) affects 1 in every 1000 pregnant women. It's an autoimmune disease that can attack your body's joints and/or organs. During pregnancy, symptoms may improve and even disappear. Nearly 75% of women with RA feel better when they're pregnant. Less pain may mean you need less medication.

Some medicines used to treat RA can be dangerous to a pregnant woman, but many are safe. Be sure to talk to your healthcare provider about any medicine you take for your rheumatoid arthritis *before* you get pregnant.

Acetaminophen is OK to use throughout pregnancy. However, NSAIDs should not be used in later pregnancy because they may increase the risk of heart problems in baby. Prednisone is usually acceptable, although methotrexate should *not* be used because it may cause miscarriage and birth defects.

Enbrel is one of the newer medications used to treat RA. Don't use this medication without checking first with your healthcare provider.

RA may not affect your labor and delivery; however, 25% of women with RA have a preterm birth. It may be harder to find comfortable labor positions if you have joint restrictions.

Your symptoms may return a few months after baby is born. See your rheumatologist within 4 weeks of having your baby. He or she may want you to restart medicine you stopped taking during pregnancy. If you breastfeed, discuss the choice of medications with your healthcare provider before resuming them.

Dad Tip

Around this time, your partner may have an ultrasound exam of your growing baby. Your partner's healthcare provider does one to learn many things. You might want to be there for this fun test—it's the first time you can actually see baby moving! Ask your partner to consider your schedule when making the appointment for her ultrasound.

How Your Actions Affect Your Baby's Development

Sexual Relations

Pregnancy can be an important time of growing closer to your partner. As you get larger, sexual intercourse may become difficult because of discomfort for you. With some imagination and different positions (ones in which you aren't on your back and your partner isn't directly on top of you), you can continue to enjoy sexual relations.

If you feel emotional pressure from your partner—either his concern about the safety of intercourse or requests for frequent sexual relations—discuss it openly with him. Ask your partner to come to a prenatal visit to discuss these things with your healthcare provider.

If you're having problems with contractions, bleeding or complications, you and your partner should talk with your healthcare provider. Together you can decide whether you should continue to have sexual relations. If your healthcare provider advises against sex, ask whether this means no intercourse or no orgasm.

You May Be Sexier than You Think

Pregnancy is sexy! We know many men think their pregnant partner is more beautiful and sexier than ever before, especially during this middle part of pregnancy. Below are reasons men have given us as to why they think their pregnant partner is sexy.

- Your skin may be smoother and softer because you use more lotions and oils.
- You ask for massages and back rubs, which may lead to further massage and sexual intimacy.
- Discovering different ways to make love can be fun.
- Sex during pregnancy often requires some creative thinking on both your parts.
- Your pregnancy makes him walk like a man. For many men, their partner's pregnancy is a source of pride.
- You may have more cleavage (or cleavage when you've never had it before).
- Your hair may be luxurious, nails may be long and skin glowing.
- You may be feeling very sexy due to increased blood flow to your pelvic area.
- Your curves can be sexy.
- Pregnancy hormones may increase your sexual desire.
- Your changing figure, such as enlarging breasts, may turn him on.
- The level of commitment you feel toward your partner may intensify your intimacy, both sexually and nonsexually. Having a child together may be the ultimate act of trust.
- You're carefree because you don't have to worry about birth control.

Body Art

We have seen an increase in piercings and tattoos of women. These types of body art may lead to situations during pregnancy that must be dealt with, so an understanding of some of the problems that may occur may help you understand where your healthcare provider is coming from if he or she has a concern.

Body piercing has been around since ancient civilization and is popular again. The most popular form of piercing is pierced earlobes—many women have pierced ears. This is a low-risk type of piercing your healthcare provider won't be concerned about.

However, other places on the body may be pierced, including the eyebrow, nostril, nasal septum, lips, tongue, nipples, navel, labia and clitoral hood; these piercings may cause your healthcare provider concern. With oral piercing, there's a chance for various infections and for swallowing jewelry. Nipple piercing can damage milk ducts, which could interfere with breastfeeding. Navel jewelry must be removed after about 3 or 4 months of pregnancy due to the stretching tummy. Leaving jewelry in the navel could lead to ripping or tearing. With any type of piercing, there's the possibility of scar-tissue formation. This is especially common with people of African descent.

If you have any oral piercings, your healthcare provider may discuss removing them before delivery. In some cases, anesthesiologists are concerned about keeping your airway open if jewelry is not removed. This situation isn't common, but no one can predict what labor and delivery will involve, so it may be safer to remove the jewelry as you get closer to your due date.

If you have any piercings (other than earlobes), bring them to the attention of your healthcare provider. Discuss any suggestions for removing jewelry, if you're concerned.

Like body piercing, *tattoos* have been part of many cultures for thousands of years. Today, many people have tattoos; the most common sites are the arms, chest, back, abdomen and legs. Some problems pregnant women with tattoos have include infection, allergic reaction, formation of scar tissue at the tattoo site, stretch marks in the area of the tattoo and removal of an unwanted tattoo.

Do not be surprised to see a change in your tattoo if it's located on a body part or in an area that can be affected by pregnancy. For example, the cute little butterfly on your abdomen may grow very large during pregnancy. In addition, stretch marks may run through it. After pregnancy, skin may remain stretched, and the cute little butterfly droops and sags until skin returns to "normal" after pregnancy, which may not be like "normal" before pregnancy.

Feeling unattractive during pregnancy? Help yourself feel beautiful by keeping pretty things around you, like flowers or a beautiful picture. You may also help yourself by *telling* yourself you're beautiful. Buy some sexy lingerie that makes you feel sexy. Boy shorts will flatter your legs, and floaty tops can camouflage your tummy.

Tattoo removal during pregnancy is not recommended. Neither is getting a new tattoo. You don't want to increase your chances of getting an infection, which is a risk when you get a tattoo. Wait until after baby's birth to receive or to remove a tattoo.

There have been rumors that women who have tattoos on their lower backs can't have regional anesthesia, such as epidurals and spinal anesthesia. However, no studies have shown this to be true. Discuss any concerns you have about anesthesia and your tattoos with your healthcare provider.

Your Nutrition

Many women use sugar and/or artificial sweeteners before pregnancy. Are they safe during pregnancy?

Caloric sweeteners include processed and unprocessed sugars, such as granulated sugar, brown sugar and corn syrup. Unprocessed sugars include honey, agave nectar and raw sugar. Caloric content ranges from 16 to 22 calories per teaspoon. If you use caloric sweeteners, you're adding empty calories to your meal plan.

Artificial (noncaloric) sweeteners help a woman cut calories. Some common artificial sweeteners include aspartame, acesulfame K, sucralose, stevia and saccharin. Can a pregnant woman use artificial sweeteners?

Aspartame is used in many foods and beverages to help reduce calories and is sold under the brand names Nutrasweet and Equal. It's a combination of two amino acids—phenylalanine and aspartic acid. If you suffer from phenylketonuria, you can't use aspartame. You must follow a low-phenylalanine diet or your baby may be adversely affected.

Sucralose, sold under the brand name Splenda, is made from sugar and is found in a variety of products. It passes through the body without being metabolized. Your body doesn't recognize it as a sugar or a carbohydrate, which makes it low calorie.

Stevia is a product made from the leaves of the stevia plant. It's been sold for decades in other parts of the world. It was approved for use in the United States in 2008 and is sold under the brand names PureVia and Truvia. Ask your healthcare provider for information about using it during pregnancy.

Saccharin is an artificial sweetener used in many foods and beverages. Although it is not used as much today as in the past, it still appears in many foods, beverages and other substances. Saccharin is also added to many foods and beverages.

Research has determined that artificial sweeteners are probably safe to use in small amounts during pregnancy. However, if you can avoid them, it's best *not* to use them during pregnancy. Eliminate any substance you don't really need from the foods you eat and the beverages you drink. Do it for the good of your baby.

Grandma's Remedy

If you want to avoid using medication, try a folk remedy. If you experience foot odor, spray some antiperspirant on your feet—it helps reduce odor and may prevent skin cracking.

You Should Also Know

Hearing Your Baby's Heartbeat

It may be possible to hear your baby's heartbeat with a stethoscope at 20 weeks. Before we had doppler equipment to hear the heartbeat and ultrasound to see the heart beating, a stethoscope helped the listener hear the baby's heartbeat. This usually occurred after quickening for most women.

The sound you hear through a stethoscope may be different than what you're used to hearing at the office. It isn't loud. If you've never listened through a stethoscope, it may be difficult to hear at first. It does get easier as the baby gets larger and sounds become louder.

If you can't hear your baby's heartbeat with a stethoscope, don't worry. It's not always easy for a healthcare provider who does this on a regular basis!

If you hear a swishing sound (baby's heartbeat), you have to differentiate it from a beating sound (mother's heartbeat). A baby's heart beats rapidly, usually 120 to 160 beats every minute. Your heartbeat or pulse rate is slower, in the range of 60 to 80 beats a minute. Ask your healthcare provider to help you distinguish the sounds.

Could You Have Osteoporosis?

Osteoporosis is a bone disease in which bones lose density and the spaces within them grow larger, resulting in increased chance of breakage. It's typically diagnosed in older, postmenopausal women. However, it's now being diagnosed in younger women.

We believe low-calorie diets, excessive exercise and drinking lots of diet soda may be possible causes. In addition, low body weight, anemia and amenorrhea (menstruation stops) may add to the problem. Your lifestyle may put you at risk. Women who smoke or drink a lot of alcohol may increase that risk.

Osteoporosis at a young age can be serious. Bones may become so thin they actually break. In later years, osteoporosis may be severe.

If you believe you may have a problem, talk to your healthcare provider about it. If you do have osteoporosis, it could have an effect on you during your pregnancy.

❧ *West Nile Virus (WNV)*

West Nile virus (WNV) is spread to humans by mosquito bites. If you get WNV, you may have no symptoms; 80% of those with West Nile virus *never* develop symptoms. Or you may get West Nile fever or severe West Nile disease. It's estimated that 20% of people who become infected with WNV will develop West Nile fever.

Symptoms appear within 3 to 14 days after being bitten and include fever, headache, fatigue, swollen lymph nodes and body aches. A skin rash on the torso appears occasionally. While the illness can be as short as a few days, even healthy people have reported being sick for several weeks.

Symptoms of severe disease, also called *West Nile encephalitis* or *meningitis* or *West Nile poliomyelitis*, include headache, high fever, neck stiffness, stupor, disorientation, coma, tremors, convulsions, muscle weakness and paralysis. These symptoms may last several weeks.

We don't know what percentage of WNV infections during pregnancy result in infection of the unborn child or medical problems in newborns. The CDC and state and local health departments record birth effects among women who had West Nile virus during pregnancy.

There is no treatment for WNV infection. If the illness is diagnosed, a detailed ultrasound can be done to evaluate the fetus for structural abnormalities. This should be done 2 to 4 weeks after onset of the illness.

If you're pregnant and live in an area with WNV, use caution to lower your risk. Avoid mosquito-infested areas, use screens on windows and doors, wear protective clothing and use an EPA-registered repellent (one that has been reviewed for safety by the U.S. Environmental Protection Agency). You can use insect repellent containing DEET. There have been no reported harmful events following use of repellents containing DEET in women or their babies. The CDC also recommends using picaridin on skin and clothing, and permethrin on clothing. Oil of lemon eucalyptus is another recommended option, but it isn't as long-lasting.

If you become ill, call your healthcare provider. If he or she believes you may have contracted the illness, diagnostic testing can be done. After baby's birth, if you have symptoms of West Nile virus, don't breastfeed.

Exercise for Week 20

Kneel on your hands and knees, with your wrists directly beneath your shoulders and your knees directly beneath your hips. Keep your back straight. Contract your tummy muscles, then extend your left leg behind you at hip height. At the same time, extend your right arm at shoulder height. Hold 5 seconds, and return to the kneeling position. Repeat on your other side. Start with 4 repetitions on each side, and gradually work up to 8. *Strengthens buttocks muscles, back muscles and leg muscles.*

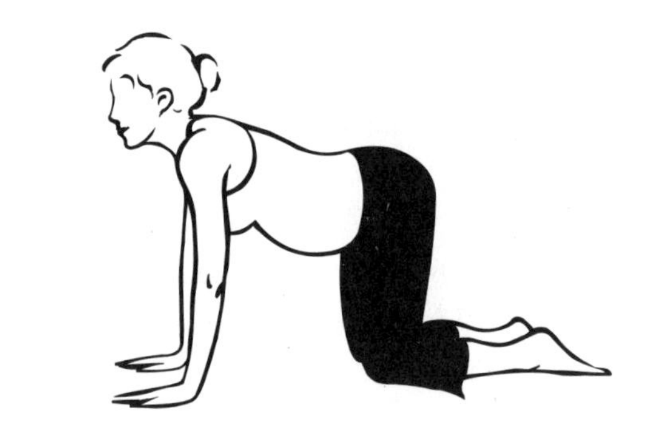

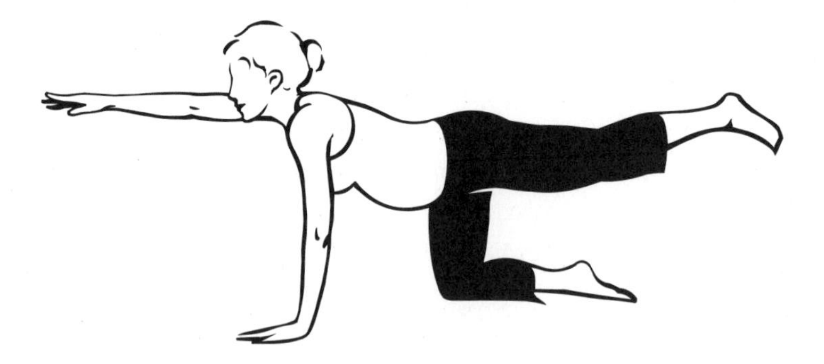

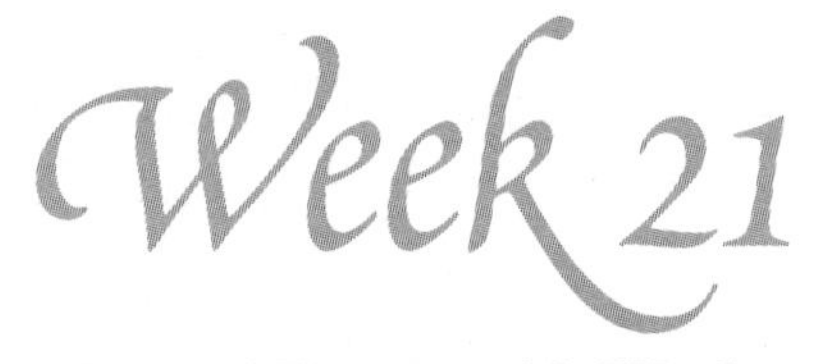

Age of Fetus—19 Weeks

How Big Is Your Baby?

Your baby now weighs about 10½ ounces (300g); its crown-to-rump length is about 7¼ inches (18cm). It's about the size of a large banana.

How Big Are You?

When your healthcare provider measures your uterus, it's almost 8½ inches (21cm) from the pubic symphysis. Your weight gain should be between 10 and 15 pounds (4.5 and 6.3kg).

By this week, your waistline is definitely gone. Your friends and relatives—and strangers—can tell you're pregnant. It would be hard to hide your condition!

How Your Baby Is Growing and Developing

Rapid growth rate of your baby has slowed. However, the baby continues to grow and to develop as different organ systems within the baby mature.

Baby's digestive system is functioning in a simple way, and baby swallows amniotic fluid. Researchers believe swallowing may help develop the digestive system. It may also condition the digestive system to function after birth. After swallowing fluid, baby absorbs much of the water and passes unabsorbed matter as far as the large bowel. With ultrasound, you can see the baby swallowing.

Studies indicate full-term babies may swallow as much as 17 ounces (500ml) of amniotic fluid in a 24-hour period. It contributes a small amount to baby's caloric needs and may contribute essential nutrients to the developing baby.

Meconium

During pregnancy, you may hear the term *meconium* and wonder what it means. It refers to undigested stuff in baby's digestive system. Meconium is made mostly of cells from the lining of baby's gastrointestinal tract and swallowed amniotic fluid.

It is a greenish-black to light-brown substance. It passes from baby's bowels before delivery, during labor or after birth. If present during labor, meconium may be an indication of fetal stress.

If a baby passes meconium into amniotic fluid, he or she may swallow the fluid. If meconium is inhaled into the lungs, baby could develop pneumonia or pneumonitis. For this reason, when meconium is found at delivery, an attempt is made to remove it from baby's mouth and throat with a small suction tube.

Changes in You

Swelling

You may notice swelling in various parts of your body, especially in your lower legs and feet, particularly at the end of the day. If you're on your feet a lot, you may notice less swelling if you can rest during the day.

Swelling often begins around week 24. Seventy-five percent of all pregnant women suffer from swollen fingers, ankles and feet. If your feet

> Your face may look fuller during pregnancy because of the weight you are supposed to gain and from water retention, which can cause some swelling in the facial area.

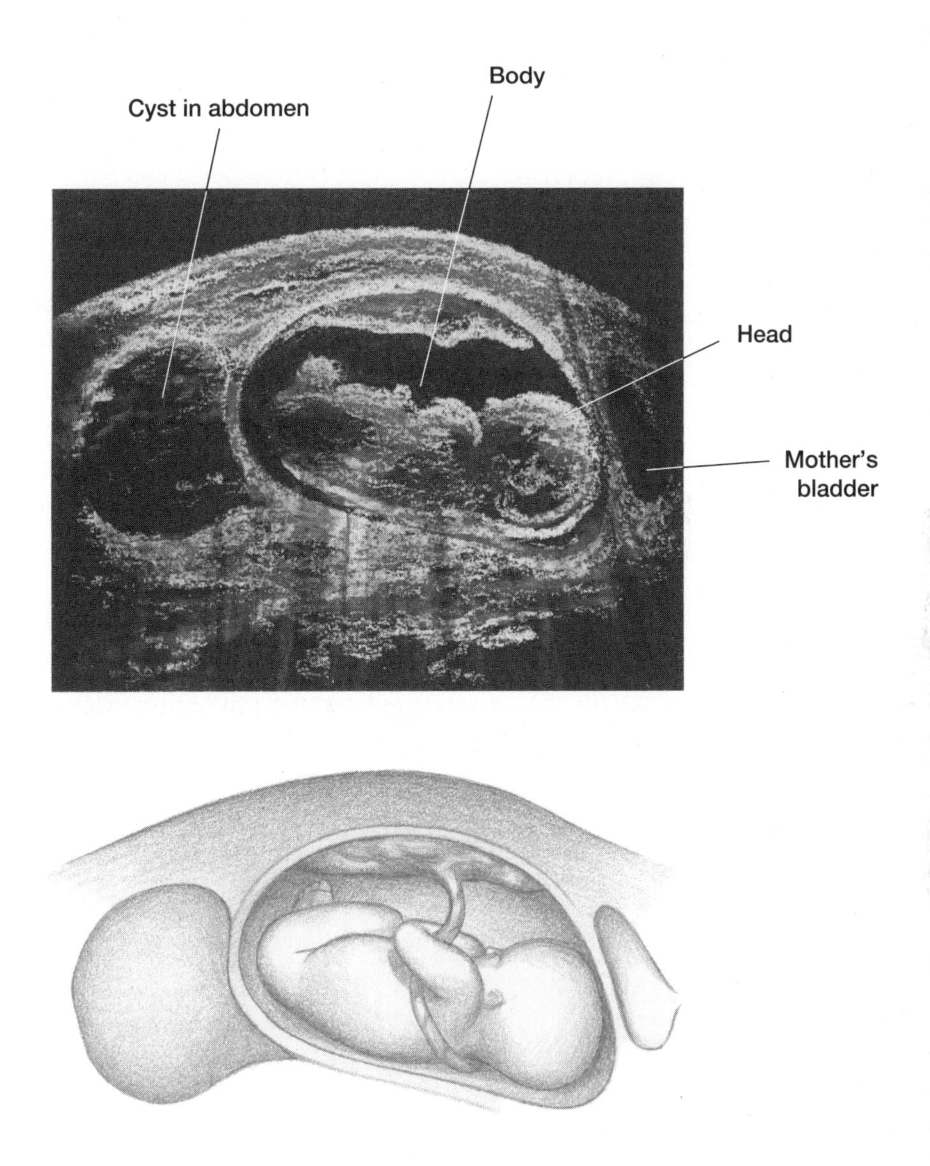

Ultrasound may be used to detect problems. In this ultrasound of a baby in utero, there is a cyst in the mother-to-be's abdomen. The interpretive illustration clarifies the ultrasound image.

swell, it can help to wear pregnancy support stockings to avoid blood from pooling in your feet. Ask your healthcare provider about them.

There are some things you can try to help control swelling. Prenatal massage may be good. Eat plenty of raisins and bananas; both are high in potassium. A potassium deficiency may allow your cells to fill with water, increasing swelling. Flexing your feet and ankles during the day helps keep blood circulating. You can also try standing on your tiptoes—it helps pump blood back to the heart. When sitting, press your toes down as if you were pushing on the gas pedal of your car to accomplish the same thing.

Blood Clots in the Legs

A serious complication of pregnancy is a blood clot in the legs or groin. Symptoms include swelling of the legs accompanied by leg pain and redness or warmth over the affected area in the legs.

This problem has many names, including *venous thrombosis, thromboembolic disease, thrombophlebitis* and *deep-vein thrombosis.* The problem is not limited to pregnancy, but pregnancy is a time when it may be more likely to occur due to blood flow slowing in the legs and changes in blood-clotting mechanisms.

The most probable cause during pregnancy is decreased blood flow, also called *stasis.* If you have had a previous blood clot—in your legs or any other part of your body—tell your healthcare provider at the beginning of your pregnancy. It's important information.

Help protect yourself from developing the problem by exercising, not sitting for longer than 2 hours, not smoking and not wearing tight clothing at or below your waist. Surgical stockings may help prevent the problem; heparin may be recommended in severe cases.

Superficial and Deep-Vein Thrombosis (DVT). Superficial thrombosis and deep-vein thrombosis are different conditions. *Superficial thrombosis* is a blood clot in veins close to the surface of the skin. You can see and feel these veins. This situation is not as serious and is treated with a mild pain reliever, elevation of the leg, support of the leg with an Ace bandage or support stockings, and occasionally heat.

Superficial thrombosis does not result in pulmonary embolism (PE). Pulmonary embolism is blockage of blood flow in the lungs; it results in failure of the lungs to work. If the condition doesn't improve rapidly, deep-vein thrombosis must be considered. DVT is more serious because a clot can travel from the legs to the lungs and cause PE.

Deep-vein thrombosis (DVT) affects nearly 2 million Americans every year; a very small percentage of them are pregnant women. Although it's a serious complication, it can often be avoided with early treatment. If you've had *any* blood clot in the past, see your healthcare provider early in pregnancy. Tell him or her at your first prenatal visit about any previous blood clots.

DVT is a blood clot that forms in the large veins in your legs. It's caused by blocked blood flow and changes in blood clotting during pregnancy. Onset can be rapid, with severe pain and swelling of the leg and thigh.

Symptoms of deep-vein thrombosis in the lower leg can differ, depending on the location of the clot and how bad it is. Symptoms include swelling in the leg, worsening cramp or pain in one leg, discoloration of the leg, including turning red, blue or purple, and/or a feeling of warmth in the affected leg. Often skin over the affected veins is red. There may even be streaks of red on the skin over veins where blood clots have occurred. If you have any of these symptoms, call your healthcare provider immediately.

Squeezing the calf or leg may be extremely painful, and it may be equally painful to walk. One way to tell if you have deep-vein thrombosis is to lie down and flex your toes toward your knee. If the back of the leg is tender, it can be a sign of the problem; this is called *Homan's sign.* (This type of pain may also occur with a strained muscle or a bruise.) Check with your healthcare provider if this occurs.

Ultrasound is usually used to diagnose the problem. Most major medical centers offer it, but the test is not available everywhere.

Treating DVT. Treatment usually consists of hospitalization and heparin therapy. Heparin and Lovenox (enoxaparin) are both anticoagulants. They are given intravenously and are safe to use during pregnancy.

While heparin is being administered, the woman is required to stay in bed. The leg may be elevated and heat applied. Mild pain medicine is often prescribed.

Recovery time, including hospitalization, may be 7 to 10 days. The woman will need to take heparin until delivery. Following pregnancy, she will need to continue taking an anticoagulant for up to several weeks, depending on the severity of the clot.

If a woman has a blood clot during one pregnancy, she will probably need heparin during her next pregnancies. If so, heparin can be given by an in-dwelling I.V. catheter or by daily injections the woman gives herself under her healthcare provider's supervision.

An oral medication used to prevent or to treat deep-vein thrombosis is warfarin (Coumadin). It is not given during pregnancy because it can be harmful to the baby. Warfarin is usually given to a woman after pregnancy to prevent blood clots. It may be prescribed for a few weeks or a few months, depending on the severity of the clot.

How Your Actions Affect Your Baby's Development

Safety of Ultrasound

On page 299 is an illustration of an ultrasound exam, accompanied by an interpretive illustration. These show a baby inside a uterus; the mother-to-be also has a large cyst in her abdomen.

Many women wonder about the safety of ultrasound exams. Medical researchers agree ultrasound exams don't pose any risk to you or your baby. Researchers have looked for potential problems for many years without finding evidence of any.

Ultrasound is an extremely valuable tool in diagnosing problems and answering some questions during pregnancy. The information ultrasound testing provides can be reassuring to the healthcare provider and the pregnant woman.

If your healthcare provider has recommended ultrasound for you and you're concerned about it, discuss it with him or her. He or she may have an important reason for doing an ultrasound exam. It could affect the well-being of your developing baby.

Eating Disorders—How Can They Affect Pregnancy?

About 7 million women in the United States have some type of eating disorder, and eating disorders are becoming more recognized in pregnant women. Experts believe as many as 1% of all pregnant women suffer from some degree of eating disorder. The two primary eating disorders are anorexia nervosa and bulimia nervosa. Other eating disorders include restricting calories or food, and weight obsession, but those afflicted with them don't meet the anorexia or bulimia criteria.

Women with *anorexia* usually weigh less than 85% of what is normal for their age and height. They are often very fearful of becoming fat, have an unrealistic body image, purge with laxatives or by vomiting, and binge. *Bulimia* is characterized by repeated binging and purging; a woman may feel a lack of control over the situation. A bulimic binges and purges at least twice a week for a period of 3 months or more.

It's often difficult for any woman to see her body gain the weight that is normal with a pregnancy. It may be even harder for a woman with an eating disorder to see the pounds add up. It may take a lot of hard work and effort to accept these extra pounds, but you must try to do it for your good health and the good health of your baby.

Eating disorders may worsen during pregnancy. However, some women find their eating disorder gets better during pregnancy. For some, pregnancy is the first time they can let go of their obsessions about their bodies.

If you believe you have an eating disorder, try to deal with it *before* you get pregnant. An eating disorder affects you *and* your baby! Problems associated with an eating disorder during pregnancy include:

- a weight gain that is too low
- a low-birthweight baby
- miscarriage and an increased chance of fetal death
- intrauterine-growth restriction (IUGR)
- baby in a breech presentation (because it may be born too early)
- high blood pressure in the mother-to-be
- depression during and after pregnancy
- birth defects
- electrolyte problems in the mother-to-be
- decreased blood volume
- low 5-minute Apgar scores, after baby's birth

Your body is designed to provide your baby with the nutrition it needs, even if it has to take it from your body stores. For example, if your calcium intake is low, your baby will take the needed calcium from your bones. This could lead to osteoporosis for you later in life.

Tip for Week 21

A good way to add calcium to your diet is to cook rice and oatmeal in skim milk instead of water.

Sometimes visualizing what baby looks like at a particular time can help you. If it does, look at the illustrations of baby that accompany many of our weekly discussions. Each week read how baby is developing. Use this information to imagine how big your baby is and what it looks like at a certain time.

More frequent prenatal visits and monitoring during pregnancy are often recommended for a woman with an eating disorder. Researchers speculate eating disorders may disrupt the way nutrients are delivered to the baby, which could result in problems. Your healthcare provider will want to keep close tabs on how baby is growing. Antidepressants may also be used to help treat the problem. An eating disorder can also increase the risk of postpartum depression.

Talk to your healthcare provider about your problem as soon as possible. It's serious and can be harmful to you and your baby.

Your Nutrition

Cravings

Some women experience food cravings during pregnancy. Food cravings have long been considered a nonspecific sign of pregnancy. We don't understand all the reasons you might crave a food while you're pregnant, but we believe hormonal and emotional changes add to the situation. Some experts believe cravings may indicate your body needs the nutrients a particular food contains.

Craving a particular food can be both good and bad. If the food you crave is nutritious and healthful, eat it in moderation. Don't eat food that isn't good for you.

What Foods Do Pregnant Women Crave?

Research indicates three common cravings among pregnant women.

- 33% crave chocolate
- 20% crave sweets of some sort
- 19% crave citrus fruits and juices

If you crave foods that are high in fat and sugar or loaded with empty calories, be careful. Take a little taste, but don't let yourself go. Try eating another food, such as a piece of fresh fruit or some cheese, instead of indulging in your craving.

Be careful what you eat when you're tired. You may crave a snack that isn't healthy for you. Try eating a small healthy snack first, and wait for a bit. See if you really want the unhealthy food. Some cravings are emotional—you may be tired and out of sorts, and you crave a hot-fudge sundae. It may be that you are craving comfort, not food.

When you crave something sweet, eat a cherry tomato or some broccoli pieces to help curb your sweet tooth. These foods may help reduce cravings. Or replace high-calorie fare with low-calorie ones, such as lowfat pudding, lowfat frozen yogurt or a smoothie. If you crave the same nonnutritious treat over and over again, buy single-serve portions, and keep them in the freezer. Eat one at a time.

If you're having trouble with sugar cravings, try chewing sugar-free gum in the afternoon. Or go out for a treat you crave. If you have to go out, you may change your mind. Understand when you indulge your cravings for high-fat, sugary foods, you may actually *increase* your cravings for them!

Food Aversions

On the opposite side of cravings is food aversion. Some foods you have eaten without problems before pregnancy may now make you sick to your stomach. It's common. Again, we believe the hormones of pregnancy are involved. In this case, hormones affect the gastrointestinal tract, which can affect your reaction to some foods.

Pica—Nonfood Cravings

Some women experience *pica* during pregnancy. They crave nonfood items, such as dirt, clay, laundry starch, chalk, ice, paint chips and other things. We don't know why pregnant women develop these cravings. Some experts believe it may be caused by an iron deficiency. Others think pica may be the body's attempt to get vitamins or minerals not being supplied in the food the woman eats. Still others speculate pica cravings may be caused by an underlying physical or mental illness.

Pica cravings may be harmful to your baby and you. Eating nonfood items could interfere with nutrient absorption of healthy foods and result in a deficiency.

If you have pica cravings, don't panic. Call your healthcare provider immediately. He or she will develop a plan with you to help deal with the cravings.

If you have food aversions, try to substitute foods to get the nutrients you need. For example, drink calcium-fortified juice if you can't drink milk. Meat making you ill? Try eggs, beans or nuts.

You Should Also Know

Will You Get Varicose Veins?

Varicose veins are large, distended veins deep under the skin. They are caused by blood-flow blockage in the veins, aggravated by pregnancy.

You may also experience *spider veins.* They are small groups of dilated blood vessels near the skin surface. You see them most commonly on face and legs.

Varicose veins, also called *varicosities* or *varices,* occur to some degree in most pregnant women. There seems to be an inherited tendency to get varicose veins during pregnancy. It can be worsened with increased age and pressure caused by standing for a long time. Most women actually begin to develop varicose veins in their 20s.

Problems usually occur in the legs but may also be present in the vulva and rectum (hemorrhoids). The change in blood flow and pressure from the uterus can make problems worse and cause discomfort. In most instances, varicose veins become more noticeable and more painful as pregnancy progresses and may get worse as you gain more weight (especially if you stand a lot).

Symptoms vary. For some, the main symptom is a blemish or purple-blue spot on the legs with little or no discomfort, except maybe in the evening. Other women have painful bulging veins that require elevation at the end of the day. Varicose veins may also cause itching. The following measures may help keep your veins from swelling as much.

- Wear medical support hose; many types are available. Ask your healthcare provider for a recommendation.
- Wear clothing that doesn't restrict circulation at the knee or groin.
- Spend as little time on your feet as you can. Lie on your side or elevate your legs when possible. This enables veins to drain more easily.
- Wear flat shoes when you can.
- Exercise regularly to help improve blood flow through the veins.
- Drink citrus juice or eat citrus fruit; the vitamin C helps keep capillary and vein walls strong.
- Consider eating spinach, broccoli and asparagus, as these foods may help lessen the severity of varicose veins. These foods are high in vitamin K, which may help relieve symptoms.
- Don't cross your legs. It cuts off circulation and can make problems worse.

The type of exercise you choose may make the problem worse. High-impact exercise, such as step aerobics or jogging,

Dad Tip

It's not too early to start thinking about baby names. Did you know nearly 50% of all Americans are named after a family member? Sometimes partners have very different ideas about names for their child. There are many books available to help you. Do you plan to honor a close friend or relative by using their name? Will you use a family name? What problems could arise if you choose a peculiar, difficult-to-say or hard-to-spell name? Find out what a name means—it could help you make a decision. What do the initials spell out? What nicknames go with the name? Start thinking about it now, even if you decide you won't pick a name until after you meet your baby.

can damage veins. Low-impact exercises, such as biking, prenatal yoga or using an elliptical trainer, may be a better choice.

Following pregnancy, swelling in the veins should go down, but varicose veins probably won't completely disappear. After-pregnancy treatment methods include laser treatment, injection and surgery.

Vaginitis

Vaginitis covers a lot of conditions that cause annoying vaginal symptoms, such as itching, burning, irritation and abnormal discharge. The most common causes of vaginitis are bacterial vaginosis, vulvovaginal candidiasis and trichomoniasis. Bacterial vaginosis is the most common of the conditions and is discussed below.

Bacterial Vaginosis (BV). It's estimated that more than 15% of all pregnant women have bacterial vaginosis (BV) during pregnancy. It is the most common vaginal infection in women of childbearing age. Some experts believe it may be caused by douching and sexual intercourse. It is also more common in women who have an IUD.

BV is caused by an imbalance or overgrowth of several types of bacteria that exist in the vagina. Bacterial vaginosis can cause problems for pregnant women.

It may be difficult to diagnose BV because bacteria can also be found in healthy individuals. Nearly half of the women infected have no symptoms. For those who do, they may experience symptoms similar to those of a yeast infection, including itching, a vaginal odor that is "fishy," painful urination and a gray-white vaginal discharge.

Your healthcare provider can detect the problem by testing vaginal discharge for BV-causing bacteria. Antibiotics are used to treat the problem. Seven days of metronidazole (Flagyl) is the treatment of choice.

If left untreated, BV can cause you problems. If you have BV, be sure it is treated.

Fibromyalgia

Fibromyalgia affects between 3 and 6 million Americans every year; 80% are women. It causes muscles all over the body to ache, burn and twitch. If you suffer from it, you probably ache all over, especially in the arms, lower back, shoulders and neck. You may also feel tingling in the fingers and toes. Severe fatigue, headaches, sleep problems, abdominal pain and gastrointestinal problems may also be present. Some sufferers experience anxiety and depression.

The problem usually begins during early adulthood or middle age and causes chronic pain and other symptoms. Symptoms can come and go throughout a person's life. Although fibromyalgia is believed to be genetic, it may lie dormant until triggered by a trauma, such as childbirth.

Fibromyalgia can be hard to diagnose, and a person may suffer for a long time before finding help. It is more common if a person also suffers from irritable bowel syndrome, celiac disease or lactose intolerance.

Fibromyalgia and Pregnancy. We don't know a lot about fibromyalgia during pregnancy. We *do* know fibromyalgia won't harm your baby. Pregnancy can be a time of high stress, and physical and emotional stress are known triggers for fibromyalgia.

During pregnancy, your body produces many hormones, which may affect your disease. Studies have found some women experience more severe symptoms during pregnancy. The third trimester may be the worst, and symptoms may last as long as 3 months after birth.

Other researchers believe pregnancy helps lessen fibromyalgia symptoms. Some women have said they felt better during pregnancy. This may be the result of the production of the hormone relaxin. Relaxin supplements have been found to help ease symptoms in many women with fibromyalgia. During pregnancy, the amount of relaxin in a woman's body increases up to 10 times!

If you suffer from fibromyalgia, bring it up at your first prenatal visit. At this time, there is no cure, and treatment is limited. The FDA has approved the drug Lyrica to help manage pain. Antidepressants and pain suppressants may also be used to treat symptoms. Discuss the use of any of these medicines with your healthcare provider. To help ease pain, acetaminophen is safe to use during pregnancy.

Exercise may offer relief. Some types of exercise to consider include yoga, exercising in the water, Pilates and stretching. Massage therapy may also help—look for a massage therapist with experience treating fibromyalgia pain who can safely perform massage on a pregnant woman.

It may help to apply moist heat to the affected area twice a day. A warm shower or bath is a good way to apply moist heat.

Exercise for Week 21

Like the Kegel exercise, you can do this exercise just about anywhere. Standing or sitting, take a deep breath. While exhaling, tighten your tummy muscles as though you were zipping up a pair of tight jeans. Repeat 6 or 8 times. *Strengthens tummy muscles.*

Do this second exercise after you've been sitting a long time, such as at your desk or in a car or on a plane, or when you have to stand for long periods. When you're forced to stand in one place for a long time, step forward slightly with one foot. Place all your weight on that foot for a few minutes. Do the same with the other foot. Alternate the leg you begin with each time. *Stretches leg muscles.*

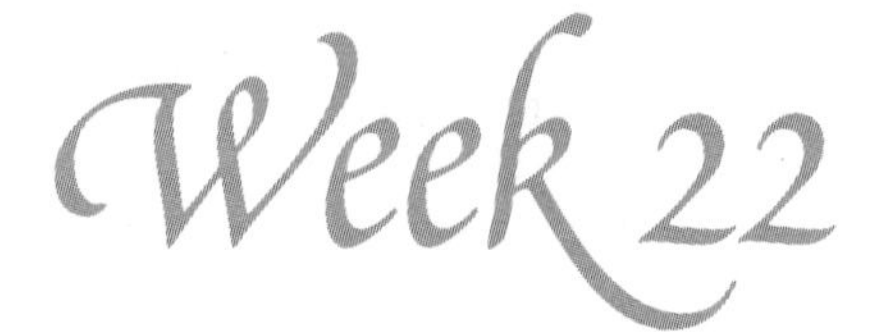

Week 22

Age of Fetus—20 Weeks

How Big Is Your Baby?

Your baby weighs about 12¼ ounces (350g). Crown-to-rump length at this time is about 7⅔ inches (19cm).

How Big Are You?

Your uterus is about ¾ inch (2cm) above your bellybutton. Your growing tummy doesn't get in your way much; you may feel pretty good. You're still able to bend over and to sit comfortably. Walking shouldn't be an effort. Morning sickness has probably passed. It's kind of fun being pregnant now!

How Your Baby Is Growing and Developing

Your baby's body grows every day. As you can see by looking at the illustration on page 314, eyelids and eyebrows are developed. Fingernails are also visible.

Your baby's organ systems are becoming specialized for their particular functions. Consider the liver. The function of the fetal liver is different from that of an adult. Chemicals are made in an adult liver that are important in various body functions. In the fetus, chemicals are present but in lower amounts.

An important function of the liver is managing bilirubin, which is produced by the breakdown of blood cells. The life span of a fetal red blood cell is shorter than that of an adult. Because of this, a baby makes more bilirubin than an adult does.

The fetal liver has a limited capacity to change bilirubin and remove it from baby's bloodstream. Bilirubin passes from fetal blood through the placenta to your blood. Your liver helps get rid of it. A premature baby may have trouble processing bilirubin because its own liver is not ready to take over this function. Full-term babies can also have this problem.

A newborn baby with high bilirubin may exhibit *jaundice.* Jaundice in a newborn usually occurs when bilirubin being handled by the mother's system must now be handled by the baby it on its own. The baby's liver can't keep up.

Changes in You

Fetal Fibronectin (fFN)

It can be hard to determine if a woman is at risk of delivering a preterm baby. Many symptoms of preterm labor are similar to various discomforts of pregnancy. A test is available that can help healthcare providers.

Fetal fibronectin (fFN) is a protein found in the amniotic sac and fetal membranes. However, after 22 weeks of pregnancy, fFN is not normally present until around week 38.

When found in cervical-vaginal secretions of a pregnant woman after 22 weeks (before week 38), it means there is a higher risk for preterm delivery. If not found, risk of premature labor is low, and the woman probably won't deliver within the next 2 weeks. fFN can rule out early delivery with 99% accuracy.

The test is similar to a Pap smear. A swab of vaginal secretions is taken from the top of the vagina, behind the cervix. It is sent to the lab, and results are available within 24 hours.

What Is Anemia?

There is a fine balance in your body between the production of red blood cells that carry oxygen to the rest of your body and the destruction of

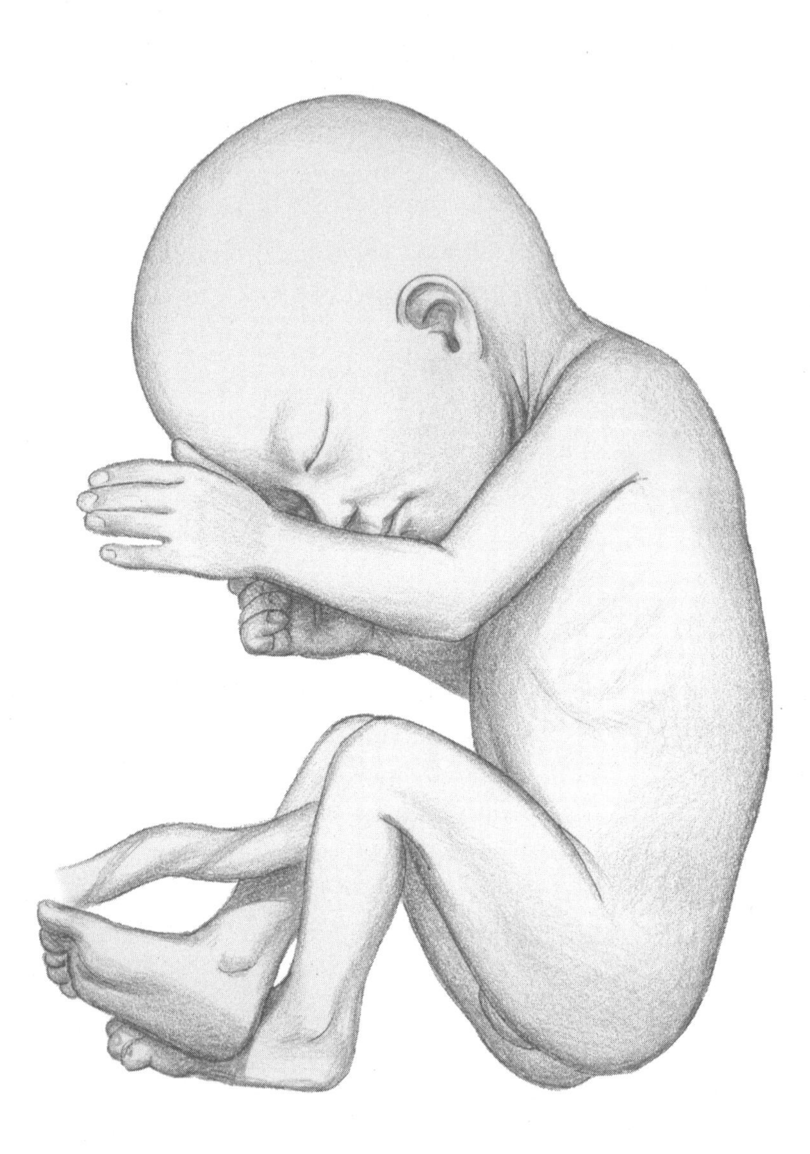

By the 22nd week of pregnancy (fetal age—20 weeks), your baby's eyelids and eyebrows are well developed. Fingernails now cover the fingertips.

these cells. *Anemia* is the condition in which the number of red blood cells is low. If you're anemic, you don't have enough red blood cells.

During pregnancy, the number of red blood cells increases. The amount of *plasma* (liquid part of the blood) also increases but at a higher rate. Your healthcare provider keeps track of these changes with a *hematocrit* reading, a measure of the percentage of the blood that is red blood cells. This is usually done at the first prenatal visit.

If your temperature rises above 100F, contact your healthcare provider. A temperature above 102F may indicate an infection is bacterial.

Your *hemoglobin* level is also tested. Hemoglobin is the protein component of red blood cells. If you're anemic, your hematocrit is lower than 37, and your hemoglobin is under 12. The test may be repeated once or twice during pregnancy and is done more often if you're anemic. If you suffer from anemia during pregnancy, you won't feel well, you'll tire easily and you may experience dizziness. Treatment is important for you and your baby.

There is always some blood loss at delivery. If you're anemic when you go into labor, you may need a blood transfusion after your baby is born.

Follow your healthcare provider's advice about diet and supplementation if you have anemia. For a discussion of sickle-cell disease and thalassemia, two types of inherited anemia, see page 320.

Iron-Deficiency Anemia. The most common type of anemia seen in pregnancy is *iron-deficiency anemia*. During pregnancy, your baby uses some of the iron stores you have in your body. If you have iron-deficiency anemia, your body doesn't have enough iron left to make red blood cells because the baby has used some of your iron for its own blood-cell production. It's important to treat the problem. Iron deficiency has been tied to increased risks.

Most prenatal vitamins contain iron, but it's also available as a supplement. If you can't take a prenatal vitamin, you may be given 300 to 350mg of ferrous sulphate or ferrous gluconate 2 or 3 times a day. Iron is the most important supplement to take during pregnancy and is required in almost all pregnancies.

Some women develop iron-deficiency anemia during pregnancy even if they take iron supplements. Several factors may make a woman more likely to have this condition in pregnancy, including:

- bleeding during pregnancy
- multiple fetuses
- previous surgery on the stomach or part of the small bowel
- antacid overuse that causes a decrease in iron absorption
- poor eating habits

The goal in treating iron-deficiency anemia is to increase the amount of iron you take in. Iron is poorly absorbed so you need to take it every day. It can be given as an injection, but it's painful and may stain the skin.

Side effects of taking iron supplements include nausea and vomiting, with stomach upset. If this occurs, you may have to take a lower dose. Taking iron may also cause constipation.

If you can't take an iron supplement, eat more foods that are high in the mineral. Liver or spinach are good choices. Ask your healthcare provider for information on what types of foods you should include in your diet.

How Your Actions Affect Your Baby's Development

It's possible you could have diarrhea or a cold during pregnancy, as well as other viral infections such as the flu. These problems may raise concerns for you.

- What can I do when I feel ill?
- What medicine or treatment is OK?
- If I'm sick, should I take my prenatal vitamins?
- If I'm sick and unable to eat my usual diet, what can I do?

If you become sick during pregnancy, call the office. Get your healthcare provider's advice about a plan of action. He or she can advise you about what medicine to take to help you feel better. Even if it's only a cold or the flu, your healthcare provider wants to know when you're feeling ill. If any further measures are needed, your healthcare provider can recommend them.

Is there anything you can do to help yourself? Yes. If you have diarrhea or a possible viral infection, increase your fluid intake. Drink a lot of water, juice and other clear fluids, such as broth. To help you retain fluid, add 1 teaspoon of sugar to a cup of water or tea; the glucose in table sugar helps the intestines absorb water instead of releasing it. A bland diet without solid food may help you feel a little better.

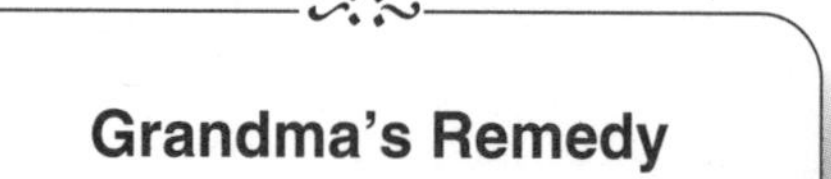

Grandma's Remedy

If you want to avoid using medication, try a folk remedy. If you have allergies, try some local honey. Made by bees in the area, it contains very tiny amounts of the pollen that causes your sneezes and sniffles. Eating very small amounts of it can work like allergy shots by helping you tolerate a pollen. Start with ¼ teaspoon a day, and very slowly increase up to 2 teaspoons a day.

Going off your regular diet for a few days won't hurt you or baby, but you do need to drink plenty of fluids. Solid foods may be difficult to handle and can make diarrhea a bigger problem. Milk products may also make diarrhea worse. If diarrhea continues beyond 24 hours, call your healthcare provider. Ask what medicine you can safely take for diarrhea during pregnancy.

When you're sick, it's OK to skip your prenatal vitamin for a few days. However, begin taking it again when you're able to keep food down. Don't take any medicine to control diarrhea without first consulting your healthcare provider. Usually a viral illness with diarrhea is a short-term problem and won't last more than a few days. You may have to stay home from work or rest in bed until you feel better.

Your Nutrition

You need to drink water during pregnancy—lots of it! Fluid helps you in a lot of ways. You may feel better during your pregnancy if you drink more water than you normally do.

When you don't drink water, you can become dehydrated. If you're dehydrated, you can tire more easily. Once you're dehydrated, it may reduce the amount of nutrients baby receives from you. Your blood thickens, making it harder to pass nutrients to baby. Dehydration may also increase your risk of problems.

Our bodies contain 10 to 12 gallons of water. Studies show that for every 15 calories your body burns, you need about 1 tablespoon of water. If you burn 2000 calories a day, you need to drink well over 2 quarts of water! As calorie needs increase during pregnancy, so does your need for water.

New guidelines suggest you should drink 101 ounces of fluid a day during pregnancy. Water should account for at least 50 ounces of this intake. Water in food can make up another 20 ounces. The other 30+ ounces should come from milk, juice and other beverages. Sip water and other fluids throughout the day. If you decrease your consumption later in the day, you may save yourself some trips to the bathroom at night.

Keep the consumption of caffeinated beverages low. Tea, coffee and cola may contain sodium and caffeine, which act as diuretics. They essentially *increase* your water needs.

Some of the common problems women experience during pregnancy may be eased by drinking water. Headaches, uterine cramping and bladder infections may be less of a problem when you drink lots of water.

Check your urine to see if you're drinking enough. If it's light yellow to clear, you're getting enough fluid. Dark-yellow urine is a sign to increase your fluid intake. Don't wait till you get thirsty to drink something. By the time you get thirsty, you've already lost at least 1% of your body's fluids.

Dad Tip

When you ride together in the car with your partner, ask if you can help her in any way. You may offer to assist her getting in and out of the car. Ask if she needs help adjusting her seat belt or the car seat. Try to make riding and driving as easy and accessible as possible for her. You may propose trading vehicles (if you have more than one), if it's more comfortable for her to drive the other car.

Your Drinking Water

Fitness waters may benefit you if you're very active. Ask you healthcare provider for more information.

Water supplies in the United States are some of the least-contaminated in the world. Most of our country has high-quality drinking water. Most experts agree tap water in the United States is safe to drink. Often tap water contains minerals that have been removed from bottled water.

Drinking water contaminated with chemical byproducts from chlorine may not be safe for you to drink. Chlorine is often added to drinking water to disinfect it. When added to water that contains organic matter, such as from farms or lawns, it can form unhealthy compounds (for pregnant women), such as chloroform. Check with your local water company if you're concerned.

Do *not* rely on bottled water as safer than tap water. One study showed nearly 35% of over 100 brands of bottled water were contaminated with chemicals or bacteria. However, tap water must meet certain minimum standards if it is supplied by a municipal water company, so you know it's safe to drink. In addition, some bottled water contains sugar, caffeine and/or herbs.

You Should Also Know

Appendicitis

Appendicitis can happen at any time, even during pregnancy. Acute appendicitis is the most common condition requiring surgery during pregnancy.

Pregnancy can make diagnosis difficult because some symptoms can be typical in a normal pregnancy, such as nausea and vomiting. Pain in the lower abdomen on the right side may be credited to round-ligament pain or a urinary-tract infection. Diagnosis may be difficult because as the uterus grows, the appendix moves upward and outward, so tenderness and pain are located in a different place than normal. See the illustration on page 321.

Treatment of appendicitis is immediate surgery. This can be major abdominal surgery, with a 3-or 4-inch incision; it requires a few days in the hospital. Laparoscopy, with smaller incisions, is used in some situations, but laparoscopy may be harder to do during pregnancy because of the large uterus.

Rupture of a pregnant woman's appendix occurs up to 3 times more often because acute appendicitis is not diagnosed soon enough. Most physicians believe it's better to operate and remove a "normal" appendix than to risk infection of the abdominal cavity if an infected appendix bursts. Antibiotics are administered; many antibiotics are safe to use during pregnancy.

Sickle-Cell Disease

Sickle-cell disease is the most common hemoglobin disorder in the United States. About 8% of Black/African Americans carry the sickle-hemoglobin gene. However, it is also found in people of Arabic, Greek, Maltese, Italian, Sardinian, Turkish, Indian, Caribbean, Latin American and Middle-Eastern descent. In the United States, most cases of sickle-cell disease occur among Black/African Americans and Latino/Hispanics. About one in every 500 Black/African Americans has sickle-cell disease.

Sickle-cell disease is inherited. Normally, red blood cells are round and flexible, and flow easily through blood vessels. In sickle-cell disease, abnormal hemoglobin causes red blood cells to become stiff. Under the microscope, they may look like the C-shaped farm tool called a *sickle.*

Because they are stiffer, these red blood cells can get stuck in tiny blood vessels and cut off the blood supply to nearby tissues. This causes a great deal of pain (called *sickle-cell pain episode* or *sickle-cell crisis*) and may damage organs. These abnormal red blood cells die and break down more quickly than normal red blood cells, which results in anemia.

A person who inherits the sickle-cell gene from one parent and the normal type of that gene from the other parent is said to have *sickle-cell trait.* Carriers of the sickle-cell gene are usually as healthy as non-carriers. Sickle-cell trait cannot change to become sickle-cell disease.

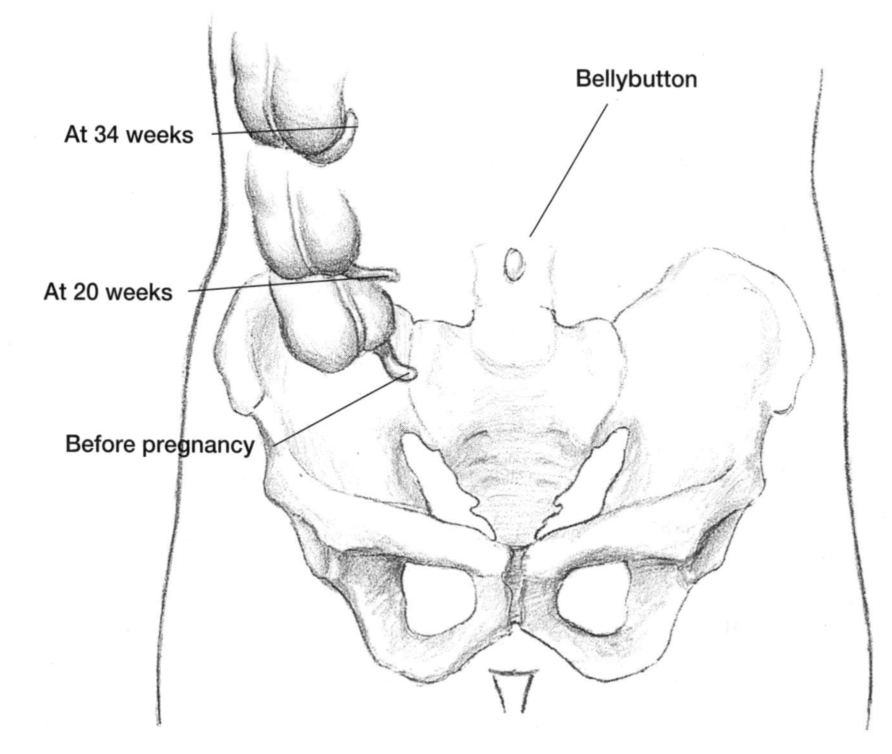

Location of the appendix at various times during pregnancy.

When two people with sickle-cell trait have a child, there is a one-in-four chance their child may inherit two sickle-cell genes (one gene from each parent) and have the disorder. There is a two-in-four chance the child will have the trait. There is a one-in-four chance the child will have neither the trait nor the disease. These chances are the same in each pregnancy. If only one parent has the trait and the other doesn't, there is *no* chance their children will have sickle-cell disease. However, there is a 50–50 chance of each child having the trait.

> ### *Tip for Week 22*
> **Drink extra fluids (water is best) throughout pregnancy to help your body keep up with the increase in your blood volume. You'll know you're drinking enough fluid when your urine looks almost like clear water.**

Sickle-cell disease can also affect biracial children. To what degree depends on the ethnic group of each parent and his or her genetic makeup. A union of a Caucasian and a Black/African American will not result in a child with sickle-cell disease because Caucasians are not carriers of the sickle-cell gene. However, the union of a Black/African American and a person of Mediterranean or Latino/Hispanic descent *could* result in a child with sickle-cell disease if both parents carry the sickle-cell gene. In addition, if both parents are biracial, they could pass the disease to their children if each parent carries the gene. The risk of both biracial partners being carriers is lower, but the risk is still there and depends on each person's genetic background and makeup.

Pregnancy and Sickle-Cell Disease. A woman with sickle-cell disease can have a safe pregnancy. However, if you have the disease, your chances are greater of having problems that can affect your health and your baby's health.

During pregnancy, the disease may become more severe, and pain episodes may be more frequent. You will need early prenatal care and careful monitoring throughout pregnancy.

Until 1995, there was no effective treatment, other than blood transfusions, to prevent the sickling of the blood that causes a pain crisis. The medication, hydroxyurea, was found to reduce the number of pain episodes by about 50% in some severely affected adults. At this time, we do not recommend hydroxyurea for pregnant women. However, researchers continue to study new drug treatments to help reduce complications of the disease.

A blood test can reveal sickle-cell trait. There also are prenatal tests to find out if a baby will have the disease or carry the trait. Most children with sickle-cell disease are now identified through newborn screening tests.

Your healthcare provider will pay close attention to your sickle-cell disease during pregnancy. Work with your healthcare team to stay as healthy as possible.

Thalassemia

Thalassemia, also called *Cooley's anemia,* is not just one disease. It includes a number of different forms of anemia. The thalassemia trait is found all over the world but is most common in people from the Middle East, Greece, Italy, Georgia (the country, not the state), Armenia, Viet Nam, Laos, Thailand, Singapore, the Philippines, Cambodia, Malaysia, Burma, Indonesia, China, East India, Africa and Azerbaijan. It affects about 100,000 babies each year.

There are two main forms of the disease—alpha thalassemia and beta thalassemia. The type depends on which part of an oxygen-carrying

Eating Dark Chocolate

Eating dark chocolate (at least 70% cocoa content) may be good for you. A daily dose of 30g of dark chocolate has been associated with lower blood pressure and a reduced risk of anemia. Chocolate also helps relax and dilate blood vessels to help lower blood pressure. Antioxidants found in dark chocolate may be healthy for you. Keep in mind the following when choosing dark chocolate.

- Chocolate should be 70% or more cocoa.
- Don't eat more than 3 ounces a day.
- Dark chocolate should replace other sweets.

protein (the hemoglobin) is lacking in red blood cells. Most individuals have a mild form of the disease. The effects of beta thalassemia can range from no effects to very severe.

A carrier of thalassemia has one normal gene and one thalassemia gene; this is called the *thalassemia trait.* Most carriers lead completely normal, healthy lives.

When two carriers have a child, there is a one-in-four chance their child will have a form of the disease. There is a two-in-four chance the child will be a carrier like its parents and a one-in-four chance the child will be completely free of the disease. These odds are the same for each pregnancy when both parents are carriers.

Various tests can determine whether a person has thalassemia or is a carrier. Chorionic villus sampling (CVS) and amniocentesis can detect thalassemia in a fetus. Early diagnosis is important so treatment can begin at birth to prevent as many complications as possible.

Having the thalassemia trait doesn't usually cause health problems, although women with the trait may be more likely to develop anemia during pregnancy. Healthcare providers may treat this with folic-acid supplementation.

Most children born with thalassemia appear healthy at birth, but during the first or second year of life they develop problems. They grow slowly and often develop jaundice.

Treatment of thalassemia includes frequent blood transfusions and antibiotics. When children are treated with transfusions to keep their hemoglobin level near normal, many complications of thalassemia can be prevented. However, repeated blood transfusions may lead to a buildup of iron in the body. A drug called an *iron chelator* may be given to help rid the body of excess iron.

Certified Nurse-Midwives, Advance-Practice Nurses and Physician Assistants

In today's obstetric-and-gynecology medical practices, you may find many types of highly qualified people helping to take care of you. These people—mostly women, but not all!—are on the forefront in guiding women through pregnancy to delivery. They may even help deliver their babies!

A *certified nurse-midwife* (CNM) is an advance-practice registered nurse (RN). He or she has received additional training delivering babies and providing prenatal and postpartum care to women. A CNM works closely with a doctor or team of doctors to address specifics about a particular pregnancy, and labor and delivery. Often a CNM delivers babies.

A certified midwife can provide many types of information to a pregnant woman, such as guidance with nutrition and exercise, ways to deal with pregnancy discomforts, tips for managing weight gain, dealing with various pregnancy problems and discussions of different methods of pain relief for labor and delivery. A CNM can also address issues of family planning and birth control and other gynecological care, including breast exams, Pap smears and other screenings. A CNM can prescribe medications; each state has their own specific requirements.

A *nurse practitioner* is also an advance-practice registered nurse (RN). He or she has received additional training providing prenatal and postpartum care to women. A nurse practitioner may work with a doctor or work independently to address specifics about a woman's pregnancy, and labor and delivery.

A nurse practitioner can provide many types of information to a pregnant woman, such as guidance with nutrition and exercise, ways to deal with pregnancy discomforts, tips for managing weight gain, dealing with various pregnancy problems and discussions of different methods of pain relief for labor and delivery. He or she can also address issues of family planning and birth control and other gynecological care, including breast exams, Pap smears and other screenings. In some cases, a nurse practitioner may prescribe medications or provide pain relief during labor and delivery (as a certified registered nurse anesthetist [CRNA]).

A *physician assistant (PA)* is a qualified healthcare professional who may take care of you during pregnancy. He or she is licensed to practice medicine in association with a licensed doctor. In a normal, uncomplicated pregnancy, many or most of your prenatal visits may be with a PA, not the doctor. This may include labor and delivery. Most women find this is a good thing—often these healthcare providers have more time to spend with you answering questions and addressing your concerns.

(continues)

A PA's focus is to provide many health-care services traditionally done by a doctor. They care for people who have conditions (pregnancy is a condition they see women for), diagnose and treat illnesses, order and interpret tests, counsel on preventive health care, perform some procedures, assist in surgery, write prescriptions and do physical exams. A PA is *not* a medical assistant, who performs administrative or simple clinical tasks.

We are fortunate to have these dedicated professionals working in OB/GYN practices and clinics. The care they provide is crucial to the medical community and makes quality medical care for women something every woman can look forward to.

Exercise for Week 22

Lie on your left side on the sofa, with your left knee bent. Bend your left arm, and place it under your head. Lower your right foot to the floor while keeping your leg straight. Hold for 10 seconds, then lift the straightened leg to a 45° angle; hold for 5 seconds. Do 5 complete repetitions with each leg. *Helps ease sciatica; strengthens hips and upper buttocks muscles.*

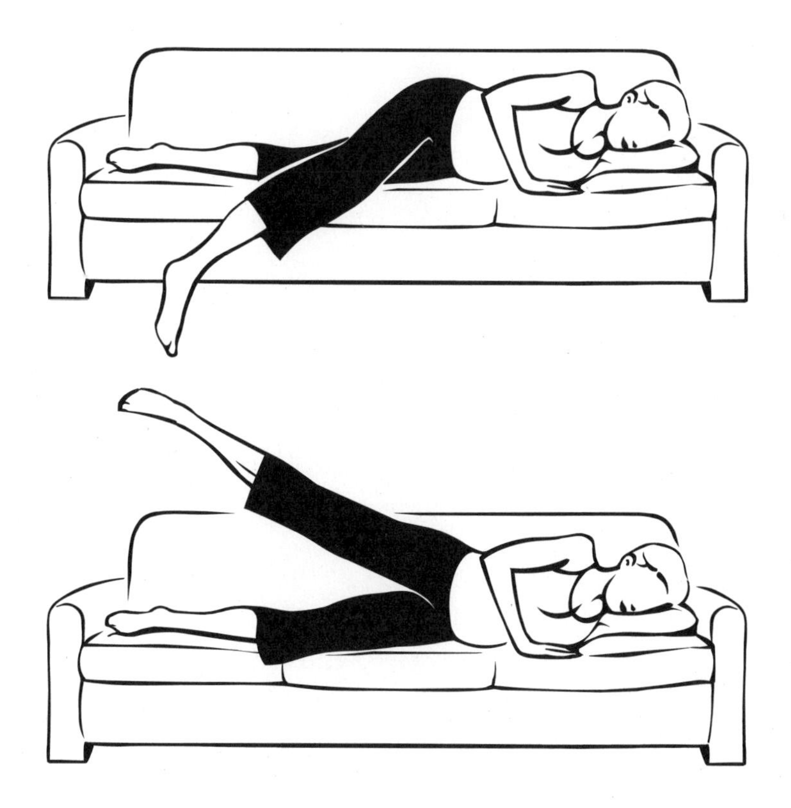

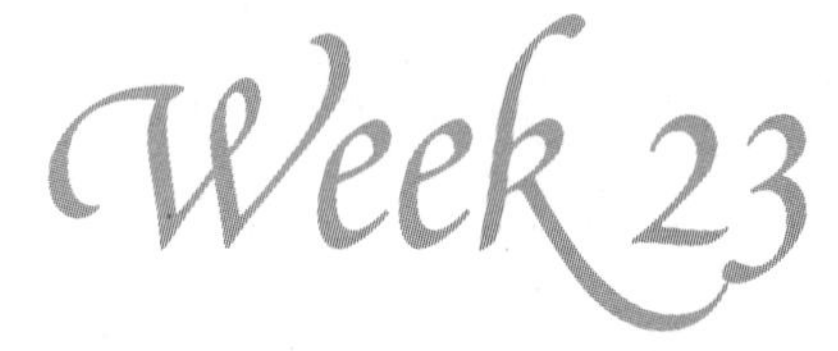

Week 23

Age of Fetus—21 Weeks

How Big Is Your Baby?

By this week, baby weighs almost 1 pound (455g)! Its crown-to-rump length is 8 inches (20cm). Your baby is about the size of a small doll.

How Big Are You?

Your uterus extends about 1½ inches (3.75cm) above your bellybutton or about 9¼ inches (23cm) from the pubic symphysis. Your total weight gain should be between 12 and 15 pounds (5.5 and 6.8kg).

How Your Baby Is Growing and Developing

Baby's body is getting plumper but skin is still wrinkled; see the illustration on page 330. Lanugo hair on the body occasionally turns darker at this time. The baby's face and body begin to assume more of the appearance of an infant at birth.

Your baby's pancreas is important in insulin production. Insulin is necessary for the body to break down and to use sugar. When the fetus is exposed to high blood-sugar levels from the mother-to-be, its pancreas responds by increasing the blood-insulin level. Insulin has been identified in a fetal pancreas as early as 9 weeks of pregnancy and in fetal blood as early as 12 weeks.

Blood-insulin levels are generally high in babies born to diabetic mothers. This is one reason your healthcare provider may monitor you for development of gestational diabetes.

Twin-to-Twin Transfusion Syndrome (TTTS)

Twin-to-twin transfusion syndrome (TTTS) occurs only in identical twins who share the same placenta. The syndrome is also called *chronic intertwin transfusion syndrome.* The condition can range from mild to severe and can occur at any point during pregnancy, even at birth.

TTTS cannot be prevented; it's not a genetic disorder nor a hereditary condition. We believe it occurs in 5 to 10% of all identical-twin pregnancies. TTTS occurs when twins share a placenta. These problems do not occur in twins who each have a placenta.

In TTTS, twins also share some of the same blood circulation. This allows the transfusion of blood from one twin to the other. One twin becomes small and anemic. Its body responds by partially shutting down blood supply to many of its organs, especially the kidneys, which results in reduced urine output and a small volume of amniotic fluid.

> **Dad Tip**
>
> Are you also having pregnancy symptoms? Studies show as many as 50% of all fathers-to-be experience physical symptoms of pregnancy when their partner is pregnant. *Couvade*, a French term meaning "to hatch," is used to describe the condition in a man. Symptoms for an expectant father may include nausea, weight gain and cravings for certain foods.

The other twin grows large, overloaded with blood. It produces excessive amounts of urine so it is surrounded by a large volume of amniotic fluid. Because the recipient twin has more blood, it urinates more and has more amniotic fluid. Its blood becomes thick and difficult to pump through its body; this can result in heart failure.

The twins are often very different in size. There can also be a large difference in their weights. TTTS is a progressive disorder, so early treatment may prevent complications.

Symptoms of TTTS. There are symptoms of the syndrome your healthcare provider looks for. If your abdomen enlarges quite rapidly over a 2- to 3-week period, it may be caused by the buildup of amniotic fluid in the recipient twin. The result can be premature labor and/or premature rupture of membranes. If one twin is small for its gestational age or one is big for its gestational age, it may indicate TTTS. In addition, your

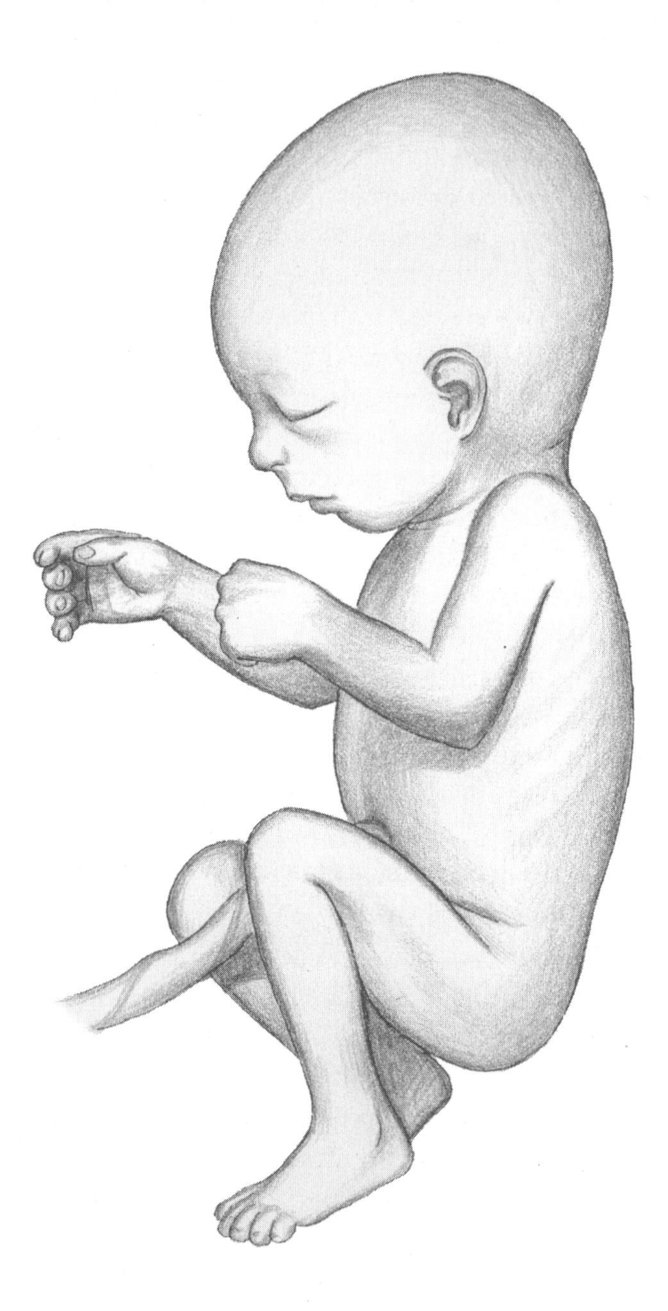

By the 23rd week of pregnancy (fetal age—21 weeks), your baby's eyelids and eyebrows are well developed.

healthcare provider may suspect TTTS if any of the following is seen during an ultrasound:

- large difference in the size of fetuses of the same gender
- difference in size between the two amniotic sacs
- difference in size of the umbilical cords
- one placenta
- evidence of fluid buildup in the skin of either fetus
- indications of congestive heart failure in the recipient twin

An additional problem may develop in either twin. With this condition, fluid accumulates in some part of the fetus, such as in the scalp, abdomen, lungs or heart.

Diagnosing and Treating TTTS. Report any of the following to your healthcare provider, especially if you know you're expecting twins:

- rapid growth of your uterus
- abdominal pain, tightness or contractions
- sudden increase in body weight
- swelling in the hands and legs in early pregnancy

The syndrome may also be detected with ultrasound examination of the uterus. It's important to find out whether twins share the same placenta, preferably in the first trimester because in the second trimester it can be harder to learn whether they share one placenta.

If the syndrome is mild or undetected on ultrasound, the appearance of the twins at birth may identify it. A complete blood cell count done after birth will show anemia in one twin and excess red blood cells in the other.

If diagnosed, the Twin to Twin Transfusion Syndrome Foundation recommends weekly ultrasounds after 16 weeks till the end of the pregnancy to monitor TTTS. They recommend this be done even if the warning signs of TTTS have decreased.

The most common treatment for TTTS is amnioreduction, in which large volumes of amniotic fluid are drained from the sac of the larger twin. A needle is placed through the mother's abdomen, and fluid is drained. The procedure is repeated, if necessary.

In another procedure, a hole punched between the two amniotic sacs can help equalize the fluid between the sacs. However, neither of these procedures stops the twin-to-twin transfusion.

Some cases of TTTS do not respond to amnioreduction. A small-scope laser procedure may be done to seal off some or all of the blood vessels the twins share. Usually only one procedure is necessary during the pregnancy. Survival rates are also about 60% with this procedure. This treatment is most successful if done before 26 weeks of pregnancy.

With the laser treatment, a detailed ultrasound exam is done first to help locate the abnormal connection. Then a thin fiber-optic scope is placed through the mother's abdomen, through the wall of the uterus and into the amniotic cavity of the larger twin. By looking directly at the placenta, blood connections can be found and sealed by directing a laser beam at them. This separates the circulation of the fetuses and ends twin-to-twin transfusion. However, this requires doing the procedure while the babies are still in the womb and may cause serious complications.

The most conservative treatment is to watch and to wait. The pregnancy is followed closely with frequent ultrasound examinations, with the choice of delivering the twins by Cesarean delivery if medically necessary.

Newborns with twin-to-twin transfusion syndrome may be critically ill at birth and require treatment in a neonatal intensive care unit. The smaller twin is treated for anemia, and the larger twin is treated for excess red blood cells and jaundice.

If you would like further information, resources are available. Contact the TTTS Foundation at www.tttsfoundation.org or call their headquarters at 800-815-9211.

Changes in You

Your healthcare provider will measure you at every visit after this point. He or she may use a measuring tape or his or her fingers to measure by finger breadth. As baby grows larger, your uterus will be checked to see how much it has grown since your last visit. Within limits, changing measurements are a sign of baby's well-being and growth.

You will also be weighed and your blood pressure checked at each visit. Your healthcare provider is watching for changes in your weight gain and the size of your uterus. What's important is continual growth and change.

Loss of Fluid

Your uterus grows larger and gets heavier. In early pregnancy, it lies directly behind the bladder, in front of the rectum and the lower part of the colon, which is part of the bowel. Later in pregnancy, the uterus sits on top of the bladder. As it grows, it can put a lot of pressure on your bladder. You may notice times when your underwear is damp.

You may be unsure whether you've lost urine or if you're leaking amniotic fluid. It may be difficult to tell the difference. When your membranes rupture, you usually experience a gush of fluid or a continual leaking from the vagina. If you experience this, call your healthcare provider immediately!

Emotional Changes Continue

Do you find your mood swings are worse? Are you still crying easily? Do you wonder if you'll ever be in control again? Don't worry. These emotions are typical at this point in pregnancy. Most experts believe hormonal changes are the culprit.

There's not much you can do about moodiness. If you think your partner or others are suffering from your emotional outbursts, talk about it with them. Explain these feelings are common in pregnant

> When shopping, pick up some healthy convenience foods, such as low-sodium canned vegetables, frozen fruits and veggies, all-natural applesauce or marinara sauce, instant brown rice, quick-cooking oatmeal, whole-wheat tortillas and pitas, and low-fat cottage cheese and yogurt.

women. Ask them to be understanding. Then relax, and try not to get upset. Feeling emotional is a normal part of being pregnant.

How Your Actions Affect Your Baby's Development

Diabetes and Pregnancy

Diabetes is one of the most common medical complications of pregnancy. It occurs in 7 to 8% of all pregnancies. It was once a very serious problem during pregnancy, but today many diabetic women go through pregnancy safely.

Diabetes is defined as a lack of insulin in the bloodstream. Insulin is important for breaking down sugar and transporting it to the cells. Pregnancy increases the body's resistance to insulin. If you don't have insulin, you will have high blood sugar and a high sugar content in your urine.

With the use of insulin and the development of various ways to monitor a fetus, it's uncommon to have a serious problem. Of those women who have diabetes during pregnancy, 10% are type-1 or type-2 diabetics and 90% are gestational diabetics. Gestational diabetes is discussed on page 336.

Type-1 diabetes causes the body to stop making insulin; *type-2* causes the body to use insulin ineffectively. Type-2 diabetes is becoming more common in pregnant women. The result of either type is that too much sugar circulates in the woman's blood.

Pregnancy is well known for its tendency to reveal women who are predisposed to diabetes. Women who have trouble with high blood-sugar levels during pregnancy are more likely to develop diabetes in later life. Symptoms of diabetes include more-frequent urination, blurred vision, weight loss, dizziness and increased hunger.

Some experts recommend screening pregnant women at risk for diabetes during the first trimester. Others recommend testing all pregnant women at 28 weeks. Tests used most often are the glucose-tolerance test (GTT) or a 1-hour glucose challenge test.

If you have diabetes or know members of your family have diabetes, tell your healthcare provider. This is important information.

Diabetes and Pregnancy. Diabetes can cause various problems during pregnancy. Your chances of developing postpartum depression doubles. Birth defects may be more common and can occur as early as 5 to 8 weeks after the last menstrual period. That's one reason it's important to take care of diabetes *before* pregnancy. Your risk for having a very large baby (macrosomia) increases; it may require a Cesarean delivery.

If your diabetes is not controlled during pregnancy, the baby is at greater risk. Women with poorly controlled diabetes are 3 to 4 times more likely to have a baby with heart problems or neural-tube defects.

One way to maintain steady blood-sugar levels is *never* to skip meals and to get enough exercise. Regular exercise can help keep blood-sugar levels in check and may reduce your need for medicine.

Insulin is the safest way to control diabetes during pregnancy. If you already take insulin, you may need to adjust your dosage or the timing of your dosage. You may also have to check your blood-sugar levels 4 to 8 times a day. You must balance your eating plan and your insulin at all times so your glucose levels don't climb too high. Avoid long-lasting insulin during pregnancy. It may also help if you take in more folic acid; discuss it with your healthcare provider and endocrinologist.

Some diabetic women inject less insulin than they need in an effort to try to lose weight. It is sometimes called *diabulimia.* Insulin helps glucose leave the bloodstream and enter the body's cells to nourish them. If you have type-1 diabetes and reduce the amount of insulin you're supposed to receive, your body can't process glucose. Glucose will build up in the blood, which can increase your risk of problems.

Some women take diabetes pills; some oral antidiabetes medications taken during pregnancy may cause problems for the developing baby. There are safe oral medications for diabetes in pregnancy. You may have to adjust the amount of oral medication you take, and you may need to switch to insulin shots. Your healthcare provider can advise you.

Talk to your healthcare provider about getting an ultrasound of the baby's heart. A special ultrasound, called a *fetal echocardiogram,* can show if the baby has a problem. Some babies need surgery soon after they are born.

If you have type-1 diabetes, you may experience a delay in your milk coming in. You'll need to keep your breasts well stimulated to protect your milk supply.

Gestational Diabetes

Some women develop diabetes only during pregnancy; it is called *gestational diabetes.* It occurs when pregnancy hormones affect the way your body makes or uses insulin, a hormone that converts sugar in food into energy the body uses.

If your body doesn't make enough insulin or if it doesn't use the insulin appropriately, sugar in the blood rises to an unacceptable level. This is called *hyperglycemia* and means you have too much sugar in your blood. Occasionally, hormones made by the placenta can alter the actions of insulin, and gestational diabetes occurs. Several other factors can affect your blood-sugar levels, including stress, the time of day (glucose values are often higher in the morning), the amount of exercise you do and the amount of carbohydrates in your diet.

Gestational diabetes affects about 10% of all pregnancies. After birth, nearly all women who experience the problem return to normal, and it disappears. However, if gestational diabetes occurs with one pregnancy, there's almost a 90% chance it will happen in future pregnancies. In addition, some women who develop gestational diabetes may develop type-2 diabetes within 10 years. Your best protection is to stay within the recommended weight-gain limits your healthcare provider gives you.

We believe gestational diabetes occurs for two reasons. One is the mother's body produces less insulin during pregnancy. The second is the mother's body can't use insulin effectively. Both situations result in high blood-sugar levels. Risk factors for developing gestational diabetes include:

- over 30 years old
- obesity
- family history of diabetes
- gestational diabetes in previous pregnancy
- previously gave birth to baby who weighed over 9½ pounds

- previously had a stillborn baby
- being Black/African American, Latina/Hispanic, Asian, Native American or Pacific Islander

A woman's weight when she was born may also be an indicator of her chances of developing gestational diabetes. One study showed women who were in the *bottom 10th percentile* of weight when they were born were 3 to 4 times more likely to develop gestational diabetes during pregnancy.

Symptoms and Treatment for Gestational Diabetes. Good control of gestational diabetes is important. If left untreated, it can be serious for you and your baby. You will both be exposed to a high concentration of sugar, which is not healthy for either of you. You might experience *polyhydramnios* (excessive amounts of amniotic fluid). This may cause premature labor because the uterus becomes overdistended. Symptoms of gestational diabetes include:

- blurred vision
- tingling or numbness in hands and/or feet
- excessive thirst
- frequent urination
- sores that heal slowly
- excess fatigue

If you have gestational diabetes, you're at higher risk of problems. If your blood-sugar level is high, you may get more infections during pregnancy. You are also more likely to develop gum disease, which may raise your resistance to insulin. Treating it may help lower your risk of developing pregnancy complications.

Experts believe a woman with gestational diabetes may overfeed her fetus and cause baby to store more fat after birth. Treating the problem may help reduce your baby's risk of being obese in later life. You may also have a long labor because baby is big. Sometimes a baby can't fit through the birth canal, and a Cesarean delivery is required.

Treatment of gestational diabetes includes regular exercise and increased fluid intake. Diet is essential in handling the problem. If your gestational diabetes is controlled by diet alone, monitor yourself very closely. Controlling your gestational diabetes can lower the risk of delivering an oversize infant.

Your healthcare provider will probably recommend a six-meal, 2000- to 2500-calorie-per-day eating plan. You may also be referred to a dietitian. Research shows women who receive dietary counseling, blood-sugar monitoring and insulin therapy (when needed) do better during pregnancy than women who receive routine care.

Eating a diet low in fat and high in fiber may help reduce your risk of getting gestational diabetes. If your intake of vitamin C is low, it may increase your risk.

Insulin therapy is the first choice when medicine is necessary to treat the problem. In some cases, oral medications, such as glyburide or Metformin, are used.

Your Nutrition

You may need to be careful with your sodium intake during pregnancy. Taking in too much sodium may cause you to retain water, which can contribute to swelling and bloating. However, you do need *some* every day to help deal with your increased blood volume. Aim for between 1500 and 2300mg of sodium a day.

Tip for Week 23

Keeping your consumption of sodium to 2 grams (2000mg) or less a day may help you reduce fluid retention.

Eat potassium-rich foods, such as raisins and bananas; potassium helps the body get rid of sodium faster. Avoid foods that contain lots of sodium or salt, such as salted nuts, potato chips, pickles, canned foods and processed foods.

Read food labels. They list the amount of sodium in a serving. Some books list the sodium content of foods without labels, such as fast foods. Check them out. You'll be surprised how many milligrams of sodium a fast-food hamburger contains!

Sodium Content of Various Foods

Food	Serving Size	Sodium Content (mg)
American cheese	1 slice	322
Asparagus	14½-oz. can	970
Big Mac hamburger	1 regular	963
Chicken á la king	1 cup	760
Cola	8 oz.	16
Cottage cheese	1 cup	580
Dill pickle	1 medium	928
Flounder	3 oz.	201
Gelatin, sweet	3 oz.	270
Ham, baked	3 oz.	770
Honeydew melon	½	90
Lima beans	8½ oz.	1070
Lobster	1 cup	305
Oatmeal	1 cup	523
Potato chips	20 regular	400
Salt	1 teaspoon	1938

Look at the chart above; it lists some common foods and their sodium content. You can see foods that contain sodium don't always taste salty. Check available information before you eat!

You Should Also Know

Sugar in Your Urine

Sugar in the urine is called *glucosuria*. It's common during pregnancy, especially in the second and third trimesters. It occurs because of changes in sugar levels and how sugar is handled in the kidneys, which control the amount of sugar in your system. If extra sugar is present, you will lose it in your urine.

Many healthcare providers test every pregnant woman for diabetes, usually around the end of the second trimester. Testing is important if you have a family history of diabetes. Blood tests used to diagnose diabetes are a fasting blood-sugar test and a glucose-tolerance test (GTT).

For a *fasting blood-sugar test,* you eat a normal meal the evening before the test. In the morning, before eating anything, you go to the lab and have a blood test done. A normal result indicates diabetes is unlikely. An abnormal result (a high level of sugar in the blood) needs further study.

Further study involves the *glucose-tolerance test (GTT).* Again you must fast after dinner the night before this test. In the morning at the lab, you are given a solution to drink that has a measured amount of sugar in it. It is similar to a bottle of soda pop but doesn't taste as good. After you drink the solution, blood is drawn at certain intervals, usually 30 minutes, 1 hour and 2 hours, and sometimes even 3 hours. Drawing blood at intervals reveals how your body handles sugar. If you need treatment, your healthcare provider can devise a plan for you.

Teen Pregnancy

Teen pregnancy impacts our society in many ways and costs the United States about $7 billion each year. *Teen pregnancy* is defined as pregnancy in young women between the ages of 13 and 19 years of age. Young women in the 18- to 19-year-old range have the highest pregnancy rate among teens. The United States continues to have the highest rates of teenage pregnancy/births in the western world. Some ethnic groups in our country are at higher risk.

Teenage births have dropped by nearly a third since the early 1990s. Some experts believe this drop in number has occurred because the *overall birth rate* in the United States has fallen.

Thirteen percent of all U.S. births are to teens; 24% of births to unmarried women are to teenage moms. About 65% of all teen pregnancies are unplanned. An unplanned pregnancy is defined as a pregnancy that was mistimed or unwanted at the time of conception.

Pregnancy in a teenager can be difficult for the mother-to-be for many reasons. Many teens do not seek prenatal care until the second trimester. Many teenage mothers-to-be have poor eating habits, and often they don't take their prenatal vitamins. A large number of teens continue to drink alcohol, use drugs and/or smoke during pregnancy. In fact, teens have the highest smoking rate of all pregnant women.

Studies show pregnant teens are often underweight when they enter pregnancy and often do not gain enough weight during pregnancy. This can lead to low-birthweight babies. Teen mothers are also more likely to give birth to premature babies. Other problems include anemia and high blood pressure. Depression during pregnancy has also been reported to be higher in teens. Babies born to teen moms may also have more birth defects.

Sexually transmitted diseases may be a problem for pregnant adolescents. Over 25% of all cases of STDs reported every year occur in teenagers.

A teenager who is pregnant will do herself and her baby a favor by paying attention to the following:

- eating a healthy diet
- gaining the correct amount of weight, as determined by her healthcare provider
- not smoking
- not drinking alcohol
- staying away from drugs
- getting early prenatal care
- keeping all her prenatal appointments
- addressing any health care problems immediately, such as taking care of an STD
- following her healthcare provider's recommendations when dealing with problems
- avoiding all prescription and over-the-counter medicines, unless her healthcare provider tells her to take them
- asking for help when she needs it

Exercise for Week 23

Sit on the edge of a chair, and place both feet flat on the floor. Relax your shoulders, and curve your arms over your head. Keeping your back straight, hold in your tummy muscles while you extend one leg out in front. Using your thigh muscles only, lift your leg about 10 inches off the floor. Hold for a count of 5, then slowly lower your foot. Repeat 10 times with each leg. *Tones thigh, hips and buttocks muscles.*

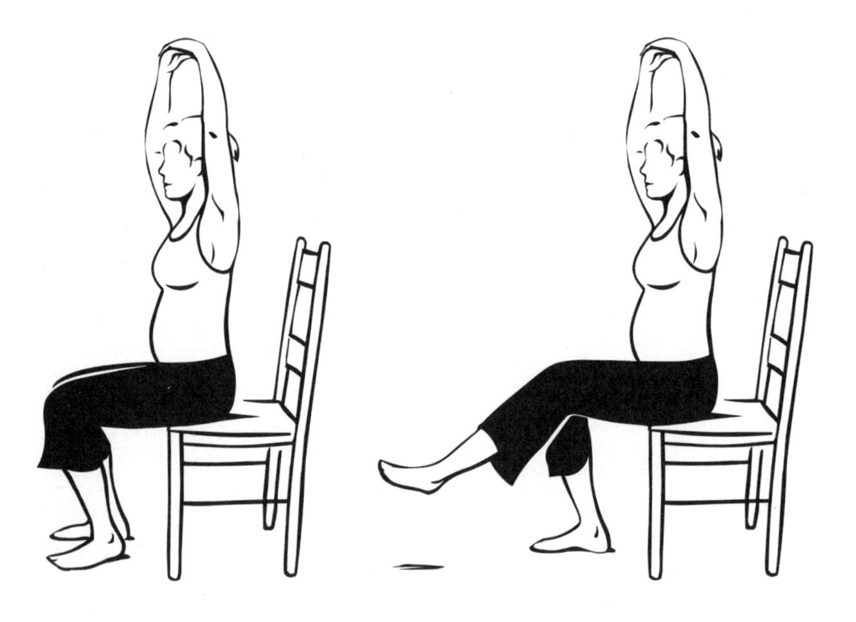

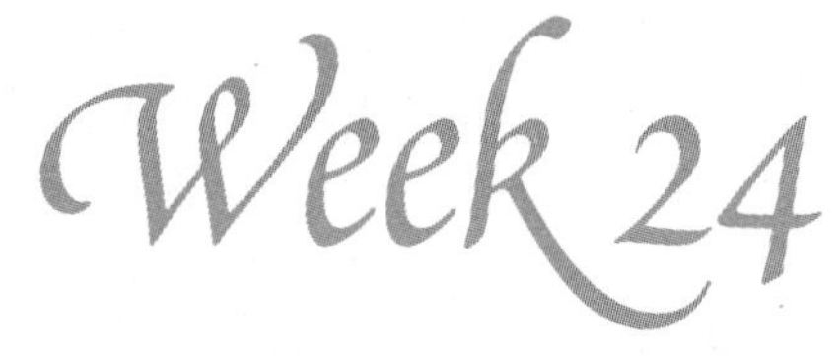

Week 24

Age of Fetus—22 Weeks

How Big Is Your Baby?

By this week, baby weighs about 1¼ pounds (540g). Its crown-to-rump length is about 8½ inches (21cm).

How Big Are You?

Your uterus is now about 1½ to 2 inches (3.8 to 5.1cm) above the belly-button. It measures almost 10 inches (24cm) above the pubic symphysis.

How Your Baby Is Growing and Developing

Your baby is filling out. Its face and body look more like that of an infant at the time of birth. Although it weighs a little over 1 pound at this point, it is still very tiny.

The baby grows in amniotic fluid inside the amniotic sac. See the illustration on page 345. Amniotic fluid has several important functions. It provides an environment in which the baby can move easily and cushions the fetus against injury. It regulates temperature. It also provides a way of assessing the health and maturity of the baby.

Amniotic fluid increases rapidly from an average volume of 1½ ounces (50ml) by 12 weeks of pregnancy to 12 ounces (400ml) at midpregnancy. The volume of amniotic fluid continues to increase as your due date approaches until a maximum of about 2 pints (1 liter) of fluid is reached at 36 to 38 weeks gestation.

Makeup of amniotic fluid changes during pregnancy. During the first half of pregnancy, it's similar to the fluid in your blood without blood cells, except it has a much lower protein content. As baby grows, fetal urine adds to the amount of amniotic fluid present. Amniotic fluid also contains old fetal blood cells, lanugo hair and vernix.

The fetus swallows amniotic fluid during much of pregnancy. If it can't swallow the fluid, you may develop a condition of excess amniotic fluid, called *hydramnios* or *polyhydramnios*. If the fetus swallows but doesn't urinate (for example, if the baby lacks kidneys), the volume of amniotic fluid surrounding the fetus may be very small. This is called *oligohydramnios*.

Changes in You

Nasal Problems

Some women complain of stuffiness in their nose or frequent nosebleeds during pregnancy. Some experts believe these symptoms occur because of circulation changes caused by hormonal changes during pregnancy. Mucous membranes of your nose and nasal passageways swell and bleed more easily.

A few decongestants and nasal sprays can be used during pregnancy. Some brands to consider include chlorpheniramine (Chlor-Trimeton) decongestants and oxymetazoline (Afrin, Dristan Long-Lasting) nasal sprays. Before you begin using any product, discuss it with your healthcare provider.

It may also help to use a humidifier, particularly during winter months when heating may dry out the air. Some women get relief from increasing their fluid intake and/or using a gentle lubricant in their nose, such as petroleum jelly.

Depression

Depression can occur at any time during a person's life. Many things can contribute to depression, including chemical imbalances in the body, stressful life events and situations that cause anxiety and tension. If you

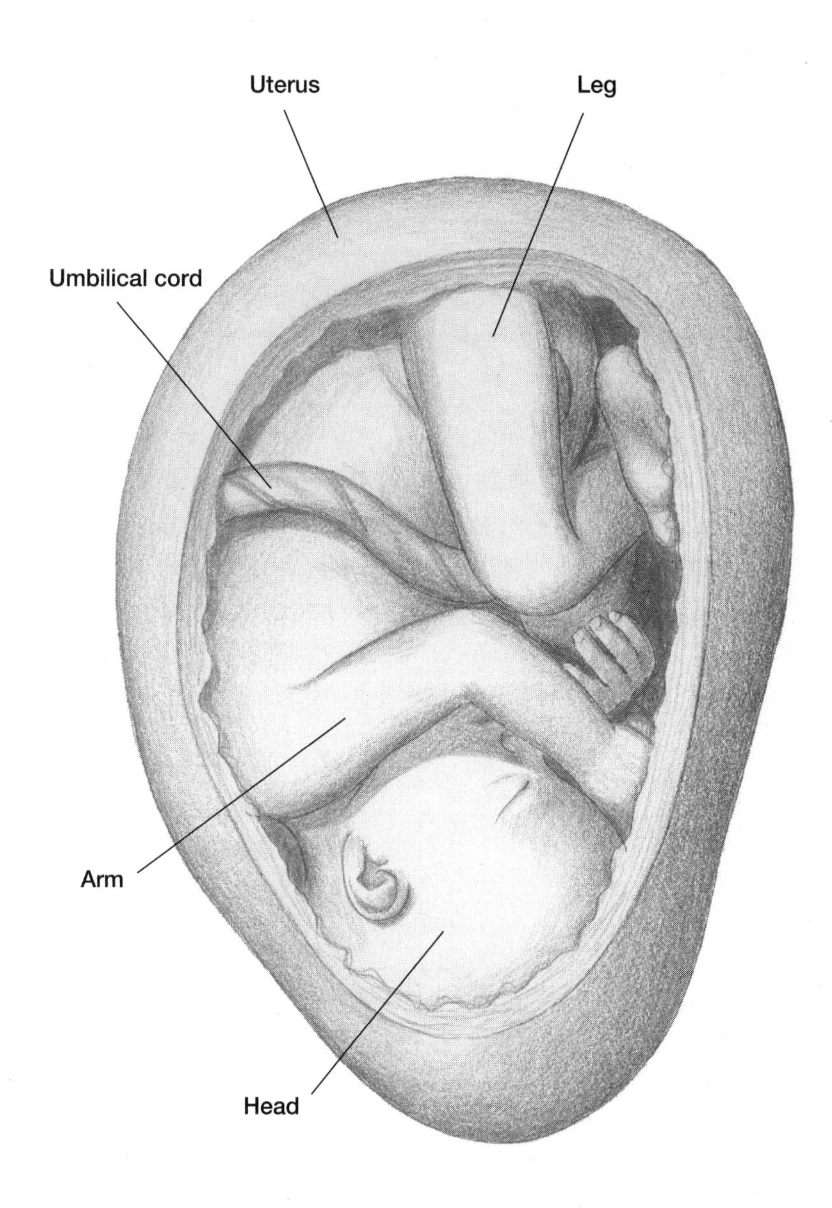

The fetus doesn't appear to have a great deal of room to move in the uterus by the 24th week. As the weeks pass, space gets even tighter.

have a history of major depression, you're at increased risk of depression occurring during pregnancy. In fact, between 3 and 5% of all women experience a major depression during pregnancy. It's estimated another 15% have some degree of depression.

If you're being treated for depression when you get pregnant, it's important to continue treatment. Treating depression is as important as treating any other problem.

If you take antidepressants, don't stop unless advised by your healthcare provider to do so. Studies show up to 70% of women who stop taking antidepressants during pregnancy relapse into depression. Stopping your medication can raise stress hormones, which increases your risks of problems during pregnancy. The risks to you and your baby from depression may be greater than your risk of taking antidepressants. We know depression can be difficult to manage without using drug therapy.

There may be a very small increased risk of birth defects with some medicines used to treat depression when taken during the first trimester. It may help to switch to an antidepressant that is safer during pregnancy, including fluoxetine (Prozac), citalopram and escitalopram (Lexapro). Pregnancy may affect your body's ability to use lithium. If you take an SSRI, the dose may need to be increased during the third trimester to maintain your normal mood. Talk to your healthcare provider as soon as you confirm your pregnancy.

There is continued concern about the safety of Paxil during pregnancy. Research suggests using the drug in the first trimester of pregnancy may be tied to an increased risk of heart problems in baby. However, do *not* stop taking your antidepressant medicine without first consulting your healthcare provider.

If you're feeling depressed, your level of vitamin D may be low. Talk about it with your healthcare provider. Other suggestions for dealing with depression include getting some exercise and being sure you get enough B vitamins, folic acid and omega-3 fatty acids. Taking about 3.5g of omega-3 fatty acids every day has been shown to help fight depression.

Additional therapies include massage and reflexology. Another option is light therapy, similar to the type of treatment given to those who suffer from "seasonal affective disorder."

Depression during Pregnancy. Depression *during* pregnancy does occur. Experts believe it's one of the most common medical problems seen in pregnant women. Studies show up to 25% of all moms-to-be experience some degree of depression, and nearly 10% will experience a major depression. And if left untreated, 50% of women who are depressed during pregnancy will experience postpartum depression.

Treating depression during pregnancy is important for your health and baby's health. This is one of the many reasons healthcare providers today make treating depression a priority.

Dad Tip

Now's a good time to explore prenatal classes in your area. Encourage your partner to find out how many classes there are, when and where to register, and the registration cost. You may be able to take classes at the hospital or birthing center where your partner plans to deliver. Try to complete the classes at least 1 month before baby is due.

Depression is actually more common during pregnancy than after giving birth. (For a discussion of depression after pregnancy, see Appendix F, page 616.) If you have a family history of depression, you may be at higher risk during pregnancy. If you don't have enough serotonin, researchers believe you may be at higher risk. If you've been struggling with infertility or miscarriage, you may also be more prone to depression.

If you're depressed, you may not take good care of yourself. Babies born to depressed women may be smaller or born prematurely. Some women use alcohol, drugs and cigarettes in an attempt to ease their depression. You may also have trouble bonding with your baby after birth.

Consider the following to measure your risks of being depressed. You may be at higher risk if:

- you experienced mood changes when you took oral contraceptives
- your mother was depressed during pregnancy
- you have a history of depression
- you feel sad or depressed longer than 1 week
- you're not getting enough sleep and rest
- you have bipolar disorder—pregnancy can trigger a relapse, especially if you stop taking your mood-stabilizing medications

Symptoms and Treatment. It may be hard to differentiate between some of the normal pregnancy changes and signs of depression. Many symptoms of depression are similar to those of pregnancy, including fatigue and sleeplessness. The difference is how intense the symptoms are and how long they last. Some common symptoms of depression include:

- overpowering sadness that lasts for days, without an obvious cause
- difficulty sleeping, or waking up very early
- wanting to sleep all the time or great fatigue (this can be normal early in pregnancy but usually gets better after a few weeks)
- no appetite (as distinguished from nausea and vomiting)
- lack of concentration
- thoughts of harming yourself

Women who are depressed are more likely to develop diabetes, and women who develop diabetes are more likely to be depressed. This is also true for pregnant women. If you have diabetes and untreated depression, then become pregnant, it can be serious if you don't get help. You may have a difficult time caring for yourself. This could lead to difficulties in controlling weight and sugar levels. Your risk of addictive-substance abuse, such as alcohol use and cigarette smoking, may increase. And you may not be able to meet the nutritional demands of your pregnancy.

Research shows it's better for baby if only one medicine is used during pregnancy to treat a woman's depression.

Babies born to mothers with untreated depression can have many problems. They often cry a lot, have difficulty sleeping, are fussier and are difficult to soothe.

If you have symptoms and they don't get better in a few weeks or every day seems to be bad, seek help as soon as you recognize you might be depressed. Call your healthcare provider, or bring it up at your next prenatal visit. There are steps to take to help you feel better again. It's important to do it for yourself and your baby!

How Your Actions Affect Your Baby's Development

Outside Noises Can Affect Baby

Can a baby hear sounds from outside its mom's body while inside the uterus? From various studies, we know sounds penetrate amniotic fluid and reach your baby's developing ears. In fact, ultrasounds done around this time have shown babies reacting to loud noises.

If you work in a noisy place, you may want to request a quieter area. Data suggests chronic loud noise and short, intense bursts of sound may cause hearing damage to the baby before birth.

It's OK to expose your growing baby to loud noises, such as a concert, every once in a while. But if you're repeatedly exposed to noise that is so loud it forces you to shout, it may be dangerous for your growing baby.

Moving during Pregnancy

Moving to a new city at any time can be stressful; when you're pregnant, it can also be challenging. How can you find a new healthcare provider? What hospital will you use?

Before you leave your old home, find a hospital in the area you're moving to that you want to use, then find a healthcare provider (who is accepting new patients) who delivers at that hospital. Do this as soon as you learn you're moving because it may take some time to get in to see the new healthcare provider for your first appointment.

A real-estate agent should be able to help in this situation. Ask about a hospital with a level-2 or level-3 nursery. These hospitals are better able to deal with various complications of pregnancy and birth. Even if you haven't had any problems, you'll rest easier knowing the hospital can handle an emergency.

When you've chosen the hospital, call the labor-and-delivery department and ask to speak with a supervisor. Explain your situation, and ask for recommendations for three or four good obstetricians who deliver at the hospital, who are accepting new patients.

When you have the names, call each office and explain your situation. Request information about fees and insurance coverage. Ask if you can get an appointment for the first week you're in town. Then make your decision about which healthcare provider you want to use, and call back and confirm your appointment.

After you decide on someone, go to the healthcare provider you now see, and ask for copies of your medical records. Be sure they include results of any tests you've had. Take everything with you. If the office says they'll send them to the new healthcare provider, tell them that's fine, but you must also have copies to take with you. Sending records can take a long time.

If you haven't had your alpha-fetoprotein test or a triple-screen test done, and you are between 15 and 19 weeks of pregnancy, ask your current healthcare provider to order them and have the results sent to you at your new address. It can take several weeks to get the results of these two tests, and it will be helpful for your new healthcare provider to have the results when you go to see him or her. Ask your healthcare provider to write a short letter of introduction that you can give to your new healthcare provider. This is a brief summary of your pregnancy, current health and health concerns.

Your Nutrition

Many pregnant women are concerned about eating out. Some want to know if they can eat certain types of food, such as Mexican, Vietnamese, Thai or Greek food. They're concerned spicy or rich foods could be harmful to the baby. It's OK to eat out, but you might find certain foods don't agree with you.

The best types of food to eat at restaurants are those you tolerate well at home. Chicken, fish, fresh vegetables and salads are usually good choices. Eating foods at restaurants that feature spicy foods or unusual cuisine may cause stomach or intestinal distress. You may even notice an increase in weight from water retention after eating at a restaurant.

Avoid restaurants that serve highly salted food, food high in sodium or food loaded with calories and fat, such as gravies, fried food, junk food and rich desserts. It may be difficult to control your calorie intake at specialty restaurants.

Another challenge of eating out is maintaining a healthy diet if you work outside the home. It may be necessary to go to business lunches or to travel for your company. Be selective. If you can choose off the menu, look for healthy or low-fat choices. Ask about preparation—maybe a dish can be steamed instead of fried. On a business trip, take along some of your own food. Choose healthy, nonperishable foods, such as fruits and vegetables, that don't need refrigeration.

You Should Also Know

Crohn's Disease and Pregnancy

Crohn's disease is a chronic illness in which the intestine or bowel becomes inflamed and scarred with sores; it usually affects the part of the small intestine called the *ileum*. However, Crohn's can occur in any part of the large or small intestine, stomach, esophagus or even the mouth.

Crohn's disease is part of a group of diseases called *inflammatory bowel disease* or *IBD*. See the discussion of IBD in Week 18. Crohn's disease most commonly occurs between ages 15 and 30. Sufferers experience periods of severe symptoms followed by periods with no symptoms. Symptoms include chronic diarrhea, rectal bleeding, weight loss, fever, abdominal pain and/or tenderness and a feeling of fullness in the lower-right abdomen.

> *Tip for Week 24*
>
> Overeating and eating before going to bed at night are two major causes of heartburn. Eating five or six small, nutritious meals a day and skipping snacks before bedtime may help you feel better.

If you have active Crohn's disease, getting pregnant may be more difficult. An active disease raises the risk of problems. A flare-up may occur during pregnancy, most often in the third trimester, but flare-ups are often mild and respond to treatment.

> ### *Is Food Hot Enough to Be Safe?*
>
> Don't rely on a taste test to determine if food is hot enough to be safe to eat. When reheating leftovers, use a quick-reading thermometer to make sure food has reached an interior temperature of 165F. This is the temperature at which harmful bacteria are killed.

Symptoms may be less severe because pregnancy alters the immune system. Being pregnant may also protect against future flare-ups and may reduce the need for surgery. During pregnancy, your body produces the hormone relaxin. Researchers believe relaxin may also curb the formation of scar tissue.

You probably won't need to change your medicines during pregnancy. Sulfasalazine, mesalamine, balsalazide and olsalazine don't hurt the baby. Infliximab (Remicade) and adalimumab (Humira) may be necessary during pregnancy and breastfeeding. Avoid methotrexate during pregnancy.

You may need various tests during pregnancy. Experts believe it's safe to have a colonoscopy, sigmoidoscopy, upper endoscopy, rectal biopsy or abdominal ultrasound during pregnancy. Avoid X-rays and CT scans. Ask your pregnancy healthcare provider about an MRI if one is recommended.

If you've had a bowel resection, you probably won't have problems during pregnancy. An ileostomy may decrease fertility. If you develop an abnormal opening near your rectum or in the vaginal area, you may need a Cesarean delivery.

The type of delivery you have depends on the condition of the tissues around the vagina and anus. A Cesarean may be recommended if you develop a fistula or to reduce your risk of developing fistulas.

Many women suffer flare-ups immediately after birth. Healthcare providers believe this is due to the hormonal changes after pregnancy.

How Pregnancy Affects Your Sexual Desire

Pregnancy and sex. Has your sexual desire increased? Is sex the last thing on your mind? Generally, women experience one of two sex-drive patterns during pregnancy. One is a lessening of desire in the first and third trimesters, with an increase in the second trimester. The second is a gradual decrease in desire for sex as pregnancy progresses.

During the first trimester, you may experience fatigue and nausea. In the third trimester, your weight gain, enlarging abdomen, tender breasts and other problems may make you desire sex less. This is normal. Tell your partner how you feel, and try to work out a solution that pleases you both. Tenderness and understanding can help.

Pregnancy enhances the sex drive for some women. A woman may experience orgasms or multiple orgasms for the first time during pregnancy. This is due to heightened hormonal activity and increased blood flow to the pelvic area.

When to Avoid Sexual Activity

Some situations should alert you to refrain from sexual activity. If you have a history of early labor, your healthcare provider may warn against intercourse and orgasm; orgasm causes mild uterine contractions. Chemicals in semen may also stimulate contractions, so it may not be advisable for a woman's partner to ejaculate inside her.

If you have a history of miscarriage, your healthcare provider may caution you against sex and orgasm. However, no data actually links sex and miscarriage. Your healthcare provider may advise no sex if you have certain pregnancy problems.

Some sexual practices should be avoided when you're pregnant. Don't insert any object into the vagina that could cause injury or infection. Blowing air into the vagina is dangerous because it can force a potentially fatal air bubble into a woman's bloodstream. (This can occur whether or not you are pregnant.) Nipple stimulation releases oxytocin, which causes uterine contractions; discuss this practice with your healthcare provider.

An Incompetent Cervix

An incompetent cervix refers to painless premature dilatation (stretching) of the cervix, which usually results in delivery of a premature baby. Usually the problem doesn't happen until after the 16th week of pregnancy. The woman doesn't realize the cervix has dilated until the baby is delivering; it often occurs without warning. Diagnosis is usually made after one or more deliveries of a premature infant without any pain before delivery. Fortunately, an incompetent cervix is relatively rare.

If this is your first pregnancy, there's no way to know whether you have the problem. The cause of cervical incompetence is usually unknown. Some experts believe it occurs because of previous injury or surgery to the cervix, such as dilatation and curettage (D&C) for an abortion or a miscarriage. If you've had problems in the past or have had premature deliveries and have been told you might have an incompetent cervix, share this important information with your healthcare provider.

Ultrasound may be used to measure the cervix. If a woman's cervix is shorter than normal, the condition is sometimes described as a *short cervix* or *shortened cervix.*

Treatment for an incompetent cervix is usually surgical. The weak cervix is closed with a *McDonald cerclage.* A suture, similar to a "purse-string," is stitched around the cervix to keep it closed. The procedure is usually performed in a hospital operating room or in labor and delivery. General anesthesia or I.V. sedation is given. The procedure takes about 30 minutes; after it's over, you'll probably be monitored for a few hours before you can go home. It's normal to have a little bit of spotting or bleeding afterward.

Treat Yourself Well

Be good to yourself during your pregnancy. Light some candles and soak in the tub. Go to your hairdresser for some pampering. Download some of your favorite music to your iPod or MP3 player. Rent a tear-jerker movie, and cry your eyes out. Buy yourself flowers. Get a pedicure even if you can't see your feet anymore.

At about 36 weeks or when you go into labor, the stitch is removed, and baby can be born normally. The suture is removed in labor and delivery without anesthesia. It takes about 5 minutes. Labor does not necessarily happen immediately after it's removed; it can occur in a few days to a few weeks.

Exercise for Week 24

Stand with your right side against the back of the sofa or a sturdy chair. Hold onto the back with your right hand. Bend your knee, and bring your left foot up behind your bottom. Grasp your foot with your left hand. Keeping your right knee slightly bent, hold for 10 seconds. Repeat for your right leg. *Strengthens quadriceps.*

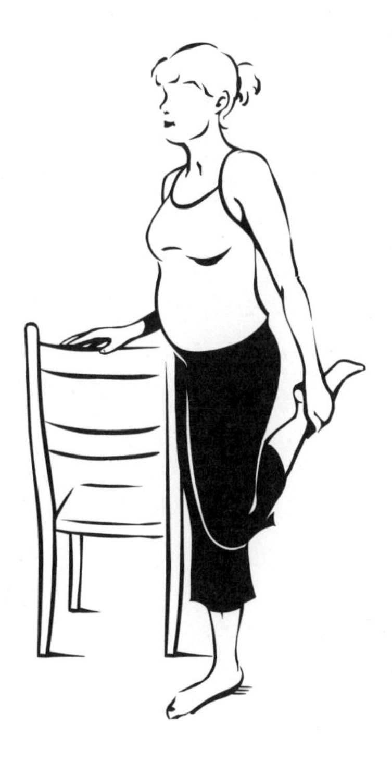

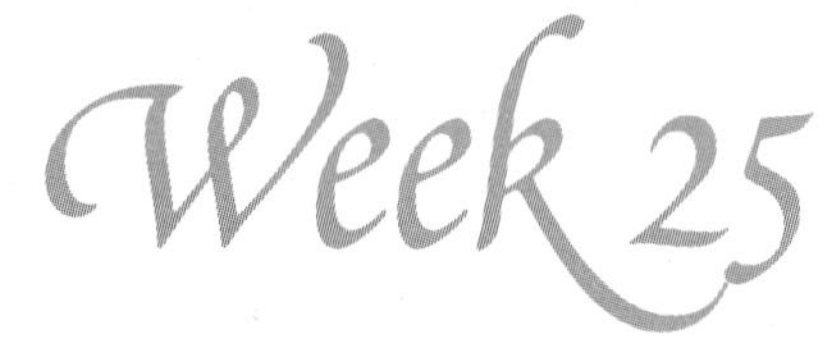

Week 25

Age of Fetus—23 Weeks

How Big Is Your Baby?

Your baby now weighs about 1½ pounds (700g), and crown-to-rump length is about 8¾ inches (22cm). These are average lengths and weights, and can vary from one baby to another and from one pregnancy to another.

How Big Are You?

Look at the illustration on page 358. Your uterus has grown quite a bit and is about the size of a soccer ball. When you look at a side view, you're much bigger. During pregnancy, your baby will have growth spurts, which may slightly affect your weight gain at certain times.

Measurement from the pubic symphysis to the top of the uterus is about 10 inches (25cm). The uterus is about halfway between your belly-button and the lower part of your sternum (the bone between your breasts where the ribs come together). If you were seen around 20 weeks of pregnancy, you've probably grown about 1½ inches (4cm).

How Your Baby Is Growing and Developing

Survival of a Premature Baby

It may be hard to believe, but if your baby were delivered now, it would have a chance of surviving. A baby born at this time probably weighs less than 2 pounds and is extremely small. Survival can be difficult, and the baby would probably spend several months in the hospital. See the discussion of Premature Labor in Week 29.

Is Baby a Boy? A Girl?

One of the most common questions we hear is, "What is the sex of our baby?" For many couples, not knowing is part of the fun of having a baby.

Amniocentesis can definitely determine baby's sex. Ultrasound may predict baby's sex but is not foolproof. Some at-home tests claim to be able to determine baby's gender, but don't count on it. Some people believe a baby's heartbeat rate can indicate its sex. Unfortunately, there is no scientific proof of this.

> Although this book is designed to take you through pregnancy by examining one week at a time, you may want specific information. Because the book can't include *everything* you need *before* you know you're looking for it, check the index, beginning on page 655, for a particular topic. We may not cover the subject until a later week.

A more reliable source might be a mother, mother-in-law or someone who can look at you and tell by how you're carrying the baby if it is a boy or girl. Although we make this statement with our tongues placed firmly in our cheeks, many people believe it's true. Some people claim they're never wrong about guessing or predicting the sex of a baby before birth. Again, there is no scientific basis for this method.

Your healthcare provider is more concerned about the health and well-being of you and your baby. He or she will concentrate on making sure you both are progressing through pregnancy safely and you both get through pregnancy, labor and delivery in good health.

Changes in You

Itching

Itching (pruritus gravidarum) is a common symptom during pregnancy. There are no bumps or lesions on the skin; it just itches. Nearly 20% of all pregnant women suffer from itching, often in the last weeks

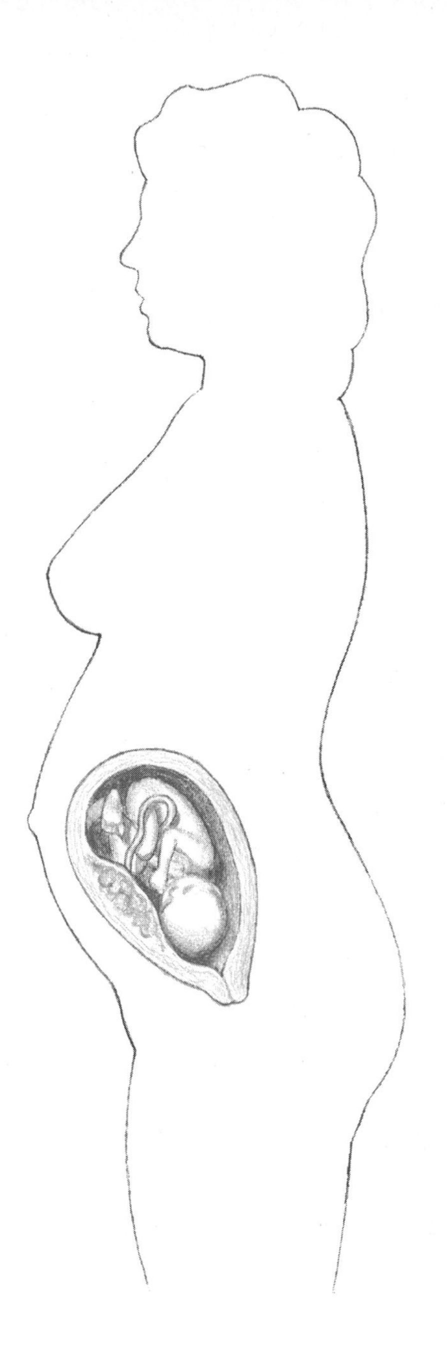

Comparative size of the uterus at 25 weeks of pregnancy (fetal age—23 weeks). The uterus can be felt about 2 inches (5cm) above your umbilicus (bellybutton).

of pregnancy, but it can occur at any time. It may occur with each pregnancy and may also appear when you use oral contraceptives. The condition isn't harmful to you or baby.

> **Tip for Week 25**
>
> **Pregnancy can be a time of communication and personal growth with your partner. Listen when he talks. Let him know he is an important source of emotional support for you.**

As your uterus has grown and filled your pelvis, your skin and muscles have stretched. Itchiness may be a consequence. Lotions are OK to use to help reduce itching. Try not to scratch and irritate your skin—that can make it worse! Ask your healthcare provider about taking antihistamines or using cooling lotions containing menthol or camphor. Often no treatment is needed.

Stress during Pregnancy

Feeling stress is common during any woman's life. *Stress* is what you feel in situations that are dangerous, difficult or menacing. *Chronic stress* is stress caused by ongoing situations or problems, such as unemployment, deployment of your partner, financial problems. *Anxiety* is magnified worry and is greater than justified.

> Many experts believe stress in you can affect the health of your baby, including causing gastric disorders, such as colic, and later in life, reading difficulties and/or behavioral problems.

Pregnancy is stressful! Studies show pregnancy ranks #12 on a list of life's most stressful events. Normal stress probably won't hurt you or baby, but major stress may increase your risk of premature birth. Learning to manage stress can go a long way in making your life more manageable—when you're pregnant and when you're not!

During pregnancy, stress can be caused by many things. Hormone changes can cause you to react in ways that aren't normal for you, which can be stressful. Your body is changing, which stresses many women.

You may have worked very hard to get and/or to maintain your figure—now that you're pregnant, there's not much you can do about it.

Eating well and exercising can help you feel better and may relieve some stress. You may be thinking about being a good parent—the prospect of parenthood can be stressful for anyone. You may not be feeling very well, which adds to the problem. You may feel stress from working or other obligations.

Relax, and take it easy! There are many things you can do to help relieve stress. Try them, and encourage your partner to try them if he's also feeling stressed out.

- Get enough sleep each night. Lack of sleep can make you feel stressed.
- Rest and relax during the day. Read or listen to music during a quiet period. Slow down in your daily activities.
- When you feel stressed, stop and take a few slow, deep breaths. This can help turn off the stressed part of your nervous system.
- Exercise can help you work off stress. Take a walk or visit the gym. Put on an exercise video for pregnant women. Do something active and physical (but not too physical) to relieve stress. Ask your partner to join you.
- It may sound corny, but think "happy thoughts." When you turn your thoughts to good things, it actually sends a chemical message to your brain that flows through your entire body and helps you relax.
- Eat nutritiously. Having enough calories available all through the day helps you avoid "lows."
- Be positive. Sometimes deciding to be more positive can affect you. Smiling instead of frowning can help ease stress—put on a happy face.
- Do something you enjoy, and do it for you.
- If smells are important to you, make sure you include them in your life. Burn scented candles, or buy fragrant flowers to help you relax.
- Don't be a loner. Share your concerns with your partner, or find a group of pregnant women you can talk with.

How Your Actions Affect Your Baby's Development

Falling and Injuries from Falls

A fall is the most frequent cause of minor injury during pregnancy. Fortunately, a fall is usually without serious injury to the baby or mother-to-be. The uterus is well protected in the abdomen inside the pelvis. The baby is protected by the cushion of amniotic fluid surrounding it. Your uterus and abdominal wall also offer some protection.

If you fall, contact your healthcare provider; he or she may want to examine you. You may feel reassured if you're monitored and baby's heartbeat is checked. Baby's movement after a fall can be reassuring.

Minor injuries to the abdomen are treated as though you were not pregnant. However, avoid X-rays if possible. Ultrasound evaluation may be the test of choice after a fall. This is judged on an individual basis, depending on the severity of your symptoms and your injury.

Your balance and mobility change as you grow larger during pregnancy. Be careful during the winter when parking lots and sidewalks may be wet or icy. Many pregnant women fall on stairs; always use the handrail. Walk in well-lit areas, and try to stay on sidewalks.

> **Dad Tip**
>
> Who knew forgetfulness could be tied to pregnancy? If you find your partner just can't remember things you ask her to do or to remember something important to you, make lists for her. Approach it with humor—you may find you get a better response.

Slow down a little as you get larger; you won't be able to get around as quickly as you normally do. With the change in your balance, plus any dizziness you experience, it's important to be watchful to avoid falling.

Some signs can alert you to a problem after a fall, including bleeding, a gush of fluid from the vagina, indicating rupture of membranes, and/or severe abdominal pain. Placental abruption, premature separation of the placenta from the uterus, is one of the most serious problems caused by a fall.

Sometimes a fall or accident causes a broken bone, which may require X-rays and surgery. Treatment cannot be delayed until after pregnancy;

the problem must be dealt with immediately. If you find yourself in such a situation, insist your pregnancy healthcare provider be contacted before any test is done or treatment is started.

If X-rays are required, your pelvis and abdomen must be shielded. If they can't be shielded, the need for the X-ray must be weighed against the risk it poses to baby.

Anesthesia or pain medication may be necessary with a simple break that requires setting or pinning. It is best for you and the baby to avoid general anesthesia if possible. You may need pain medicine, but keep its use to a minimum.

If general anesthesia is required to repair a break, the baby should be monitored closely. Your surgeon and pregnancy healthcare provider will work together to provide the best care for you and your baby.

Your Nutrition

Pregnancy increases your need for vitamins and minerals. It's best if you can meet most of these needs through the foods you eat. However, being realistic, we know that can be hard to do. That's one reason your healthcare provider prescribes a prenatal vitamin for you—to help you meet your nutritional needs.

Some women do need extra help during pregnancy—supplements are often prescribed for them. These pregnant women include teenagers (whose bodies are still growing), severely underweight women, women who ate a poor diet before conception and women who have previously given birth to multiples. Women who smoke or drink may need supplements, as do some who have a chronic medical condition, those who take certain medications and those who have problems digesting cow's milk, wheat and other essential foods. In some cases, vegetarians may need supplements.

If you have a burst of energy during this trimester, use it to get out of the house.

A Balanced Meal Plan

Below is a list of some foods to choose from each group and an appropriate serving size for each. There are many different foods to choose from.

- Breads, cereals, rice, pasta and grains, 6 to 11 servings—1 slice of bread, ½ bun, ½ English muffin, ½ small bagel, ½ cup cooked pasta, rice or hot cereal, 4 crackers, ¾ cup cold cereal
- Fruit, 2 to 4 servings—¼ cup dried fruit, ½ cup fresh, canned or cooked fruit, ¾ cup juice
- Vegetables, 3 to 5 servings—½ cup cooked vegetables, 1 cup leafy salad vegetables, ¾ cup juice
- Protein sources, 2 to 3 servings—2 to 3 ounces of cooked poultry, meat or fish, 1 cup cooked beans, ¼ cup seeds or nuts, ½ cup tofu, 2 eggs
- Dairy products, 4 servings—1 cup milk (any type), 1 cup yogurt, 1½ ounces cheese, 1½ cups of cottage cheese, 1½ cups frozen yogurt, ice milk or ice cream
- Fats, oils and sweets—limit intake of these food products; concentrate on nutritious, healthy foods

Your healthcare provider can discuss the situation with you. If you need more than a prenatal vitamin, he or she will advise you. **Caution:** Never take *any* supplements without your healthcare provider's OK!

You Should Also Know

At-Home Teeth Whitening Kits

At-home teeth whitening products are very popular, and many people use them. Are they safe for pregnant women? We advise you to wait until after pregnancy to whiten your teeth.

Most whitening products contain hydrogen peroxide, which can be swallowed during the whitening process. We don't have enough information about how hydrogen peroxide and other whitening agents can affect a growing baby. The substances used in tooth whiteners may also increase irritation if your gums are sensitive.

Housecleaning and Yardwork

When you're doing housekeeping chores, avoid oven cleaners and aerosol sprays. Be careful with chlorine bleach and ammonia; use safer products, such as vinegar and dishwashing soap, to clean your house. Wear rubber gloves to protect your skin.

If you have regular manicures and/or pedicures, choose a salon with ventilation hoods that remove contaminated air from the area.

Be careful when you do yardwork, especially if you like to work in the garden. Sit on something that provides some support. Always wear gardening gloves; rubber gloves under your gardening gloves is a great idea.

Thyroid Disease

The thyroid gland produces hormones to regulate metabolism and control functions in many of your body's organs. About 2% of all pregnant women have a thyroid disorder. In fact, even if you don't have a thyroid problem before pregnancy, if there is a chance you could have a problem, it may appear during pregnancy.

If you have a history of thyroid problems, if you're now taking medication or if you've taken medication in the past, tell your healthcare provider. Discuss treatment during pregnancy.

Left untreated, thyroid disorders can be harmful to you and baby. Research shows women with a history of miscarriage or premature delivery, or those who have problems near delivery, may have problems with their thyroid-hormone levels.

You can go to parties while you're pregnant and still have a good time. A couple of things to remember—eat something before you go and practice portion control.

Thyroid hormone is made in the thyroid gland; this hormone affects your entire body and is important in metabolism. Levels may be high or low. Low levels of thyroid cause a condition called *hypothyroidism;* high levels cause *hyperthyroidism.*

Hypothyroidism is common during pregnancy. Symptoms include unusual weight gain and fatigue (both of which can be hard to determine during pregnancy), a hoarse voice, dry skin, dry hair and a slow pulse.

If you have these symptoms, tell your healthcare provider.

Hypothyroidism can affect your baby's health if you're not treated. Your baby may not receive adequate nutrition from you. Even with treatment, a baby is at risk of being born with abnormal thyroid levels. Many weigh less than babies born to mothers who didn't have hypothyroidism.

Flavors from foods eaten by a mom-to-be pass into amniotic fluid, which may promote flavor preferences *before* birth. By this time, baby can distinguish between sour, bitter and sweet. We know even unborn babies have a natural preference for sweet.

Symptoms and Treatment. Symptoms of thyroid disease may be masked by pregnancy. Or you may notice changes during pregnancy that cause your healthcare provider to suspect the thyroid is not functioning properly. These changes could include an enlarged thyroid, changes in your pulse, redness of the palms and warm, moist palms. Because thyroid-hormone levels can change during pregnancy *because* of pregnancy, your healthcare provider must be careful interpreting lab results about this hormone while you're pregnant.

The thyroid is tested primarily by blood tests (a thyroid panel), which measure the amount of thyroid hormone produced. The tests also measure thyroid-stimulating hormone (TSH). An X-ray study of the thyroid (radioactive iodine scan) should not be done during pregnancy.

With hypothyroidism, thyroid replacement (thyroxin) is prescribed. It is believed to be safe during pregnancy. Your healthcare provider may check the level during pregnancy with a blood test to make sure you're receiving enough of the hormone.

If you have hyperthyroidism, treatment is the medication propylthiouracil. It passes through the placenta to the baby, so ask your healthcare provider to prescribe the lowest possible amount to reduce risk to your baby. Blood testing during pregnancy is necessary to monitor the amount of medication needed. After delivery, it's important to test the baby and to watch for signs of thyroid problems.

Iodide is another medication used for hyperthyroidism, but it shouldn't be used during pregnancy. It can harm a developing baby.

Pregnant women with hyperthyroidism should not be treated with radioactive iodine either.

Velocardiofacial Syndrome (VCFS)

Velocardiofacial syndrome (VCFS) is a genetic condition that may be hereditary. It is known by many names, including *Shprintzen syndrome, craniofacial syndrome* and *conotruncal anomaly face syndrome.* VCFS is one of the most common syndromes in humans, second only to Down syndrome in frequency.

The term *velocardiofacial* derives from three Latin words: "velum" meaning palate, "cardia" meaning heart and "facies," having to do with the face. It is characterized by various medical problems. The immune system, endocrine system and neurological system may be involved. Symptoms do not all occur 100% of the time. Most people with VCFS exhibit a small number of problems; many problems are relatively minor.

If you have acid reflux, stay away from foods that could add to the problem. Some to avoid include acid foods, such as tomatoes and citrus fruit, and spicy and fried foods.

The exact cause of velocardiofacial syndrome is unknown; however investigators have identified a chromosomal defect in people with VCFS. Most children who have been diagnosed with this syndrome are missing a small part of chromosome 22.

Only one parent must have the chromosomal change to pass it along to a child. A parent with velocardiofacial syndrome has a 50/50 chance of having a child with it. However, it's estimated VCFS is inherited in only 10 to 15% of cases. Most of the time neither parent has the syndrome nor carries the defective gene.

The occurrence of congenital heart disease is most often the leading factor in diagnosis. Diagnosis is most frequently made using a genetic test called a *FISH analysis (fluorescent in situ hybridization),* which is almost 100% accurate. If the test shows chromosome 22 is not complete, the person has VCFS. If the test fails to show the deletion, the person does not have VCFS.

Familial Mediterranean Fever (FMF)

Familial Mediterranean Fever (FMF) occurs most often in Sephardi Jews, Armenians, Arabs and Turks. As many as one in 200 people in these populations have the disease; 20% are carriers. However, cases have occurred in other groups, particularly Ashkenazi Jews. About 50% have no family history of the disorder.

FMF is inherited and usually characterized by recurrent episodes of fever and inflammation of the abdominal membrane (peritonitis). Less frequently, pleuritis, arthritis, skin lesions and pericarditis can occur.

Onset of the disease usually occurs between the ages of 5 and 15 but may also occur during infancy or much later. Attacks have no regular pattern of recurrence and usually last 24 to 72 hours; some last for as long as a week. High fever (as high as 104F; 40C) is usually accompanied by pain. Abdominal pain occurs in nearly all sufferers and can vary in severity with each attack. Other symptoms include joint pain and a rash on the lower leg. Most people recover quickly and are OK until the next attack. Narcotics are sometimes needed for pain relief.

Grandma's Remedy

If you want to avoid using medication, try a folk remedy. If you experience leg cramps, mix together 2 teaspoons of apple-cider vinegar and 1 teaspoon of honey in a glass of warm water, and drink it before bed.

Currently, no diagnostic test for FMF is available. The problem is diagnosed more on the basis of repeated episodes. However, researchers have identified the gene for FMF and found several different gene mutations that can cause the disease. The gene is found on chromosome 16. A protein assists in keeping inflammation under control by turning off the immune response. Without this function, an attack of FMF occurs.

Researchers continue to work to develop a blood test to diagnose FMF. With more research, it may also become easier to recognize environmental triggers that lead to attacks, which may lead to new treatments for FMF.

Some Information May Scare You

In an effort to give you as much information as possible about pregnancy, we do include serious discussions throughout the book that some might find "scary." The information is not included to frighten you; it's there to provide facts about particular medical situations that may occur during pregnancy.

If a woman experiences a serious problem, she and her partner will probably want to know as much about it as possible. If a woman has a friend or knows someone who has problems during pregnancy, reading about it might relieve her fears. We also hope our discussions can help you start a dialogue with your doctor, if you have questions.

Nearly all pregnancies are uneventful, and serious situations don't arise. However, please know we have tried to cover as many aspects of pregnancy as we possibly can so you'll have all the information at hand that you might need and want. Knowledge is power, so having various facts available can help you feel more in control of your own pregnancy. We hope reading information helps you relax and have a great pregnancy experience.

If you find serious discussions frighten you, don't read them! Or if the information doesn't apply to your pregnancy, just skip over it. But realize information is there if you want to know more about a particular situation.

Exercise for Week 25

Sit tall at the edge of a straight-backed side chair. Fold your arms in front of you, at shoulder height, and slowly lean forward a bit. In this position, lift your left foot off the floor, and hold for 5 seconds; be sure you are sitting erect. Lower your left leg. Do 5 times for each leg. *Stretches and strengthens abdominal muscles, thigh muscles and lower-back muscles.*

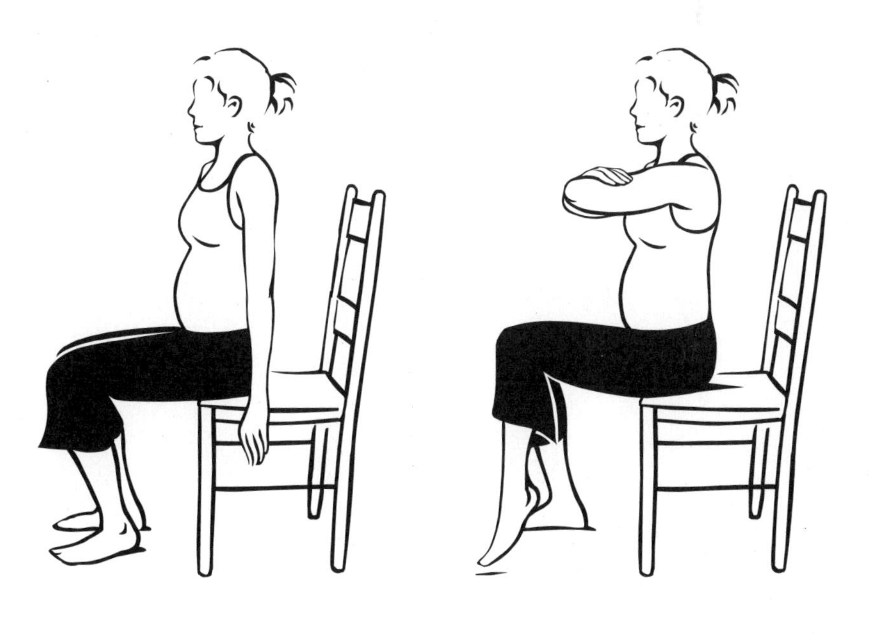

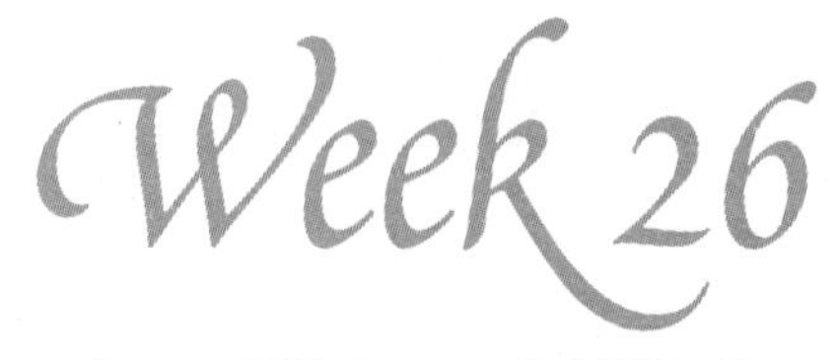

Week 26

Age of Fetus—24 Weeks

How Big Is Your Baby?

Baby now weighs almost 2 pounds (.91kg). By this week, crown-to-rump length is about 9¼ inches (23cm). See the illustration on page 372.

How Big Are You?

Your uterus is about 2½ inches (6cm) above your bellybutton or nearly 10½ inches (26cm) from your pubic symphysis. During the second half of pregnancy, you'll grow nearly ½ inch (1cm) each week. If you've been following a balanced meal plan, your total weight gain is probably between 16 and 22 pounds (7.2 to 9.9kg).

How Your Baby Is Growing and Developing

The fetus has distinct sleeping and waking cycles. You may find a pattern; at certain times of the day baby is very active, while at other times he or she is asleep. In addition, all five senses are now fully developed.

Heart Arrhythmia

By now you have heard your baby's heartbeat at several visits. When listening to your baby's heartbeat, you may be startled to hear a skipped beat. An irregular heartbeat is called an *arrhythmia.* You'll hear it as regular pulsing or pounding with an occasional skipped or missed heartbeat. Arrhythmias in a fetus are not unusual.

There are many causes of fetal arrhythmias. It may occur as the heart grows and develops. As the heart matures, the arrhythmia often disappears. It may occur in the fetus of a pregnant woman who has lupus.

If an arrhythmia is discovered before labor, you may need fetal heart-rate monitoring during labor. When an arrhythmia is detected during labor, it may be a good idea to have a pediatrician present at the delivery. He or she will make sure the baby is all right or is treated right away if a problem exists.

Tip for Week 26

Lying on your side (your left side is best) when you rest provides the best circulation to your baby. You may not experience as much swelling if you lie on your side.

Changes in You

You're getting bigger as your uterus, placenta and baby grow larger. Discomforts, such as back pain, pressure in your pelvis, leg cramps and headaches, may occur more frequently.

Time is passing quickly. You're approaching the end of the second trimester. Two-thirds of the pregnancy is behind you; it won't be long until baby is born.

How Your Actions Affect Your Baby's Development

Previous Weight-Loss Surgery

Before pregnancy, some women have weight-loss surgery to help them lose weight. *Bariatric surgery* is defined as surgery related to the prevention and control of obesity and related diseases.

Women who get pregnant after losing weight with weight-loss surgery generally have fewer risks during pregnancy than women who are morbidly obese. One study found *reduced* risks of gestational diabetes, a large baby and Cesarean delivery in women who had weight-loss surgery.

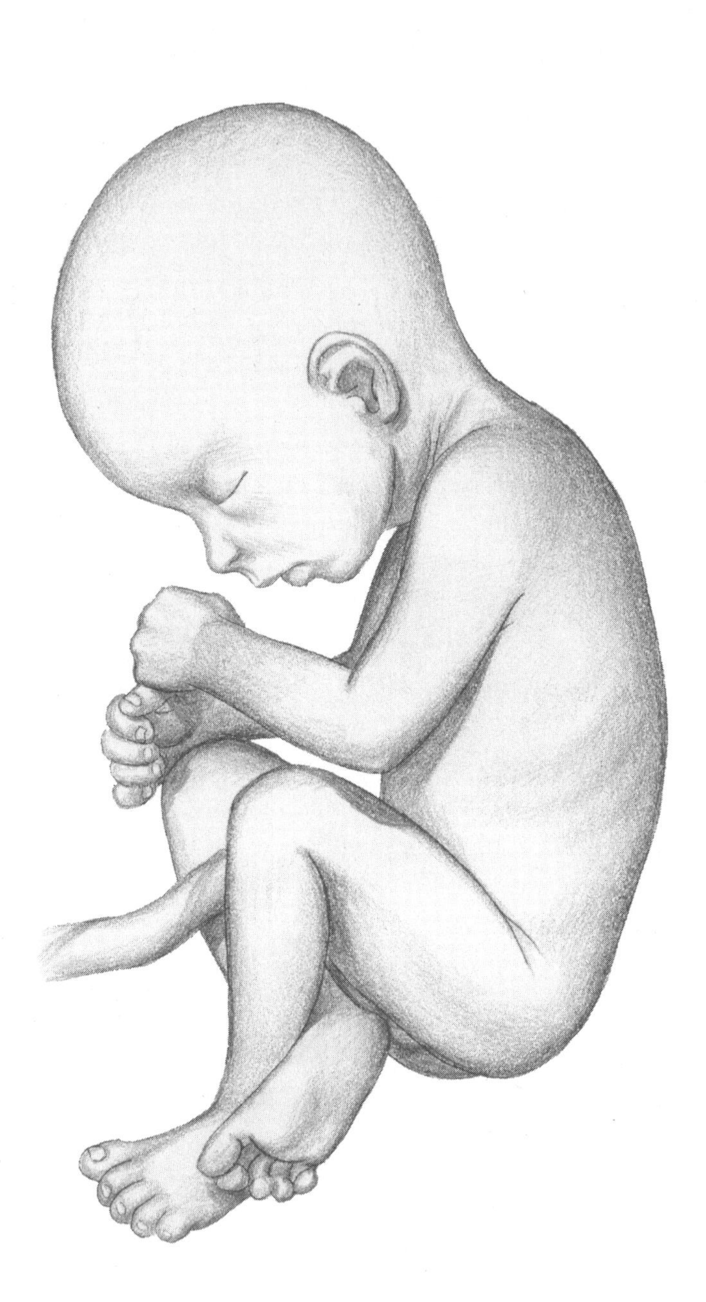

By this week, your baby weighs about 2 pounds (910g).
It is now putting on some weight and filling out.

If you had lap-band surgery, you probably know it is fully reversible. It's possible to have your stomach-outlet size enlarged so you can meet the increased nutritional needs of pregnancy. The doctor who performed the surgery can adjust the band during pregnancy so you and baby get the nutrition you both need.

If you had gastric-bypass surgery, studies show no particular problems associated with the procedure, especially if you waited 12 to 18 months after surgery to get pregnant. This time allows you to lose a lot of weight and restore lost nutrients.

Some basic safeguards should be taken when you get pregnant. You may need to be checked during pregnancy for nutritional deficiencies and may need supplements because gastric-bypass surgery makes it harder for your body to absorb enough calcium, iron and B_{12} for your good health and your baby's. Severe iron-deficiency anemia may result because you don't absorb enough of the nutrients you need.

If you've had weight-loss surgery and find out you're pregnant, call your healthcare provider immediately. You need to be seen and evaluated early in pregnancy. You and your healthcare provider can also plan a nutrition program so you and baby get the nutrients you need for a healthy pregnancy.

How to Have a Successful Labor and Delivery

It's not too early to start thinking about labor and delivery. It helps to know what makes a labor and delivery successful. Below are some things to consider as you move through pregnancy.

Become informed about pregnancy and the birth experience. Knowledge is power. When you understand what can and will occur during pregnancy, you may be able to relax more. Read our other pregnancy books, discuss questions and concerns with your healthcare provider and share information and your knowledge with your partner.

The relationships you have with your healthcare team are important. Follow medical suggestions, watch your weight, eat healthfully, take your prenatal vitamins and go to all your prenatal appointments and tests. Expect your medical team to work hard for you. Each of you should support the other.

Being able to help make decisions about your medical care, including birth positions, pain-relief methods, feeding baby and your partner's level of participation in labor and delivery, helps you feel more in control. Discuss questions and various situations with your healthcare provider at prenatal appointments. (We'll discuss prenatal classes in Week 27.)

Home Uterine Monitoring

Home uterine monitoring helps identify women with premature labor. It combines recording uterine contractions with daily telephone contact with the healthcare provider. A recording of contractions is transmitted from a woman's home by telephone to a center where they can be evaluated. Your healthcare provider may be able to view the recordings at his or her office or home.

Cost for home monitoring varies but runs between $80 and $100 a day; some insurance companies cover it. The cost can often be justified if a premature delivery is prevented—it saves a lot of money in the care of a premature baby (sometimes more than $100,000). Not everyone agrees home monitoring is beneficial or cost-effective.

It may be difficult to find out if you need this type of monitoring. It is often considered on an individual basis. Discuss it with your healthcare provider if you had preterm labor in the past or have other risk factors.

Your Nutrition

Fish Can Be Healthy during Pregnancy

Eating fish is healthy; it is especially good during pregnancy. Women who eat fish during pregnancy often have longer pregnancies and give birth to babies with higher birth weights. Studies show the omega-3 fatty acids found in fish may help protect you from premature labor and other problems. Remember—the longer a baby stays in the uterus, the better its chances are of being strong and healthy at delivery.

Many fish are safe to eat, and you should include them in your diet. Most fish is low in fat and high in vitamin B, iron, zinc, selenium and

Good Fish and Shellfish Choices

Below is a list of fish that are safe to eat if you cook them thoroughly. Don't exceed a total of 12 ounces of all fish a week!

bass	ocean perch	pollack
catfish	orange roughy	red snapper
cod	Pacific halibut	salmon
croaker	haddock	scrod
flounder	herring	sole
freshwater perch	marlin	

The following shellfish are safe to eat if they are thoroughly cooked.

clams	crab	lobster
oysters	scallops	shrimp

In addition, fish sticks and fast-food fish sandwiches are OK to eat—they are commonly made from fish that is low in mercury.

copper. Many fish choices are excellent, healthful additions to your diet (with certain limits, as discussed below). See the box above and the box on page 377 for lists of acceptable and unacceptable fish choices.

Omega-3 Fatty Acids. Omega-3 fatty acids are good for you during pregnancy. They help protect your skin by keeping it lubricated and help to reduce skin inflammation. Fish oil is important to fetal brain development.

Anchovies, herring, mullet, mackerel (*not* King mackerel), salmon, sardines and trout are some fish with a lot of omega-3 fatty acids. Omega-3 fatty acids are also found in animal foods, including grass-fed beef and eggs from hens fed special diets. If you're a vegetarian or you don't eat fish, add tofu, canola oil, flaxseed, soybeans, walnuts and wheat germ to your food plan. These foods contain linolenic oil, which is a type of omega-3 fatty acid.

Fish-oil capsules may be another option. If you buy fish-oil capsules, choose the *filtered* type because they don't contain pollutants. Don't take more than 2.4g of omega-3 fatty acids a day. Fish-oil capsules may upset your stomach. To solve the problem, freeze them or take them with meals or at bedtime.

Methyl-Mercury Poisoning. Some fish are contaminated as the result of man-made pollution. People who eat these fish are at risk of methyl-mercury poisoning.

Mercury is a naturally occurring substance and a pollution by-product. Mercury becomes a problem when it is released into the air. The worst methyl-mercury polluters are coal-burning power plants; they account for more than 40% of the methyl mercury released into the air. It settles into the oceans and from there winds up in some types of fish, where it accumulates in their muscles. Larger fish that live longer have the highest levels of mercury because they've had the longest time to accumulate it in their system.

Eating 12 ounces of fish every week during pregnancy may help your child enjoy better development during his or her early years.

Methyl mercury above a certain level in fish is dangerous for humans. We know methyl mercury can pass from mother to fetus across the placenta. Research shows 60,000 children are born each year who are at risk of developing problems linked to the seafood their mothers ate during pregnancy.

A fetus may be more at risk of methyl-mercury poisoning than an adult. Studies show one in five American women of childbearing age has mercury levels that are too high—about 8% of them have levels high enough to put a fetus at risk.

Pregnant women should limit their fish and shellfish intake to no more than 12 ounces *a week*. Twelve ounces is two to three average servings.

The amount of mercury in fish varies. Try to choose fish and shellfish that are lower in mercury. If you eat a lot of fish, a hair-mercury analysis may be recommended. This testing is often done at university medical centers.

There is debate about eating canned tuna. Talk to your healthcare provider about it at a prenatal appointment if this is a favorite of yours. The box on page 377 contains information on canned and fresh tuna.

Some freshwater fish may also be risky to eat, such as walleye and pike. Consult local or state authorities for any advisories on eating freshwater fish. Other fish to avoid include some found in warm tropical waters, especially Florida, the Caribbean and Hawaii. Avoid the following "local" fish from those areas: amberjack, barracuda, bluefish, grouper, mahimahi, snapper and fresh tuna.

Fish to Avoid

There are fish to avoid during pregnancy and breastfeeding. The FDA recommends avoiding swordfish, shark, king mackerel and tilefish. Also avoid walleye, pike, amberjack, barracuda, bluefish, grouper, mahimahi and snapper.

There are different thoughts about pregnant women eating tuna. Canned light tuna has less mercury than albacore tuna, so eat that. Don't eat more than one 6-ounce can of light tuna a week. If you want to eat a cooked tuna steak every once in awhile, keep your total tuna intake (fresh and/or canned) to no more than 6 ounces a week. If you have questions, talk to your healthcare provider.

Some Additional Cautions about Fish. Parasites, bacteria, viruses and toxins can contaminate fish. Eating infected fish can make you sick. Sushi and ceviche are fish dishes that could have viruses or parasites. Contaminated raw shellfish could cause hepatitis-A, cholera or gastroenteritis. Avoid *all* raw fish during pregnancy!

Fish can contain other environmental pollutants. Dioxin and polychlorinated biphenyls (PCBs) are found in bluefish and lake trout; avoid them.

You may want to double check tilapia. *Farm-raised tilapia* is one of the most highly consumed fish in America; however, it has low levels of omega-3 fatty acids and high levels of unhealthy omega-6 fatty acids.

We advise pregnant women not to eat sushi. However, if you're craving sushi, eat a California roll (no raw fish) or shrimp tempura. Other dishes made with *cooked* eel and rolls with *steamed* crab and veggies are OK.

If you're unsure about whether you should eat a particular fish or if you want further information, ask your healthcare provider for pamphlets about fish. Or contact the Food and Drug Administration for information.

You Should Also Know

Dreams

Are you having weird dreams during pregnancy? Are they intense and vivid? Do some of them frighten you? Do you remember more dreams when you wake up than you ever did before? This is natural. A woman often dreams a lot, in great detail, during pregnancy and remembers her dreams more easily. Dreams may be more emotional than usual.

Researchers once believed dreams were random thought patterns that occurred while you slept. Today, they consider dreams to be your body's effort to play back ideas and thoughts about what has happened in the past. They may be your subconscious mind's way of working out important feelings. Pregnancy brings a lot of stress and change in your life. When you dream, you may be attempting to deal with all that is going on. Dreams may be helping you prepare to become a mother.

What Do Your Dreams Mean?

Your Dream	What It May Mean
About your mother	You are aware of your own impending motherhood
Baby animals that are cuddly	You know the fetus is growing
Baby's appearance	Your hopes and fears about your baby
Building, factories, construction sites	You're aware of your growing baby
Carrying something heavy; having trouble walking	You know you're gaining weight
Driving a large car or truck	You feel awkward
Former boyfriends or lovers	You want to feel attractive
Large animals	Awareness the fetus is growing larger
Open door, falling, blood	You fear a miscarriage
Partner being difficult	You crave security
Partner having an affair	You feel unattractive
Water, ocean, lakes, pools	You are aware of the amniotic fluid

Dreams occur while you are in REM sleep, which is the deepest sleep phase. Most people have four to five episodes of REM sleep each night. In reality, you don't dream more dreams or dream any more often while you're pregnant.

One reason you remember your dreams more readily is you probably wake up more often during the night. It's a fact that when you wake up to try to get comfortable or to go to the bathroom while a dream is still fresh in your mind, you'll remember it more easily. Another reason you may be dreaming more is you may be getting more sleep at night because you're more tired than normal. A third reason is hormones; progesterone and estrogen may increase the amount of time you dream and your recall of dreams.

To help you come to terms with some of your dreams, it may help to keep a journal or diary of your dreams. Jot down your dream as soon as you wake up. It may be fun to share them with your child when he or she gets older.

Dream Themes. What you dream is unique to you. However, studies have found themes and ideas common in dreams, including pregnancy dreams. Many pregnant women have dreams that are similar. Let's examine some common themes.

In the first trimester, you may dream about your childhood or events that occurred in the past. It may be your mind's way of dealing with unresolved situations from your past. You may also dream about gardens, fruits and flowers, signifying the growing baby inside you. Water images may also be part of your dreams.

Second-trimester dreams may relate to how your relationship will be with your baby, such as getting to know your baby and bonding with him or her. Baby may first appear in your dreams in a formless way, becoming more definite as weeks pass. Dreaming about animals and pets can also symbolize your growing baby.

In your third trimester, dreams may help you get ready for baby's birth. Labor and delivery are common themes. In dreams, labor and delivery are pain-free! You may also dream about how your baby looks or feels to hold. You may find your dreams focusing on water; this may

Dad Tip

As pregnancy moves along, a lot of women start to feel unattractive. They may experience swelling in their hands and feet. They may find their hair and nails have changed. Their skin may not be normal for them. And their tummy is growing and growing! Try to reassure your partner that you know she's going through a lot to give your baby a healthy start in life. Take her on a date—go to dinner and a movie! Tell her she's beautiful. Take a full-view picture of her as a remembrance of how lovely she is now.

occur because water is the source of all life.

Other researchers divide dreams into categories, including relationships, identity and fear. Relationship dreams deal with the fact that many of your personal relationships will change when you become a mother. You may dream about your own parents, your partner, friends and other family members. This also includes bonding with baby.

Dreams that deal with your identity may be about your new role as a mother. You may dream about your job and your new baby or your feelings about becoming a mom. In your dreams, you may not take very good care of baby, like misplacing him or her; this may reflect some ambivalence toward becoming a mother. Don't let these types of dreams upset you—many women have them.

Dreams that cover situations, feelings or events that frighten you address the fact that you may be anxious about becoming a mother or you may be nervous about your baby's health. Many of your fears may be unrecognized or unnamed. Dreams may help you deal with these fears. Labor and delivery, especially if this is your first baby, can also be scary because it's something you've never experienced before. Your dreams may be a way to rehearse this important event. Anxiety dreams may indicate you're trying to deal with a situation or problem.

Recurrent dreams suggest you may not be dealing effectively with a situation, and it's unresolved. If your recurrent dream appears in the form of a nightmare, it may mean it is very important to you.

Dads-to-Be Dream, Too. You may not be the only one having dreams—your partner may also be having some. His dreams indicate he's experiencing fear, anxiety and hope, just as you are. Pregnancy dreams can be strong for a man. His dreams may also reflect certain themes. One common theme is being left out of what is happening or dreams about what the baby will look like. Dads-to-be may dream *they* are pregnant or giving birth. Celebrations may also be part of their dreams.

Using Retin-A

Retin-A (tretinoin), not to be confused with Accutane (isotretinoin), is a cream or lotion used to treat acne and to help get rid of fine wrinkles on the face. If you are pregnant and using Retin-A, stop using it immediately!

We don't have enough data to know if it's safe to use during pregnancy. We do know any type of medication you use—whether taken internally, inhaled, injected or spread on the skin—gets into your bloodstream. Many substances in your bloodstream can be passed to your baby.

Some medicines a mother-to-be uses become concentrated in baby. Your body can handle it, but your baby's body may not be able to. If some substances build up in the baby, they can have important effects on its development. In the future, we may know more about the effects of Retin-A on a growing baby. At this time, it's best to avoid using it for the sake of your baby.

Seizures and Epilepsy

A history of seizures—before pregnancy, during a previous pregnancy or during this pregnancy—is important information you must share with your healthcare provider. (Another term for seizure is *convulsion.*) It's estimated that about 500,000 women in the United States with a seizure disorder are of childbearing age.

Seizures can and usually do occur without warning. A seizure indicates an abnormal condition related to the nervous system, particularly the brain. During a seizure, a person often loses body control. This can be serious for mom and baby.

Be sure you get enough sleep. Sleep deprivation can cause more seizures.

If you have never had a problem with seizures, know that a short episode of dizziness or lightheadedness is *not* usually a seizure. Seizures are usually diagnosed by someone observing the seizure and noting the symptoms previously mentioned. An electroencephalogram (EEG) may be needed to diagnose a seizure.

Epilepsy. If you have epilepsy, it's important to control your disease during pregnancy because seizures can affect you and baby in many ways. One-third of women with epilepsy will see a decrease in the number of seizures they have during pregnancy. One-third will have more seizures, and one-third will see no change at all.

During pregnancy, hormonal fluctuations can affect epilepsy. You may be at higher risk of some pregnancy problems. Grand-mal seizures can put the baby at risk because they reduce blood flow to the fetus.

Seizures seldom occur during labor and delivery. More than 90% of all epileptic pregnant women give birth to healthy babies.

Medications to Control Seizures. If you take medication for seizure control or prevention, tell your healthcare provider before trying to get pregnant or at the beginning of pregnancy. Medication can be taken during pregnancy to control seizures, but some are safer than others. Ask about taking large doses of folic acid; it has proved helpful in some women.

If you have morning sickness, tell your healthcare provider about it. Nausea and vomiting can interfere with your body's ability to absorb your medications.

There are concerns regarding use of anticonvulsant medications in pregnancy. There is also concern regarding *polytherapy*—when a woman takes several medications in combination. Ask your healthcare provider to put you on the lowest dosage of *one* antiepileptic drug. Take your antiseizure medication *exactly* as it is prescribed.

Most studies show increased risk to the baby when a mom-to-be takes valproate, especially in the first trimester. There's evidence exposure of a baby to this medication increases the risk of autism. Talk to your healthcare provider about this medication before you become pregnant or as soon as you know you're pregnant. Because half of all pregnancies in the United States are unplanned, most experts recommend using another medication as a first-line drug for women of childbearing age.

Dilantin can cause birth defects in a baby. Other medications may be used during pregnancy for seizure prevention. One of the more common is phenobarbital, but there's some concern about the safety of this medicine. Lamotrigine therapy alone shows no increased risk of problems in baby.

During pregnancy, kidneys may remove greater amounts of antiepileptic drugs from your system more quickly than usual. Drug levels could decrease by as much as 50%. It's important to see your neurologist every month for blood tests to check the levels in your blood. Any dosage adjustments can be made after test results are in.

Seizures during pregnancy can be serious; you may need increased monitoring during pregnancy. If you have questions or concerns about a history of possible seizures, talk to your healthcare provider about them.

Exercise for Week 26

Sit on the floor with your knees bent and your feet flat on the ground. Keep your knees about 12 inches apart. Reach underneath each thigh with your hands, then stretch back slowly until your arms are straight. Keep your feet on the floor as you return to the starting position. Repeat 8 times. *Strengthens abdominal muscles, inner thighs and pelvic floor.*

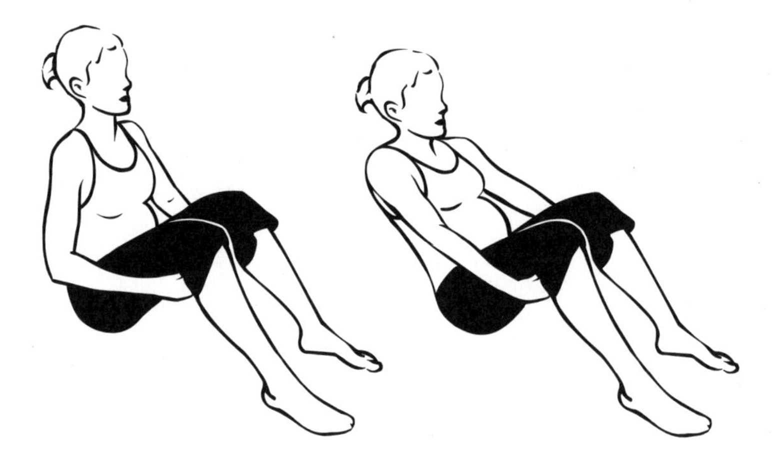

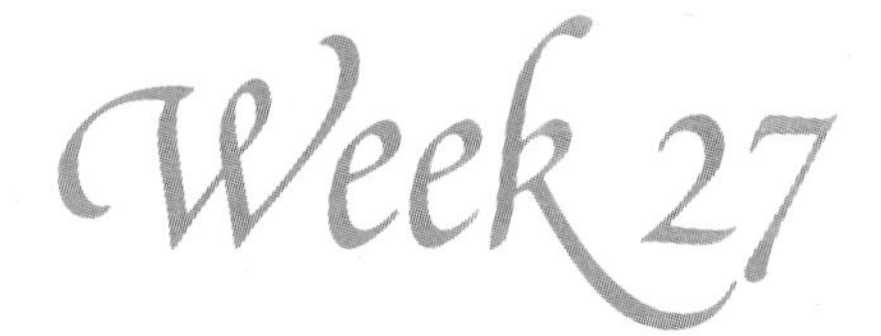

Week 27

Age of Fetus—25 Weeks

How Big Is Your Baby?

This week marks the beginning of the third trimester. Now we'll be adding total length of baby's body from head to toe. This will give you a better idea of how big your baby is during this last part of your pregnancy.

Your baby now weighs a little more than 2 pounds (875g), and crown-to-rump length is about 9⅔ inches (24cm) by this week. Total length is about 14⅓ inches (36cm). See the illustration on page 386.

How Big Are You?

Your uterus is about 2¾ inches (7cm) above your bellybutton. Measured from the pubic symphysis, it is more than 10½ inches (27cm) to the top of the uterus.

How Your Baby Is Growing and Developing

The retina, the part of the eye where light images come into focus at the back of the eye, is beginning to be sensitive to light. It develops layers around this time that receive light and light information, and transmits them to the brain for interpretation—what we know as "sight." From here on, baby will probably be able to sense bright light. If you shine a light close to your tummy, baby may react as it senses the change in luminosity.

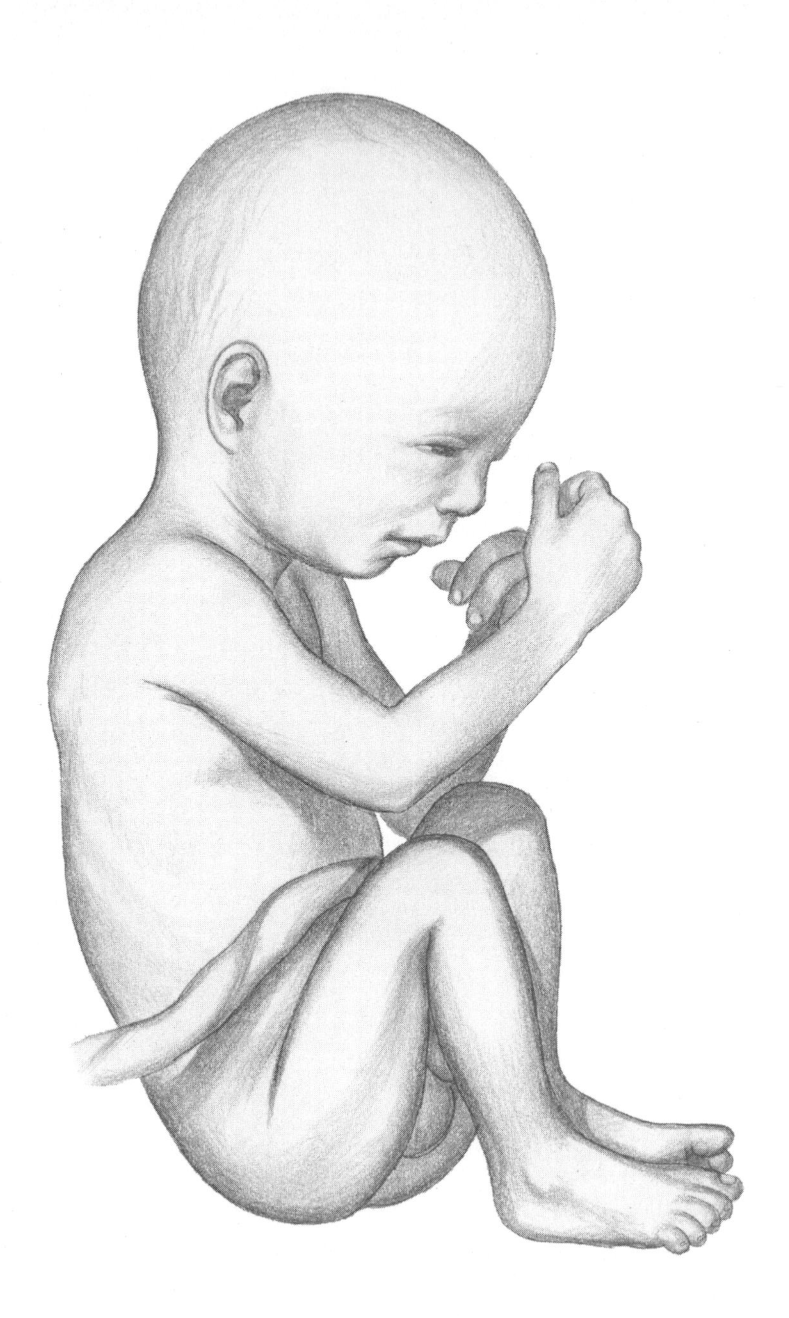

Around this time, your baby's eyelids open.
Your baby begins opening and closing its eyes
while still inside your uterus.

A *congenital cataract* is an eye problem present at birth. Most people believe cataracts occur only in old age, but they can appear in a newborn baby!

Instead of being transparent or clear, the lens that focuses light onto the back of the eye is opaque or cloudy. This problem is usually inherited. However, it has been found in children born to mothers who had German measles (rubella) around the 6th or 7th week of pregnancy.

Another congenital eye problem is *microphthalmia,* in which the overall size of the eye is too small. The eyeball may be only two-thirds its normal size. It often occurs with other eye abnormalities. It is usually the result of infections in the mom-to-be, such as cytomegalovirus (CMV) or toxoplasmosis, while baby is developing.

Changes in You

Feeling Baby Move

Feeling your baby move (quickening) is one of the more precious parts of pregnancy and can be the beginning of your bonding with baby. Many women feel they begin to connect with baby and its personality by feeling its movements. Your partner can experience and enjoy baby's movements by feeling your tummy when baby is active.

Movement can vary in intensity. It can range from a faint flutter, sometimes described as a feeling of a butterfly or a gas bubble in early pregnancy, to brisk motions or even painful kicks and pressure as baby gets larger.

Some good news about baby's movements. Studies show if your baby is active in the womb, he or she may be healthier.

Women often ask how often a baby should move. They want to know if they should be concerned if the baby moves too much or doesn't move enough. This is hard to answer because your sensation can be different from that of someone else. Each baby's movement can be different. However, studies show an active baby moves at least 10 times in 2 hours. It's usually more reassuring to have a baby move frequently. But it isn't unusual for a baby to have quiet times when there is not as much activity.

If you've been on the go, you may not have noticed baby move because you've been active and busy. It may help to lie on your side to see how much baby is moving. Many women report baby is more active at night, making it hard to sleep.

If your baby is quiet and not as active as what seems normal or what you expected, discuss it with your healthcare provider. You can always go to the office to hear baby's heartbeat if it hasn't been moving in its usual pattern. In most instances, there is nothing to worry about.

Dad Tip

Offer to do various jobs around the house that may be more difficult for your partner now. Cleaning the bathtub or the toilet can be a big help. Carry the laundry up and down stairs. Unload the dishwasher so you can put away heavy or awkward pieces. Add to her safety by putting away anything that belongs in a high or difficult-to-reach location.

Kick Count. As baby gets bigger, kicks get stronger. Toward the end of pregnancy, you may be asked to record how often you feel baby move. This test is done at home and is called a *kick count*. It provides reassurance about baby's well-being; this information is similar to that learned by a nonstress test (see Week 41).

Your healthcare provider may use one of two common methods. The first is to count how many times the baby moves in an hour. The other is to note how long it takes for baby to move 10 times. Usually you can choose when you want to do the test. After eating a meal is a good time because baby is often more active then.

Pain Under Your Ribs When Baby Moves

Some women complain of pain under their ribs and in their lower abdomen when baby moves. This type of pain isn't an unusual problem, but it may cause enough discomfort to concern you.

Baby's movement has increased to a point where you probably feel it every day, and movements are getting stronger and harder. At the same time, your uterus is getting larger and putting more pressure on all your organs. It presses on the small bowel, bladder and rectum.

If the pressure really is pain, don't ignore it. You need to discuss it with your healthcare provider. In most cases, it isn't a serious problem.

Discovering a Breast Lump

Discovering a breast lump is significant, during pregnancy or any other time. It's important for you to learn at an early age how to do a breast exam and to perform this on a regular basis (usually after every menstrual period). Nine out of 10 breast lumps are found by women examining themselves.

Your healthcare provider will probably perform breast exams at regular intervals, usually when you have your annual Pap smear. If you have an exam every year and are lump-free, it helps assure you no lumps are present before you begin pregnancy.

Finding a breast lump may be harder during pregnancy because of changes in your breasts. It may be more difficult to feel a lump. Growing breasts during pregnancy and nursing tends to hide lumps or masses in the tissue of the breast.

Continue to examine your breasts during pregnancy every 4 or 5 weeks. The first day of every month is a good time to do it.

If you find a lump, you may need a mammogram or ultrasound exam. Because a mammogram is a breast X-ray, your pregnancy must be protected during the procedure, usually by shielding your abdomen with a lead apron. Pregnancy has not been shown to accelerate the course or growth of a breast lump.

Treatment during Pregnancy. Often a breast lump can be drained or aspirated. Fluid removed from the cyst is sent to the lab to see if it contains any abnormal cells. If a lump or cyst can't be drained by needle, a biopsy may be necessary. If fluid is clear, it's a good sign. Fluid is studied under a microscope in the laboratory.

If examination of a lump signals breast cancer, treatment may begin during pregnancy. Complications during pregnancy include risks to the fetus related to chemotherapy, radiation or medication. If a lump is cancerous, the need for radiation therapy and chemotherapy must be considered, along with the needs of the pregnancy. See also the discussion of cancer in pregnancy in Week 32.

Medicine has made great strides in treating cancer in pregnant women. Today, many women are able to receive cancer treatment *and* to carry their baby to full term without harm to the baby. If you have questions, ask your healthcare provider.

How Your Actions Affect Your Baby's Development

Childbirth-Education Classes

It may be time to sign up for childbirth-education classes. Even though it's just the beginning of the third trimester, it's a good idea to sign up now so you can finish classes before you get to the end of pregnancy. And it will give you time to practice what you learn. You won't be just beginning your classes when you deliver!

> Sometimes instructors in childbirth-education classes promote the belief there is an *ideal* way to give birth (vaginally). This sets many women up to believe they have failed if they end up having a Cesarean delivery. The goal in labor and delivery is a healthy mom and a healthy baby. If various procedures are used to deliver your baby safely—even if you didn't intend to employ them—rejoice that they are available to help ensure the safe delivery of your baby. If you have concerns, talk to your healthcare provider about them.

During pregnancy, you have probably been learning what's going to happen at delivery by talking with your healthcare provider and by asking questions. You have also learned what lies ahead from reading materials given to you at prenatal visits, from our other books, such as *Your Pregnancy Quick Guide to Labor and Delivery, Your Pregnancy Questions & Answers, Your Pregnancy after 35, Your Pregnancy for the Father-to-Be* or *Your Pregnancy—Every Woman's Guide* and from other sources. Childbirth classes offer yet another way to learn about and to prepare for labor and delivery.

By meeting in class on a regular basis, usually once a week for 4 to 6 weeks, you can learn about many things that concern you and your partner. Classes often cover a wide range of subjects, including the areas that are listed below.

- What are the different childbirth methods?
- What is "natural childbirth"?
- What is a Cesarean delivery?
- What pain-relief methods are available?
- What do you need to know (and practice) for the childbirth method you choose?
- Will you need an episiotomy?
- Will you need an enema?
- When is a fetal monitor necessary?
- What's going to happen when you reach the hospital?
- Is an epidural or some other type of anesthesia right for you?

These are important questions. Discuss them with your healthcare provider, if you don't get answers in your childbirth-education classes.

Classes are usually held for small groups of pregnant women and their partners or labor coaches. This is a great way to learn. You can interact with other couples and ask questions. You'll learn other women are concerned about many of the same things you are. It's good to know you aren't the only one thinking about what lies ahead.

Prenatal classes are not only for first-time pregnant women. If you have a new partner, if it's been a few years since you've had a baby, if you have questions or if you would like a review of what lies ahead, a prenatal class can help you. Childbirth classes that deal with vaginal birth after Cesarean (VBAC) may also be available. Ask at the office for information about various classes available in your area.

Classes may help reduce any worry or address concerns you and your partner may have. And they can help you enjoy the birth of your baby even more.

Childbirth classes are offered in various settings. Most hospitals that deliver babies offer classes, often taught by labor-and-delivery nurses or by a midwife. Various classes may have different degrees of involvement. This means the time commitment or depth of the subject covered is different for each type of class that may be available.

Tip for Week 27

Childbirth-education classes are not just for couples. Classes may be offered for single mothers or for pregnant women whose partners cannot come to classes. Ask at the office about classes for you.

Classes are meant to inform you and your partner or labor coach about pregnancy, what happens at the hospital and what happens during labor and delivery. Some couples find classes are a good way to get a partner more involved and to help make him feel more comfortable. This may give him the opportunity to take a more active part at the time of labor and delivery.

If you have problems getting to a prenatal class because of cost or time or because you're on bed rest, it may be possible to take classes at home. Some instructors will come to your home for private sessions. Or you might use some videos. Check your local library or video store.

Your Nutrition

Some important vitamins you may need during pregnancy include vitamin A, vitamin B and vitamin E. Let's examine each vitamin and how it can help you.

Vitamin A is essential to human reproduction. Fortunately, deficiency in North America is rare. What's of more concern is the *excessive use* of the vitamin before conception and in early pregnancy. (This discussion concerns only the retinol forms of vitamin A, usually derived from fish oils. The beta-carotene form, of plant origin, is believed to be safe.)

The RDA (recommended dietary allowance) is 2700IU (international units) for a woman of childbearing age. The maximum dosage is 5000IU. Pregnancy doesn't change these requirements. You probably get enough vitamin A from the foods you eat, so supplementation during pregnancy isn't recommended. Read food labels to keep track of your vitamin-A intake.

B vitamins important to you in pregnancy include B_6, B_9 (folic acid/folate) and B_{12}. B vitamins help regulate the development of baby's nerves and formation of blood cells. If you don't take in enough B_{12}

during pregnancy, you could develop anemia. Taking enough may help prevent certain birth defects.

There are many good food sources of B vitamins. Some you may enjoy include milk, eggs, tempeh, miso, bananas, potatoes, collard greens, avocados and brown rice.

Vitamin E helps metabolize fats and builds muscles and red blood cells. You can usually get enough vitamin E if you eat meat. Vegetarians and women who can't eat meat may have a harder time getting enough. If you don't take in enough vitamin E, you increase the risk of your child developing asthma by age 5. But don't take megadoses of vitamin E; studies show it could cause problems.

Foods rich in vitamin E include olive oil, wheat germ, spinach and dried fruit. You may want to check with your healthcare provider or read the label on your prenatal vitamin to see if it supplies 100% of the recommended daily allowance.

Be cautious with *every* substance you take during pregnancy. If you have questions, discuss them with your healthcare provider.

You Should Also Know

Babymoons

Many parents-to-be are now scheduling a *babymoon* before the end of pregnancy. A babymoon is a prebaby vacation—a trip for expectant parents to reconnect and to enjoy each other's company before baby's birth. It usually focuses on relaxing and pampering.

A couple can plan a weekend getaway close to home or take a trip farther afield. Some hotels and resorts now offer babymoon packages. Keep in mind it's the time you spend together that's important, whether you stay in a luxury hotel close by, find a mountain lodge to cuddle up in or relax in a cottage by the sea.

A babymoon is a time to take walks, sleep in, lay by the pool, shop, eat in nice restaurants, take pictures and build memories. It's a time to enjoy each other's company before your hectic life as parents begins. Some people look forward to a babymoon so they can pamper themselves with massages and other spa treatments. Whatever you choose to do, it's a time to draw closer together.

Before You Make Plans. Be sure you discuss your plans with your healthcare provider before paying any deposits or buying any nonrefundable tickets. He or she may have valid reasons you shouldn't travel.

Baby's experiences inside the uterus impact its cognitive and sensory development.

If you get the OK to go, do some research. If you were thinking of going on a short cruise, check to see if the cruise line bans pregnant women from traveling after a particular time in pregnancy. If you're thinking about going somewhere with activities you'd like to do, check to see if there are any restrictions on pregnant women. No matter what you plan, keep it simple and casual.

Often the best time in pregnancy to travel is during the second trimester. You're usually past any morning sickness at this point, and you haven't grown too large to enjoy moving around.

If you decide to take a babymoon, relax, share time together and enjoy the baby-free environment. It won't be long until you'll both be involved in the all-encompassing days and nights of being parents!

Lupus

Lupus is an autoimmune disorder of unknown cause that occurs most often in young or middle-aged women. It is a chronic inflammatory disease that can affect more than one organ system. Those with lupus have a large number of antibodies in the bloodstream. These antibodies are directed toward the person's own tissues and various body organs and may damage organs. Affected organs include joints, skin, kidneys, muscles, lungs, the brain and the central nervous system. The most common symptom of lupus is joint pain, which is often mistaken for arthritis. Other symptoms include lesions, fever, hypertension, rashes or skin sores.

Over 1½ million people in the United States have some form of lupus. Women have lupus much more frequently than men—about nine women to every man. Nearly 80% of the cases develop in people between the ages of 15 and 45. Lupus is 2 to 3 times more common in women of color, including Black/African Americans, Latina/Hispanics, Asian American/Pacific Islanders and Native Americans/Alaska Natives.

The term *lupus* actually applies to many different forms of the same disease. There are five types of the disease: cutaneous lupus (discoid lupus, ACLE, SCLE, CCLE, DLE), systemic lupus erythematosus (SLE), drug-induced lupus (DILE), overlap lupus and neonatal lupus.

Cutaneous lupus primarily affects the skin but may involve the hair and mucous membranes. *Systemic lupus erythematosus* (SLE) can affect any body organ or system, including joints, skin, kidneys, heart, lungs or nervous system. Most often when people speak about "lupus," they are referring to this type; about 70% of all cases of lupus are SLE. SLE affects one in every 2000 to 3000 pregnancies. The effects of SLE on pregnancy are most often related to high blood pressure or kidney problems.

Drug-induced lupus can be a side effect of long-term use of some medicines. When it is stopped, symptoms often disappear completely within a few weeks. *Overlap lupus* is a condition in which a person has symptoms of more than one connective-tissue disease. In addition to lupus, a person may also have scleroderma, rheumatoid arthritis, myositis or Sjogren's syndrome.

Neonatal lupus is quite rare. A mother-to-be passes her autoantibodies to her baby, which can affect baby's heart, blood and skin. The condition is associated with a rash that appears within the first few weeks of life. It can last up to 6 months.

Lupus is diagnosed through blood tests, which look for the suspect antibodies. Blood tests done for lupus are a lupus antibody test and an antinuclear antibody test.

Treating Lupus. Steroids, short for corticosteroids, are generally prescribed to treat lupus. The most common medicines used are prednisone, prednisolone and methylprednisolone. A small amount passes to the baby. It may be unnecessary to take prednisone every day.

Dexamethasone and betamethasone pass through the placenta and are used only when it's necessary to treat the baby as well. These medications are used in preterm labor and delivery to accelerate lung maturation. This is called *antenatal corticosteroid administration.*

If you use warfarin, contact your healthcare provider; it should be replaced with heparin as soon as possible. If you have high blood pressure, you may have to switch medicines. Don't take cyclophosphamide during the first trimester. Azathioprine and cyclosporin may be continued in pregnancy.

Lupus during Pregnancy. All lupus pregnancies should be considered *high risk,* although most lupus pregnancies are completely normal. "High risk" means solvable problems may occur during the pregnancy and should be expected. More than 50% of all lupus pregnancies are completely normal, and most of the babies are normal, although babies may be somewhat premature.

About 35% of pregnant women with lupus have antibodies that interfere with the placenta's function. These antibodies may cause blood clots to form in the placenta that prevent the placenta from growing and working normally. To deal with this problem, heparin therapy may be recommended; some healthcare providers also add a small dose of baby aspirin.

The risk of complications is slightly increased in a woman with lupus. Protein in the urine may get worse. It's a good idea to see your rheumatologist every month during pregnancy. If you begin to have a flare-up or other symptoms, it can be dealt with.

If you had kidney damage from previous flare-ups, be on the lookout for kidney problems during pregnancy. Other common symptoms are arthritis, rashes and fatigue. Some women experience improvement in their lupus during pregnancy.

A "stress" steroid is often given to a woman with lupus during labor to protect her. After baby's birth, some experts believe steroids should be given or increased to prevent a flare-up of lupus in the mom. A woman with lupus can breastfeed; however, some medications, including prednisone, may interfere with milk production.

Exercise for Week 27

While standing in line at the grocery store, post office or anywhere else, use the time to do some "creative" exercises. These exercises help you develop and strengthen some of the muscles you'll use during labor and delivery.

- Rise up and down on your toes to work your calves.
- Spread your feet apart slightly, and do subtle side lunges to give your quadriceps a workout.
- Clench and relax your buttocks muscles.
- Do the Kegel exercise (see the exercise in Week 14) to strengthen pelvic-floor muscles.
- Tighten and hold in your tummy muscles.

You probably have to reach for things at home or at the office. When you do, make it an exercise in controlled breathing.

- Before you stretch, inhale, rise up on your toes and bring both arms up at the same time.
- When you're finished, drop slowly back on your heels.
- Exhale while slowly returning your arms to your sides.

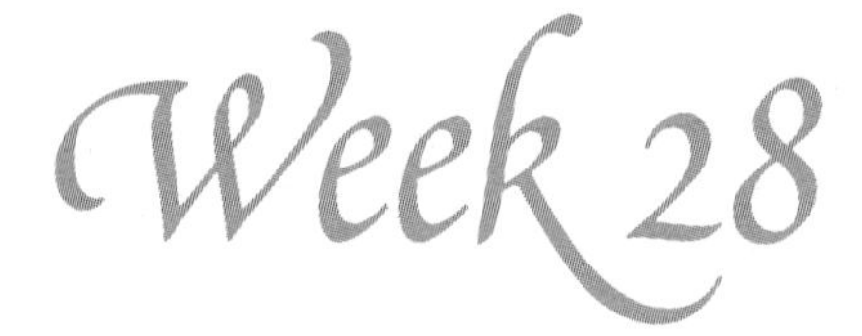

Week 28

Age of Fetus—26 Weeks

How Big Is Your Baby?

Your baby weighs nearly 2¼ pounds (1kg). Crown-to-rump length is close to 10 inches (25cm). Total length is 14¾ inches (37cm).

How Big Are You?

You continue to grow. Sometimes it seems gradual. At other times, it may seem as though changes happen rapidly, as if overnight.

Your uterus is about 3¾ inches (8cm) above your bellybutton. If you measure from the pubic symphysis, it's about 11 inches (28cm) to the top of the uterus. Your weight gain by this time should be between 17 and 24 pounds (7.7 and 10.8kg).

How Your Baby Is Growing and Developing

Until this time, the surface of baby's developing brain has appeared smooth. Around week 28, the brain begins to form characteristic grooves and indentations on the surface. The amount of brain tissue also increases.

Your baby's eyebrows and eyelashes may be present. Hair on baby's head is growing longer. The baby's body is becoming plumper and rounder because of increased fat underneath the skin. Before this time, baby had a thin appearance.

Just 11 weeks ago, baby weighed only about 3½ ounces (100g). Your baby has increased its weight more than 10 times in 11 weeks! In the last 4 weeks, from the 24th week of your pregnancy to this week, weight has doubled.

Changes in You

Changing Tastebuds

Some women complain of a bad taste in their mouth during pregnancy. It's called *dysgeusia* and is a common condition. It is probably caused by pregnancy hormones, which can alter or eliminate taste. Some women experience a metallic or bitter taste, or lose taste for certain foods. The good news is this condition usually disappears during the second trimester. If you have dysgeusia, try some of the following techniques.

- If sweets are too sweet, add a bit of salt to help cut sweetness in foods like canned fruit or jelly.
- Add lemon to water, drink lemonade or suck on citrus drops.
- Marinate fish, chicken or meat in soy sauce or citrus juice.
- Use plastic dinnerware; stainless steel utensils may increase a metallic taste.
- Brush your teeth often.
- Gargle with baking soda and water (¼ teaspoon of baking soda in 1 cup of water), which may help neutralize pH levels.

> **Tip for Week 28**
>
> **Even though delivery is several weeks away, it isn't too early to begin making plans for the trip to the hospital. This includes knowing how to reach your partner (keep all of his phone numbers with you). Also consider what you will do if he isn't near enough to take you. Who are potential drivers? How do you get hold of them? Make plans now!**

The Placenta and Umbilical Cord

The placenta plays a critical role in the growth, development and survival of the baby. The baby is attached by the umbilical cord to the placenta.

See the illustration on page 403. The umbilical cord contains two umbilical arteries and one umbilical vein.

The placenta is involved in moving oxygen and carbon dioxide to and from baby. It's also involved in nutrition and removal of waste products from the baby.

Human chorionic gonadotropin (HCG), produced by the placenta, is found in your bloodstream in measurable amounts within 10 days after fertilization. The placenta begins making estrogen and progesterone by the 7th or 8th week of pregnancy.

Two important cell layers, the amnion and the chorion, are involved in the development of the placenta and the amniotic sac. Development and function of the cell layers is complicated, and their description is beyond the scope of this book. However, the amnion is the layer around the amniotic fluid in which the fetus floats.

The placenta begins to form with cells that grow through the walls of maternal blood vessels and establish contact with your bloodstream without your blood and fetal blood mixing. (Fetal circulation is separate from yours.)

The placenta grows at a rapid rate. At 10 weeks, it weighs about ¾ ounce (20g). Ten weeks later, at 20 weeks gestation, it weighs almost 6 ounces (170g). In another 10 weeks, the placenta will have increased to 15 ounces (430g). At 40 weeks, it can weigh almost 1½ pounds (650g)!

Studies show a baby may spend a great deal of time in utero pulling and squeezing the umbilical cord.

Projections (villi) at the base of the placenta are firmly attached to the uterus. The villi absorb nutrients and oxygen from your blood and transport them to the baby through the umbilical vein in the umbilical cord. Waste products from the baby are brought through the umbilical arteries and transferred to the maternal bloodstream. In this way, baby gets rid of waste products.

At full term, a normal placenta is flat, has a cakelike appearance and is round or oval. It is about 6 to 8 inches (15 to 20cm) in diameter and ¾ to 1¼ inches (2 to 3cm) thick at its thickest part. It weighs between 17½ and 24 ounces (500 to 650g), and is a red or reddish-brown color.

Around the time of birth, the placenta may have white patches on it, which are calcium deposits. The umbilical cord attached to the placenta is about 22 inches (55cm) long and is usually white.

Placentas vary widely in size and shape. A placenta that is large (placentamegaly) may be found when a woman has syphilis or when a baby has erythroblastosis (Rh-sensitization). Sometimes it occurs without any obvious explanation. A small placenta may be found with intrauterine-growth restriction (IUGR).

The part of the placenta that attaches to the wall of the uterus has a beefy or spongy appearance. The side closest to the baby inside the amniotic sac is smooth and covered with amniotic and chorionic membranes.

In multiple pregnancies, there may be more than one placenta, or there may be one placenta with more than one umbilical cord coming from it. Usually with twins, there are two amniotic sacs, with two umbilical cords running to the fetuses from one placenta.

How Your Actions Affect Your Baby's Development

Asthma in Pregnancy

Asthma is a chronic respiratory disease that causes small airways in the lungs to narrow. It is characterized by attacks of labored breathing, wheezing, shortness of breath, chest constriction and coughing. People with asthma often have symptoms followed by symptom-free periods. The most common causes of asthma include allergens, exercise, strong odors and cold air.

The problem affects about 2% of the population in the United States and Canada. It is equally common in other countries. Asthma may occur at any age, but about 50% of all asthma cases occur before age 10. Another 33% of the cases occur by age 40. About 70% of people with asthma also suffer from allergies.

Summertime can cause asthma problems when air quality is poor. Smog can cause inflammation in the airways, coughing, wheezing and shortness of breath.

Sufferers should be careful during storm season—thunderstorms may increase the risk of an asthma attack. Research shows rain and lightning break pollen into extremely small particles, which can be more easily spread by a storm's winds.

Many asthma sufferers have heartburn; heartburn may cause asthma symptoms to worsen. Upper-respiratory infections caused by the flu may also trigger an attack.

Pregnancy's Affect on Asthma. About 8% of all pregnant women have asthma. It's 40% more common in women than in men and is one of the most common medical problems pregnant women face.

If you have asthma and are overweight when you get pregnant, your baby is more likely to have asthma.

Some pregnant women appear to get better during pregnancy, while others remain about the same. However, if you have severe asthma attacks when you aren't pregnant, you may also have severe attacks during pregnancy.

Studies show if your asthma is under control throughout pregnancy, your pregnancy outcome can be as positive as a woman who doesn't have asthma. Controlling your asthma may help lower your risk of developing some pregnancy problems. We also know asthma symptoms often improve during the last month of pregnancy due to hormonal changes.

Untreated asthma can put you and baby at risk. If you have severe, uncontrolled asthma, baby may be deprived of oxygen during your asthma attacks. If you're not getting enough air, neither is baby.

It's important to have a flu shot to reduce the risk of getting severe respiratory illness, which could make asthma attacks worse. Avoid cigarette smoke. Don't smoke, and keep away from others who smoke.

If your baby is a girl, research shows asthma attacks might worsen during pregnancy. If your baby is a boy, attacks might be better because the androgens (male sex hormones) produced by male fetuses are believed to have a protective effect on moms-to-be with asthma.

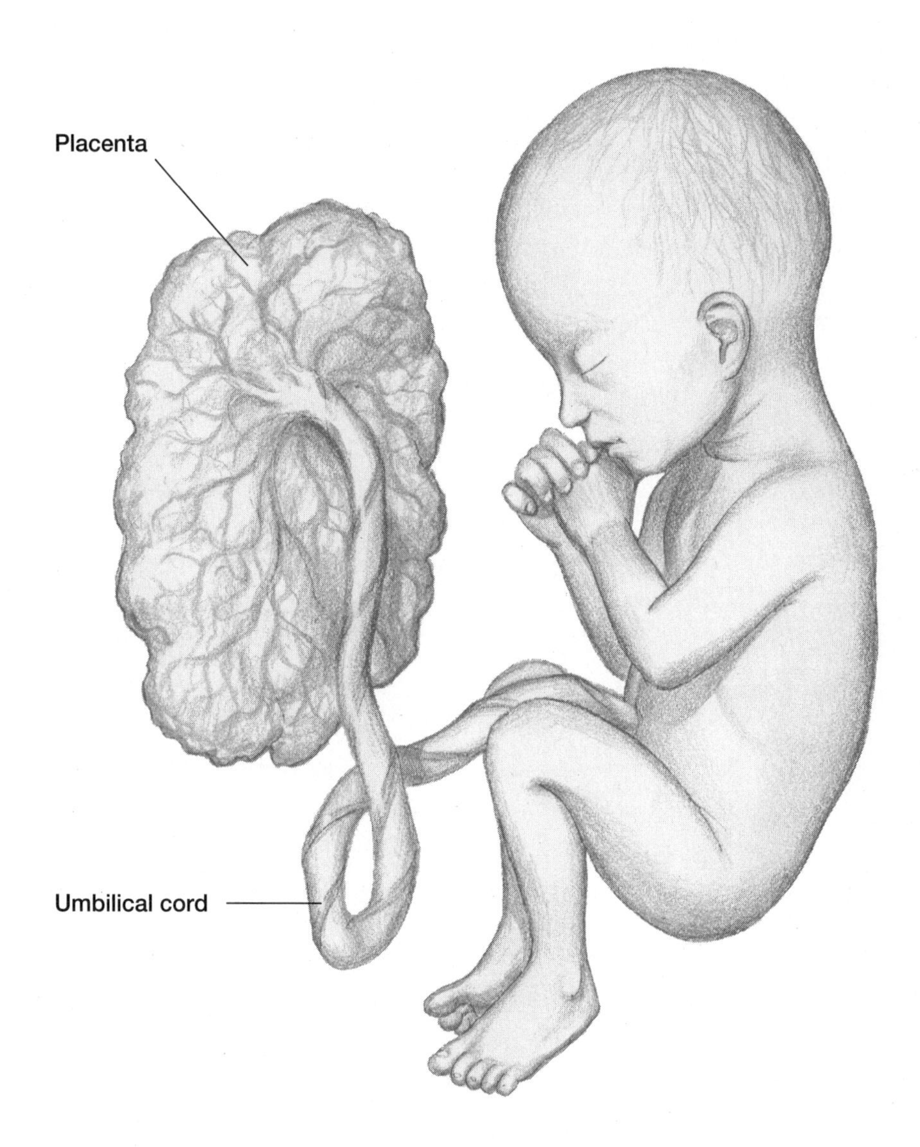

The placenta, shown here with the fetus, carries oxygen and nutrients to the growing baby. It is an important part of pregnancy.

See your allergist regularly during pregnancy for a lung-function test. This helps determine whether your medication dosage needs to be adjusted. Your allergist may also suggest you monitor your breathing with a *peak-flow meter* to find out how open your airways are.

Asthma shouldn't be a deterrent to learning breathing techniques used in labor. Talk to your healthcare provider about them.

Treating Asthma Attacks. Asthma treatment is important so baby can get the oxygen it needs to grow and to develop. During pregnancy, your oxygen consumption increases by about 25%. The treatment plan used before pregnancy often continues to be helpful.

Research shows it's better for you to take asthma medicine during pregnancy than to risk asthma attacks and their complications. Most asthma medicine appears to be safe during pregnancy; however, check with your healthcare provider before using your usual prescription medication.

Asthma medication, such as terbutaline, and steroids, such as hydrocortisone or methylprednisolone, can be used during pregnancy. Aminophylline, theophyline, metaproterenol (Alupent) and albuterol (Ventolin) are also safe to use.

Studies show inhaled steroids do not seem to affect baby's growth. Inhalers work directly on the lungs, so very little medicine enters your bloodstream. However, don't use Primatene Mist during pregnancy.

If your asthma is severe, you may be given an anti-inflammatory nasal spray, such as cromolyn sodium (Nasalcrom) or an inhaled steroid,

In addition to any medicine you take for asthma, there are a few other things you can do to help avoid attacks. Using a dust-mite-proof cover on your mattress may lower your chances of having an allergic asthma attack. One study showed eating citrus fruit—more than 46g a day (⅓ of a medium orange)—may help reduce chances of having an asthma attack. Eating spinach, tomatoes, carrots and green leafy vegetables may also reduce risk. Fish oil has been shown to improve breathing in exercise-induced asthma. Talk to your healthcare provider about how much you should eat of any of these foods.

such as beclomethasone (Vanceril). Discuss the situation at one of your early prenatal visits.

Your Nutrition

New intake guidelines have been released for vitamin D. A person should take in about 600IU each day of the vitamin. Super-high levels, such as 2000IU/day, are *not* recommended.

You can get your vitamin D from various food sources, including milk, eggs, beef liver and some fish, or by supplementation, such as vitamin-D fortified cereals. The FDA has also approved a program to

What Kinds of Foods Should You Eat?

You may be wondering what kinds of foods to eat and what to delete from your diet during this stage of your pregnancy. Look at the chart below for some guidance.

Foods to Eat	Servings per Day
Dark green or dark yellow fruits and vegetables	1
Fruits and vegetables with vitamin C (tomatoes, citrus)	2
Other fruits and vegetables	2
Whole-grain breads and cereals	4
Dairy products, including milk	4
Protein sources (meat, poultry, eggs, fish)	2
Dried beans and peas, seeds and nuts	2
Foods to Eat in Moderation	
Caffeine	200mg
Fat	limited amounts
Sugar	limited amounts
Foods to Avoid	
Anything containing alcohol	
Food additives, when possible	

allow most cheeses to be fortified with up to 20% of the daily allotment for the vitamin. Other foods are also fortified with vitamin D, such as some orange juice, yogurt and margarine. Be sure to get enough vitamin D during pregnancy—it's good for baby's bones.

You Should Also Know

Nutrisystem and Jenny Craig Meal Plans

Many women have lost weight following eating plans that provide the consumer with prepackaged foods and meals. Two of the most popular are Nutrisystem and Jenny Craig. Pregnant women want to know if they can continue to eat these foods and follow the meal plans during pregnancy.

Taking vitamin D may help relieve seasonal affective disorder (SAD), which can make you feel anxious, tired and sad during the winter months. Ask your healthcare provider about taking vitamin D during pregnancy.

Both of these programs recommend a pregnant woman not follow their food plans because calories are too restricted. The plans do not supply enough calories for you to stay healthy and for your baby to grow and to develop during your pregnancy.

After baby's birth, if you breastfeed, you need a healthful, higher-calorie diet than these plans offer because it takes extra, nutritious calories to make breast milk. If you decide not to breastfeed or when you're finished breastfeeding, one of these plans may help you lose unwanted pounds.

Third-Trimester Tests

In your third trimester, you may undergo various tests to determine how you and baby are doing as labor and delivery get nearer. Below is a list of some of the common assessment tests a healthcare provider may order. Included is the week where an in-depth discussion appears for each of these tests:

- group-B streptococcus (GBS) infection test, see Week 29
- ultrasound in the third trimester, see Week 35

- home uterine monitoring, see Week 26
- kick count, see Week 27
- Bishop score, see Week 41
- nonstress test, see Week 41
- contraction-stress test, see Week 41
- the biophysical profile, see Week 41

Twenty-eight weeks of gestation is a time when many healthcare providers initiate or repeat certain blood tests or procedures. Testing for gestational diabetes may be done at this time.

ABO Incompatibility

Blood groups are designated as types A, B, AB and O. They are sometimes called the *major blood groups.* Blood tests are performed at the beginning of pregnancy to determine ABO type and screen for the presence of antibodies (antibody screen).

ABO incompatibility is a type of blood-group difference, similar to Rh incompatibility. ABO incompatibility can cause a disease in a newborn that destroys baby's blood cells (hemolytic disease). Type A-and-B incompatibility is the most common cause of the problem in a newborn.

The situation occurs when the mother has type O blood and her partner has type A, B or AB blood, and together they conceive a baby with type A or B blood. The mother can produce antibodies that destroy the baby's blood cells. An affected baby may have jaundice or anemia when it is born; these can both be easily treated in nearly all cases.

If you are Rh-negative, you will probably receive an injection of RhoGAM at this point in pregnancy. This injection keeps you from becoming sensitized if baby's blood mixes with yours. RhoGAM protects you until delivery.

How Is the Baby Lying?

You may be wondering how your baby is lying inside the uterus. Is the baby head first? Is it bottom first (breech)? Is the baby lying sideways? It's difficult—usually impossible—at this point in pregnancy to tell just by feeling your abdomen. The baby changes position throughout pregnancy.

Is Home Birth Safe?

Home births happen. Of the 25,000 home births that occur every year in the United States, 25% (a little over 6,000) of them are unplanned. That means the other 75% (nearly 19,000) of home births *are* planned. But are home births safe?

You may have heard from friends or acquaintances they had a home birth and everything went fine. Some women want to give birth at home because they feel it's "more natural." Another factor may be the high cost of labor and delivery, especially if you don't have full insurance coverage.

But research has shown giving birth at home is an extremely risky undertaking. One study showed twice as many infant deaths and serious, dangerous complications when babies are delivered at home. What can be done at home if your baby has serious problems and needs immediate medical care that can only be provided at a hospital or birthing center staffed by professionals?

We know there are also dangers to mom. First-time pregnant women who deliver at home have nearly triple the risk of complications after baby's birth. In addition, the chance of serious problems increases when a woman suffers from various pregnancy problems. Even carrying more than one baby increases your risk.

The American College of Obstetricians and Gynecologists has firmly stated that home birthing is hazardous to a woman and her baby. Based on Dr. Curtis's own experiences with the aftermath of home births, we must concur. We advise any woman who is considering this option to talk to her healthcare provider about the safety and wisdom of delivering her baby at the hospital or a birthing center.

Dad Tip

Your partner has been feeling the baby move for a while. Around this time, you may also be able to feel it! Gently place your hand on her abdomen, and leave it there for a while. Your partner can tell you when the baby is moving.

You can feel the abdomen to try to see where the head or other parts are located. In another 3 to 4 weeks, the baby's head will be harder; it will be easier at that time for your healthcare provider to determine how the baby is lying (called *presentation of the fetus*).

Bug Sprays and Insect Repellents

If you're pregnant and live in an area where bugs are a problem, take precautions to avoid bites to reduce your risk for infections. Avoid insect-infested areas, use screens on windows and doors, and wear protective clothing. Get rid of standing water in your yard so mosquitoes and other insects don't have a place to breed.

You may be wondering if it's safe to use mosquito and other bug repellents. It's OK to use an EPA-registered repellent (one that has been reviewed for safety by the U.S. Environmental Protection Agency). The CDC recommends repellents containing DEET or picaridin on skin and clothing, and permethrin on clothing. Oil of lemon eucalyptus is another option, but it's not as long-lasting.

Grandma's Remedy

If you want to avoid using medication, try a folk remedy. If you get a sunburn, brew up some mint tea, and cool it. Wet a small towel in the tea, and apply it to your sunburned skin. It cools the burn and may prevent peeling.

Don't overdo it with bug sprays. Spray your clothing, not your skin. Bug lights and bug candles may offer some protection. Even some plants, such as citronella plants, may help repel insects.

Canavan Disease

Canavan disease, also called *Canavan sclerosis* and *Canavan-van Bogaert-Bertrand syndrome*, is a relatively common degenerative disease of the brain. Although Canavan disease may occur in any ethnic group, it's more frequent among Saudi Arabians and Ashkenazi Jews from eastern Poland, Lithuania and western Russia.

The disease is one of a group of genetic disorders called *leukodystrophies*. With Canavan disease, the white matter of the brain degenerates into spongy tissue riddled with small fluid-filled spaces. The disease causes problems in the development of the myelin sheath, the fatty covering that acts as an insulator around nerve fibers in the brain.

There is no cure, nor is there a standard course of treatment. The disease develops in infancy, and prognosis is poor. Death usually occurs before age 4, although some children have survived to their 20s.

Canavan disease can be identified by a blood test that screens for the missing enzyme or for mutations in the gene that controls aspartoacylase. Both parents must be carriers of the defective gene to have an affected child. When both parents are found to carry the Canavan gene mutation, there is a one-in-four chance with each pregnancy that the child will be affected.

Exercise for Week 28

Sit tall in a straight-backed side chair, with your knees bent, your arms relaxed at your side and your feet flat on the floor. Lift your left foot off the floor, with your leg extended. Hold for 8 seconds; be sure you are sitting erect. Lower your left leg. Do 5 times for each leg. *Stretches hamstrings, and strengthens thigh muscles.*

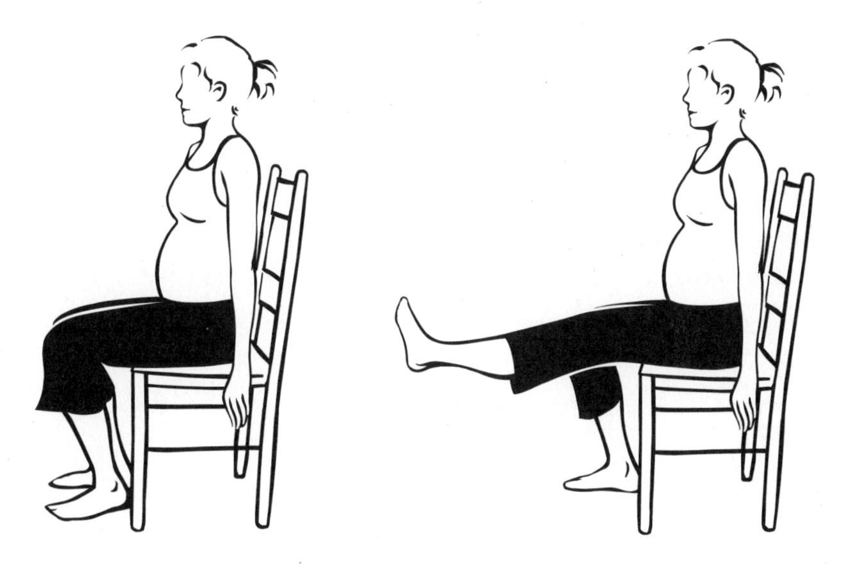

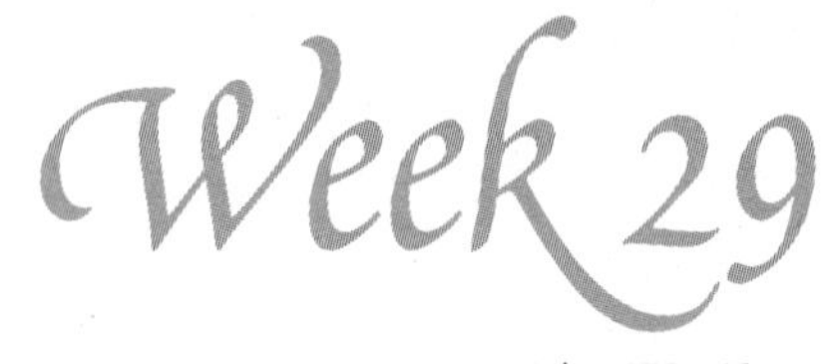

Week 29

Age of Fetus—27 Weeks

How Big Is Your Baby?

By this time, your baby weighs about 2½ pounds (1.2kg). Crown-to-rump length is almost 10½ inches (26cm). Total fetal length is 15¼ inches (38cm).

How Big Are You?

Measuring from the bellybutton, your uterus is 3½ to 4 inches (7.6 to 10.2cm) above it. Your uterus is about 11½ inches (29cm) above the pubic symphysis. Your total weight gain by this week should be between 19 and 25 pounds (8.55 and 11.25kg).

How Your Baby Is Growing and Developing

Each week, we've noted the change in your baby's size. We use average weights to give you an idea of how large baby may be at a particular time. However, these are only averages; babies vary greatly in size and weight. The average baby's birthweight at full term is 7 to 7½ pounds (3.28kg to 3.4kg).

Because growth is rapid during pregnancy, infants born prematurely may be tiny. Even a few weeks less time in the uterus can have a dramatic effect on baby's size. A baby continues to grow after 36 weeks of gestation but at a slower rate.

A couple of interesting factors about birthweight. Boys weigh more than girls. And the birthweight of an infant increases with the increasing number of pregnancies you have or the number of babies you deliver.

According to one study, adult men and women who were born prematurely have slightly lower reproduction rates than those born at term. The earlier they were born, the lower their reproductive success. Another study indicates women born prematurely are at increased risk of delivering their own babies preterm. Fourteen percent of women born between 22 and 27 weeks gestation delivered their babies prematurely. For women born between 28 and 36 weeks, 9% delivered early. Only 6% of women born at term delivered preterm.

How Mature Is Your Baby?

A baby born between the 38th and 42nd weeks of pregnancy is a *term baby* or *full-term infant*. Before the 38th week, the term *preterm* can be applied to the baby. After 42 weeks of pregnancy, your baby is overdue and the term *postdate* is used.

When a baby is born before the end of pregnancy, many people use the terms *premature* and *preterm* interchangeably. There is a difference. An infant that is 32 weeks gestational age but has mature pulmonary or lung function at the time of birth is more appropriately called a "preterm infant" than a premature infant. "Premature" best describes an infant that has immature lungs at the time of birth.

Premature Labor and Premature Birth

Many babies born in the United States are born before their due date. Statistics show nearly 13% of all babies are premature—that's over half a million babies each year! The rate of premature births has increased by over 30% since 1980.

Today, we classify premature babies into categories. The most commonly used classifications are:

- micropreemie—born before 27 weeks of pregnancy
- very premature—born between 27 and 32 weeks of pregnancy
- premature—born between 32 and 37 weeks of pregnancy
- late premature—born after 37 weeks of pregnancy

Premature birth increases the risk of problems in a baby. In 1950, the neonatal death rate was about 20 per 1000 live births. Today, the rate is less than 10 per 1000 live births. Nearly twice the number of preterm infants survive today than 60 years ago.

The higher survival rate applies mainly to babies delivered after 27 weeks or more of gestation, who weigh at least 2¾ pounds (1kg), with no birth defects. When gestational age and birthweight are below these levels, the death rate increases.

Better methods of caring for premature babies have contributed to higher survival statistics. Today, infants born as early as 25 weeks of pregnancy may survive, but long-term survival and quality of life for these babies remains to be seen as they grow older. In the lower-birthweight range, many babies had disabilities. Higher-weight babies also had disabilities, but statistics for this group were much lower. Premature babies with low birth weights are at highest risk.

The illustration on page 416 shows a premature baby with several leads attached to its body to monitor it. Many other attachments may be used, such as I.V.s, tubes and masks that provide oxygen.

It's usually best for the baby to remain in the uterus as long as possible, so it can grow and develop fully. Occasionally it's best for the baby to be delivered early, such as when baby is not receiving adequate nutrition. Nearly 25% of preterm births are a result of pregnancy complications—a baby needs to be delivered early for its health and safety.

How will you know if you are experiencing preterm labor? Signs that preterm labor may begin include the following:

- change in type of vaginal discharge (watery, mucus or bloody)
- menstruallike cramps (cramps that feel like your period)
- low, dull backache
- pelvic or lower-abdominal pressure—the feeling that your baby is pushing down hard
- unusual vaginal discharge
- increase in amount of discharge
- abdominal cramps with or without diarrhea

- ruptured membranes
- contractions every 10 minutes or more often
- bleeding

There are some actions that may help stop premature labor. Stop what you're doing and rest on your left side for 1 hour. Drink 2 to 3 glasses of water or juice. If symptoms get worse or don't go away after an hour, call your healthcare provider or go to the hospital. If symptoms go away, relax for the rest of the day. If the symptoms stop but come back, call your healthcare provider or go to the hospital.

Causes of Premature Labor and Premature Birth. In most cases, we don't know the cause of premature labor and premature birth, and finding a cause may be difficult. An attempt is always made to determine what causes it so treatment may be more effective. Half of the women who go into preterm labor have no known risk factors.

The list below contains risk factors for preterm labor. Your risk for preterm labor increases if you:

- had preterm labor or preterm birth in a previous pregnancy
- smoke cigarettes or use cocaine
- are carrying more than one baby
- have an abnormal cervix or uterus
- had abdominal surgery during this pregnancy
- had an infection while pregnant, such as a UTI or gum problems
- had any bleeding in the second or third trimester of this pregnancy
- are underweight
- have a mother or a grandmother who took DES (diethylstilbestrol; medication given to many pregnant women in the 1950s, 1960s and 1970s)
- have had little or no prenatal care
- are carrying a child with chromosomal disorders

Other risk factors have been identified, including giving birth at an older age, carrying a baby conceived from in-vitro fertilization, quickly

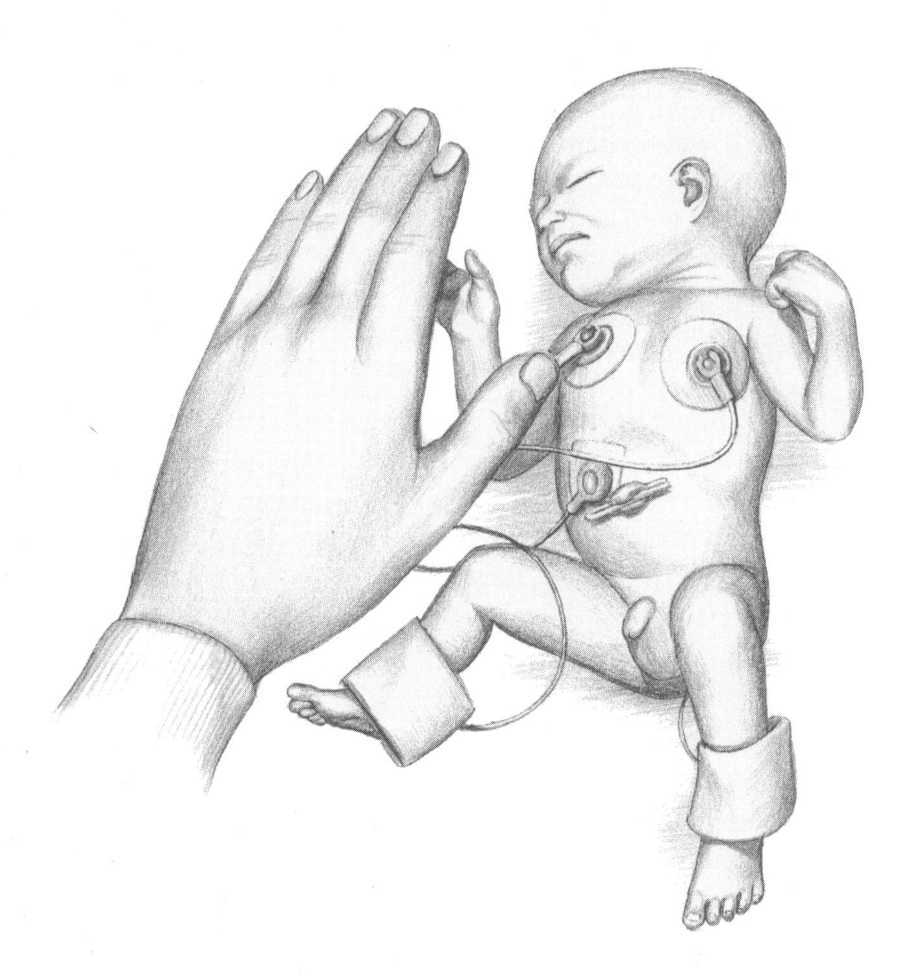

Premature baby (born at 29 weeks of pregnancy) shown with fetal monitors attached to it. Note size of adult hand in comparison.

Studies show it can be dangerous for a baby to be born even a few weeks early. The infant-mortality rate is as much as 3 times higher for babies born between 34 and 36 weeks than for babies born between 37 and 41 weeks. Babies born before 36 weeks are more likely to develop breathing difficulties, feeding problems and have trouble regulating body temperature. We once believed a baby's lungs were mature by 34 weeks, but we now know this isn't true. These findings may impact elective Cesarean deliveries and induction of labor.

getting pregnant after a previous birth (less than 9 months), you are Black/African-American or you are under 17 or over 35. Research shows if it took you longer than 1 year to get pregnant, you may have a slightly higher chance of giving birth prematurely.

Some experts believe up to half of all premature births may be tied to infections. Iron deficiency has also been linked to an increased risk. Some researchers believe taking your prenatal vitamin every day may help cut your risk by as much as 50%!

Low HDL cholesterol and elevated homocysteine levels in a mother-to-be have been shown to be key factors associated with preterm birth. When found together, the risk of premature delivery was twice as high.

One study indicates a link between preterm delivery and a mother's future risk of heart disease and stroke. The factors we know lead to stroke and heart disease were elevated in the second trimester in mothers who delivered babies prematurely.

Tests Your Healthcare Provider May Do. One test, called *SalEst,* can help determine if a woman might go into labor too early. The test measures levels of the hormone estriol in a woman's saliva. Research has shown there is often a surge in this chemical several weeks before early labor. A positive result means a woman has a 7 times greater chance of delivering her baby before the 37th week of pregnancy. Another test is fetal fibronectin (fFN). See Week 22.

Some difficult questions that must be answered when premature labor begins include those below.

- Is it better for the infant to be inside the uterus or to be delivered?
- Are the dates of the pregnancy correct?
- Is this really labor?

For a discussion of premature babies, see Appendix D, which begins on page 608.

Changes in You

Bed Rest to Treat Premature Labor

The treatment used most often for premature labor is bed rest. A woman is advised to stay in bed and lie on her side. (Either side is OK.) The term *bed rest* can cover anything from cutting back on activities to being confined to bed for 24 hours a day, getting up only to go to the bathroom and to shower. It's not uncommon to feel anger and resentment if you're advised to go on bed rest.

Even if you have symptoms of premature labor, you may not deliver early.

About 20% of all pregnant women—nearly 1 million—are advised to rest in bed at some point. However, not all experts agree on this treatment. It's OK to discuss bed rest and all of its implications with your healthcare provider if he or she recommends it. Ask if more tests, such as ultrasound or fetal fibronectin, might help or if medications are an option. Discuss getting a second opinion from a perinatologist, who deals with high-risk pregnancies.

Bed rest is often successful in stopping contractions and premature labor. If you are advised to rest in bed, it may mean you can't go to work or continue many activities. It's worth it to rest in bed if you can avoid premature delivery of your baby.

The most common reasons for ordering bed rest are premature labor, pre-eclampsia, contractions, chronic high blood pressure, incompetent cervix and placenta previa. High stress from a job or your lifestyle may also require bed rest. If serious complications arise, your healthcare provider may advise hospital treatment.

One negative to bed rest is the increased risk of a blood clot in your leg, called *deep-vein thrombosis* (see Week 21 for more on deep-vein thrombosis). Other problems include muscle weakness and/or atrophy, loss of bone calcium, weight-gain issues (gaining too much or too little weight), heartburn, constipation, nausea, insomnia, depression and family tension. Discuss with your healthcare provider exercises you can do while on bed rest, such as stretching or strength training, to prevent loss of muscle tone and strength.

Tip for Week 29

If your healthcare provider advises bed rest, follow his or her instructions. It may be difficult for you to stop your activities and sit idly by when you have lots of things to do, but remember, it's for the good health of you and your baby!

Lying down for quite a while can lead to you being out of shape. Take it easy getting back into the swing of things after baby is born. It can take some time to return to your normal level of activity. Don't rush into physical activities until you feel up to doing them.

Bed-Rest Boredom Relievers. Bed rest can mean anything from staying in bed part of the day to staying in bed 24/7. It can be pretty boring being stuck in bed. Below are some suggestions to help beat bed-rest boredom.

- Spend the day in a room other than your bedroom. Use the living-room or family-room sofa for daytime activities.
- Establish a daily routine. When you get up, change into daytime clothes. Shower or bathe every day. Comb your hair, and put on lipstick. Go to bed when you normally do.
- Don't nap during the day—it can contribute to sleeplessness at night.
- Use foam mattress pads and extra pillows for comfort.
- Keep a telephone close at hand.
- Keep reading material, the television remote control, a radio and other essentials nearby.

- A laptop with internet access can be a lifesaver. It can entertain you and keep you connected at work.
- Use the time to learn another language—many language programs are available for the computer.
- Keep food and drinks close at hand. Use a cooler to keep food and drinks cold. Use an insulated container for hot soup or herbal tea.
- Start a journal. Our book, *Your Pregnancy Journal Week by Week*, is easy to use and lets you record your thoughts and feelings to share with your partner now and your child later.
- Do some crafts that aren't messy, such as cross stitch, knitting, crocheting, drawing or hand sewing. Make something for baby!
- Use the time to plan for baby's arrival.
- Spend some time planning baby's room (someone else will have to carry through on it), deciding what you'll need for a layette and making a list of all the necessary items you'll need after baby comes home.
- Sort! Use the time to sort through recipes, to put pictures in albums, go through your coupons or make a scrapbook of information for after baby's arrival.
- Call your favorite local charity or political organization, and volunteer to make phone calls, stuff envelopes or write letters.
- If you have other children at home, day care will probably be a necessity for you.
- For support, contact other women who have been on bed rest. A national support group helps women with high-risk pregnancies. They can provide you with information and put you in touch with other women who have had the same experience. Contact *Sidelines* at 888-447-4754.

How Your Actions Affect Your Baby's Development

Most of our discussion this week has been devoted to the premature infant and treatment of premature labor. If you're diagnosed with premature labor and your healthcare provider prescribes bed rest and medicine to stop it, follow his or her advice!

If you're concerned about your healthcare provider's instructions, discuss them. If you're told not to work or advised to reduce activities and you ignore the advice, you're taking chances with your well-being and your unborn baby's. It isn't worth taking risks. Don't be afraid to ask for another opinion or the opinion of a perinatologist if you have premature labor.

Your Nutrition

Potassium-rich foods, such as raisins and bananas, may help reduce your risk of premature labor. Potassium helps the body get rid of sodium faster.

We hope you've been listening to your body during pregnancy. When you feel hungry or thirsty, eat or drink something. Eating smaller, more frequent meals provides a constant supply of nutrients to your growing baby.

Dad Tip

After the baby is born, you may want to take time off to help out at home and to be part of your baby's early development. The Family and Medical Leave Act was passed to help people take time off to care for family members. Ask your employer or supervisor now if it applies to you. If it does, and you plan to take time off, begin making arrangements soon.

Keep nourishing snacks near at hand. Dried fruit and nuts are good choices when you're on the go. Know what time of day or night hunger strikes you. Be prepared.

You can be different, if you want to be. Eat spaghetti for breakfast and cereal for lunch, if that's what appeals to you. Don't force yourself to eat something that turns you off or makes you sick. There's always an alternative. As long as you eat nourishing food and pay attention to the types of foods you eat, you help yourself and your growing baby.

You Should Also Know

Medications to Help Stop Premature Labor

Beta-adrenergic agents, also called *tocolytic agents,* may be used to suppress labor. They relax your muscles and may help decrease contractions. (The uterus is mainly muscle.)

At this time, only ritodrine (Yutopar) is approved by the FDA to treat premature labor. It is given in three different forms—intravenously, as an intramuscular injection and as a pill. It is usually first given intravenously and may require a hospital stay.

When premature contractions stop, you can be switched to oral medicine, which you take every 2 to 4 hours. Ritodrine is approved for use in pregnancies over 20 weeks and under 36 weeks gestation. In some cases, medication is used without first giving an I.V. This is done most often in women with a history of premature labor or for a woman with multiple pregnancies.

Terbutaline may also be used to halt premature labor. Although it has been shown to be effective, it hasn't been approved for this use by the FDA.

Magnesium sulfate is used to treat pre-eclampsia; it may also help stop premature labor. An additional benefit of administering magnesium sulfate during pregnancy is called *neuroprotection.* Some studies show a decreased risk of cerebral palsy and severe motor dysfunction in a baby when it is used. However, not all experts agree with using magnesium sulfate for neuroprotection.

Magnesium sulfate is usually given through an I.V. and requires hospitalization. However, it is occasionally given orally, without hospitalization. You must be monitored frequently if you take magnesium sulfate.

Some women should not receive magnesium sulfate. These include women with myasthenia gravis, those with myocardial compromise or cardiac-conduction defects and women with impaired kidney function.

Sedatives or narcotics may be used in early attempts to stop labor. A woman might receive an injection of morphine or meperidine (Demerol). This is not a long-term solution but may be effective in initially stopping labor.

Epstein-Barr Virus (EBV)

Epstein-Barr virus (EBV) is a member of the herpes virus family; it is one of the most common human viruses. Most people become infected with EBV sometime during their life. In the United States, as many as 95% of adults between 35 and 40 years of age have been infected. We don't know of any connection between an active EBV infection and problems during pregnancy. Studies of EBV during pregnancy show the virus poses little threat to the baby.

Progesterone (17-hydroxyprogesterone) may be given to a pregnant woman if her previous baby was born prematurely. Some studies indicate a woman with a short cervix may also benefit from this treatment.

Other preparations, such as vaginal creams and oral medications, are being tested. Folic-acid supplementation for at least 1 year before pregnancy has been shown to decrease the occurrence of early preterm birth.

If you have premature labor, you may need to see your healthcare provider frequently. He or she will probably monitor you with ultrasound or nonstress tests.

Exercise for Week 29

Kneel on the ground, sitting lightly on your heels with your feet tucked under you and your toes on the ground. Sit tall. Press your toes into the ground. Hold. Do 5 or 6 times, or as often as you want. *Loosens calf and foot muscles; may help prevent leg cramps.*

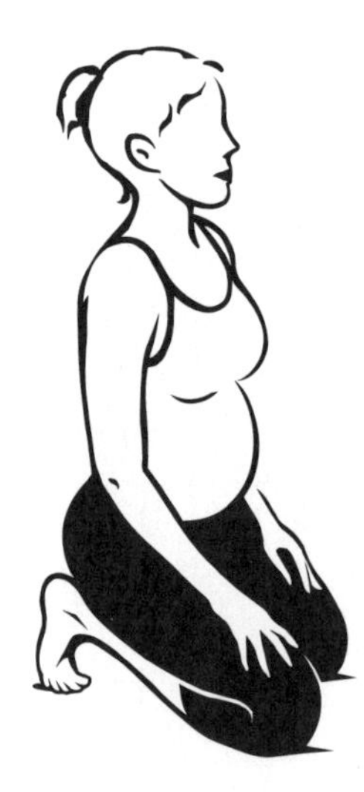

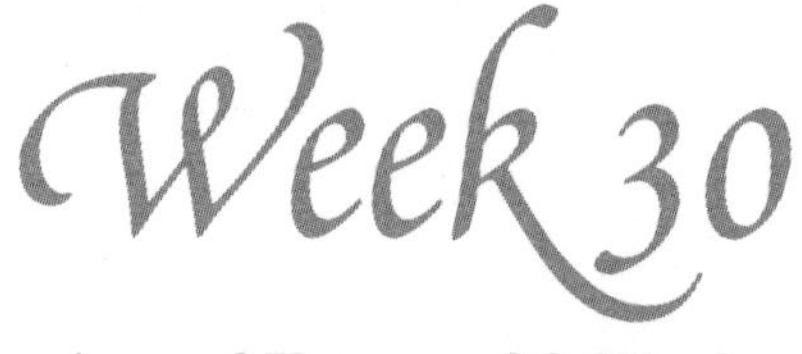

Week 30

Age of Fetus—28 Weeks

How Big Is Your Baby?

At this point, your baby weighs about 3 pounds (1.3kg). Its crown-to-rump length is a little over 10¾ inches (27cm), and total length is 15¾ inches (40cm).

How Big Are You?

It may be hard to believe you still have 10 weeks to go! You may feel like you're running out of room. Measuring from your bellybutton, your uterus is about 4 inches (10cm) above it. From the pubic symphysis, the top of your uterus measures about 12 inches (30cm).

You should be gaining about 1 pound a week. About half of this weight is concentrated in the growth of the uterus, the baby, the placenta and the volume of amniotic fluid. Growth is mostly in your abdomen and your pelvis. You may experience increasing discomfort in your pelvis and abdomen as pregnancy progresses.

How Your Baby Is Growing and Developing

The illustration on page 427 shows a fetus and its umbilical cord. Can you see the knot in the cord? You may wonder how a knot like this can occur. We do not believe the cord grows in a knot.

A baby is usually quite active during pregnancy. We believe these knots occur as the baby moves around in early pregnancy. A loop forms in the umbilical cord; the baby moves through the loop, and a knot results. Your actions do not cause or prevent this kind of complication. A knot in the umbilical cord doesn't occur often.

Changes in You

Irritable Bowel Syndrome (IBS)

Irritable bowel syndrome (IBS) is a disorder of the large intestine (colon) that causes abdominal pain and abnormal bowel movements. IBS is *not* the same as inflammatory bowel disease (IBD). It doesn't permanently damage the intestines or lead to more serious problems. We don't know what causes IBS. It may be a lifelong condition, but symptoms can often be improved or relieved with treatment.

As many as 1 in 5 American adults may have symptoms of IBS. It can occur at any age but often begins in adolescence or early adulthood; it's more common in women. IBS that occurs after an intestinal infection is called *postinfectious IBS.*

Symptoms range from mild to severe and may include abdominal pain, bloating, cramping, constipation, diarrhea, gas, depression and loss of appetite. Emotional stress may worsen symptoms. Nervous-system or colon abnormalities may cause greater-than-normal discomfort when the abdomen stretches from gas. Triggers for IBS can range from gas or pressure on your intestines to certain foods, medicines and stress.

IBS and Pregnancy. IBS symptoms may get worse during pregnancy and cause discomfort. The problem often lessens during the first

Although this book is designed to take you through pregnancy by examining one week at a time, you may want specific information. Because the book can't include *everything* you need *before* you know you're looking for it, check the index, beginning on page 655, for a particular topic. We may not cover the subject until a later week.

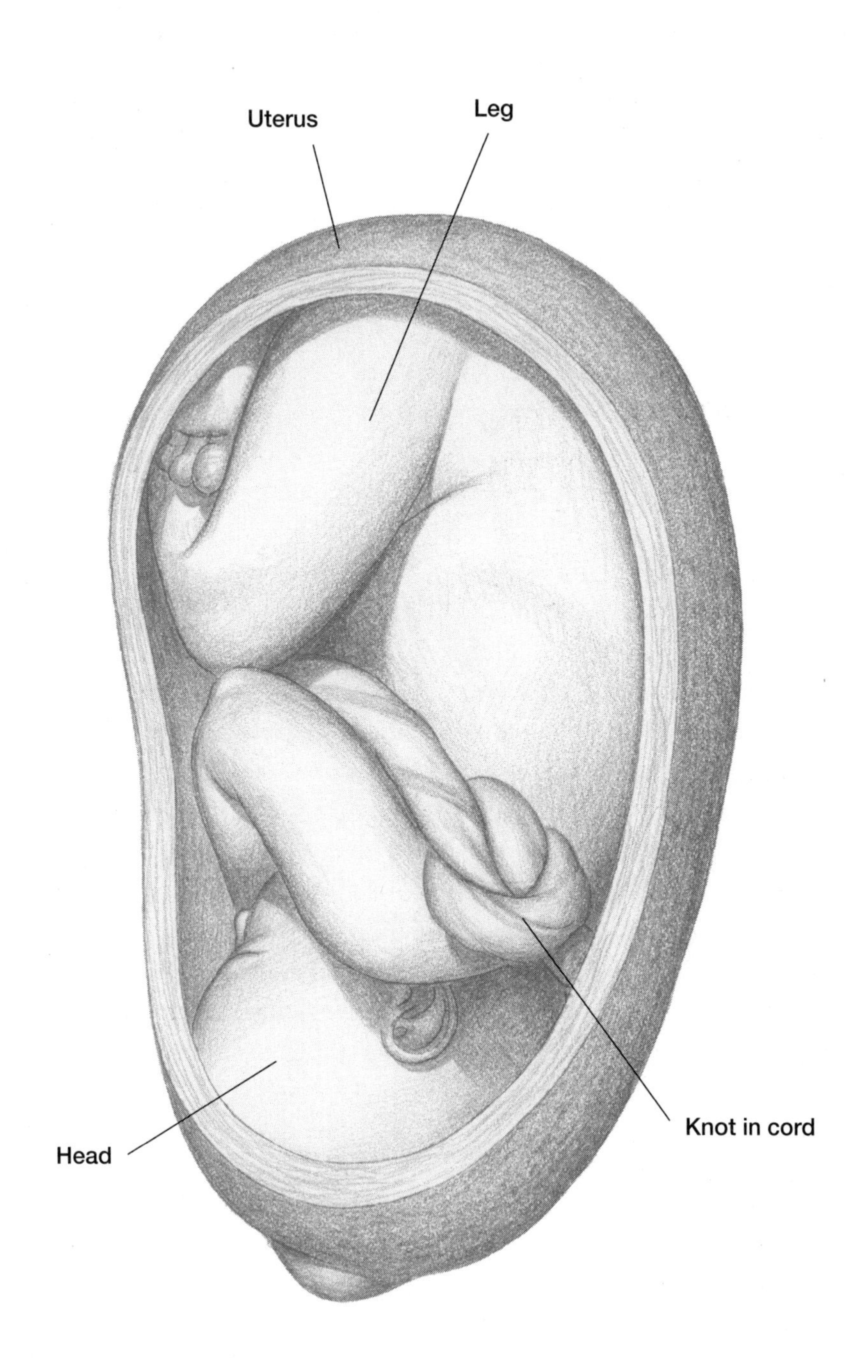

This fetus has a knot in its umbilical cord.

trimester and reappears in the second trimester. In the third trimester, symptoms often increase.

Your digestive system may slow down, causing constipation. Improper diet and lack of physical activity can also play a role in constipation. Drink plenty of water. Eat a high-fiber diet. Do moderate, safe exercise, if you have your healthcare provider's OK. Adequate rest and sleep may help. Soluble fiber supplements may reduce constipation and diarrhea.

If IBS becomes severe, you may be prescribed medication. There is no cure for the problem—the goal of treatment is to relieve symptoms. Work with your healthcare provider during pregnancy if you have IBS.

How Your Actions Affect Your Baby's Development

Bathing during Pregnancy

Many women wonder if taking a bath during pregnancy is OK. Most healthcare providers believe it's safe to bathe throughout pregnancy. They may caution you to be careful as you get in or out of the bathtub. Be sure bath water is not too hot. If you think your water has broken, don't take a bath.

Women want to know how they'll know if their water breaks while they're in the tub or shower. When your water breaks, there is usually a gush of water followed by slow leakage. If your water breaks while you're bathing, you may not notice the initial gush of fluid, but you'll probably notice the leakage of fluid, which can last for quite a while.

Choosing Where to Give Birth

It's probably time to start considering where you want to give birth. In some situations, you may not have a choice. Or in your area, you may have several choices.

Whatever birthing setup you choose, the most important considerations are the health of your baby and the welfare of you both. When you decide where to have your baby, be sure you have answers to the following questions, if you can.

When baby hears music, liquid and tissue affect the sound a great deal.

- What facilities and staff are available?
- What is the availability of anesthesia? Is an anesthesiologist available 24 hours a day?
- How long does it take to respond and to perform a Cesarean delivery, if necessary? (This should be 30 minutes or less.)
- Is a pediatrician available 24 hours a day for an emergency or problems?
- Is the nursery staffed at all times?
- In the event of an emergency or a premature baby that needs to be transported to a high-risk nursery, how is it done? By ambulance? By helicopter? How close is the nearest high-risk nursery, if not at this hospital?

These may seem like a lot of questions to ask, but the answers can help put your mind at ease. When it's your baby and your health, it's good to know emergency measures can be employed in an efficient, timely manner when necessary.

There are various hospital setups available for labor and birth. With *LDRP (labor, delivery, recovery and postpartum)*, the room you are admitted to at the beginning of labor is the room you labor in, deliver in, recover in and remain in for your hospital stay.

The concept of LDRP has evolved because many women don't want to be moved from the labor area to a delivery area, then to another part of the hospital after delivery for recovery. The nursery is usually close to labor and delivery and the recovery area. This enables you to see your baby as often as you like and to have your baby in your room for longer periods.

Another option is the *birthing room*; this generally refers to delivering your baby in the same room you labor in. Even if you use a birthing room, you may have to move to another area of the hospital for recovery and the remainder of your stay.

In many places, *labor-and-delivery suites* are available; you labor in one room, then are moved to a delivery room at the time of birth. Following this, you may go to a postpartum floor, which is an area in the hospital where you will spend the remainder of your hospital stay.

Most hospitals allow you to have your baby in your room as much as you want. This is called *rooming in* or *boarding in*. Some hospitals also have a cot, couch or chair that makes into a bed in your room so your partner can stay with you after delivery. Check the availability of various facilities in the hospitals in your area.

Your Nutrition

Some women ask if herbal teas are safe to drink during pregnancy. Some herbal teas are probably safe to drink and include chamomile, dandelion, ginger root, lemon-balm, peppermint and nettle leaf.

You may have heard warnings about drinking peppermint tea during pregnancy. Many experts agree it's OK if you only drink one or two 6- to 8-ounce cups a day to help relieve morning sickness or upset stomach. However, it may worsen heartburn and/or GERD. Look for products that contain 100% pure peppermint leaves.

Tip for Week 30

Good posture can help relieve lower-back stress and eliminate some back discomfort. Maintaining good posture may take some effort, but it's worth it if it relieves pain.

Many "pregnancy teas" contain red-raspberry leaf. Studies show you can safely drink tea made from red-raspberry leaves during pregnancy; it may help make labor a little shorter. However, many experts advise waiting until after the first trimester to drink it because it may cause uterine contractions.

Don't overuse any herbal teas, even those considered OK to drink during pregnancy. About 12 to 16 ounces *total* a day is the maximum amount of *any* tea to consume. If you have questions, check with your healthcare provider.

Avoid certain herbal teas while you're pregnant. Studies indicate those to avoid include blue cohosh, black cohosh, alfalfa, yellow-dock, penny-royal leaf, yarrow, goldenseal, feverfew, psyllium seed, mugwort, comfrey, coltsfoot, juniper, rue, tansy, cottonroot bark, large amounts

Benefits of Drinking Some Herbal Teas

chamomile	aids digestion
dandelion	helps with swelling and can soothe an upset stomach
ginger root	helps with nausea and nasal congestion
nettle leaf	rich in iron, calcium and other vitamins and minerals
peppermint	relieves gas pains and calms the stomach

of sage, senna, cascara sagrada, buckthorn, fern, slippery elm and squaw vine. We have little information on dandelion tea, stinging-nettles tea or rose hips. It may be best to avoid drinking them during pregnancy.

Green-Tea Warning

Avoid green tea during pregnancy. Studies show women who consume as little as one to two cups of green tea a day within 3 months of conception and during the first trimester *double* the risk of a baby with neural-tube defects. The antioxidant in green tea interferes with the body's use of folic acid. Folic acid in adequate amounts during the first few weeks of pregnancy has helped lower the rate of neural-tube defects.

When you're feeling good, cook ahead and freeze some meals. They'll be ready to go when you're too tired to cook.

Green tea may also interfere with blood tests; it can alter blood-sugar levels that could mess up a diabetes test. In addition, it may interfere with blood clotting. So wait until after pregnancy to have your green tea.

You Should Also Know

MRSA

Methicillin-resistant Staphylococcus aureus (MRSA; sounds like *MERSA*) is a bacteria that causes infections that are difficult to treat because antibiotics often don't work against them. The bacteria (Staphylococcus aureus, also called *staph)* are resistant to, or develop resistance to, many antibiotics. Bacteria have adapted or changed so antibiotics that were effective in the past no longer work. Staph bacteria have proved to be good at developing resistance to antibiotics.

Methicillin is a strong antibiotic that was useful in treating staph in the past but is less useful today. Besides methicillin, other antibiotics that are ineffective against MRSA include dicloxacillin, nafcillin and oxacillin. A nickname used in the media for MRSA or Staphylococcus aureus is "super-bug."

Some experts believe staph has become resistant because of overuse of antibiotics. Treating every cough, cold or earache with antibiotics gives the staph bacteria an opportunity to develop resistance. Antibiotics that *do* work against MRSA include vancomycin, doxycycline and TMP-SMZ (trimethoprim/sulfamethoxazole).

MRSA is a serious infection and may be deadly. It's passed from person to person, usually by poor hygiene. It can start as inflamed skin, with boils or pimples. The area may be red and hot to the touch. MRSA can spread through the bloodstream. When this happens, it can cause sepsis or septic shock. It's estimated that in the United States in 2005, nearly 100,000 serious infections involved MRSA, and about 19,000 people died.

A very common location of MRSA is the nose or nostrils. Other possible sites are open wounds, I.V. catheters and the urinary tract. Many hospitals and surgical centers routinely perform a nasal culture for MRSA when a patient is admitted.

Washing your hands with regular soap, alcohol-based foams or hand sanitizers works well in preventing MRSA. Don't share towels, soap or other personal items. If you have a cut or abrasion, keep it clean, dry and covered. If you develop any pimples or boils, don't pop them. Keep the area tightly covered, and call your healthcare provider immediately.

There are safe antibiotics to use during pregnancy. Evidence doesn't indicate MRSA during pregnancy causes increased risk of miscarriage or birth defects. It's very unlikely you will pass MRSA to baby during delivery. In addition, it's safe to breastfeed if you have MRSA.

Pregnant women may be at greater risk for MRSA because of decreased immunity. If either you or your partner work in a hospital or healthcare facility, prison or anyplace where you have a lot of contact with people, you could be at risk. Discuss any of your concerns with your healthcare provider. He or she can give you advice about your particular situation.

When to Call Your Healthcare Provider. Call your healthcare provider if you believe you have been exposed to MRSA. Take care of cuts and scratches. Know what a MRSA infection looks like—it usually begins as a skin infection then develops small red bumps like pimples. This can be accompanied by a fever or a rash.

Your healthcare provider can lance and clean the infected area. Cultures or rapid tests of the skin can be done. A vaccine against MRSA is being developed.

Grandma's Remedy

If you want to avoid using medication, try a folk remedy. Eat 1 teaspoon of honey before bedtime to help you sleep. Honey helps stabilize blood sugar while it increases melatonin levels and decreases stress hormones.

Group-B Streptococcus Infection (GBS)

Group-B streptococcus (GBS) is a type of bacteria found in up to 40% of all pregnant women. A GBS infection rarely causes problems in adults but can cause life-threatening infections in newborns. GBS passed to a newborn during birth can cause a blood infection, meningitis or pneumonia in the baby.

In women, GBS is most often found in the vagina or rectum. It is possible to have GBS in your system and not be sick or have any symptoms. It is recommended all women be screened for GBS between 35 and 37 weeks of pregnancy. If tests show you have the bacteria but no symptoms, you are *colonized.* If you're colonized, you can pass GBS to your baby.

The battle to eradicate GBS is one of the true medical success stories. Before the 1990s, 7500 newborns contracted the infection each year; 30% of those babies died. Today, only 1600 cases are reported each year. Much of the success has been the result of healthcare providers following the

Centers for Disease Control and Prevention (CDC) guidelines, which include the following:

- a late prenatal culture (35 to 37 weeks) for vaginal and rectal GBS colonization
- an earlier culture (earlier than 35 weeks), based on clinical risk factors
- antibiotics prescribed to all carriers—penicillin G is the antibiotic of choice, followed by ampicillin
- antibiotics prescribed for any woman who has given birth to a previous infant with proven GBS infection

If you're allergic to ampicillin or penicillin, clindamycin is usually given. In this case, tests to see if clindamycin kills the GBS bacteria can be done. If these tests aren't available, you may receive vancomycin. In some cases, cefazolin can be given.

The CDC, the American College of Obstetricians and Gynecologists (ACOG) and the American Academy of Pediatrics (AAP) have developed recommendations aimed at preventing this infection in newborns. They recommend all women with risk factors be treated for GBS. Risk factors include giving birth to a previous infant with GBS infection, preterm labor, ruptured membranes for more than 18 hours or a temperature of 100.4F (38C) immediately before or during childbirth. In addition, if you've had a bladder infection with a positive strep-B urine specimen during pregnancy, you should receive antibiotics at delivery.

Child-Care Decisions

You may think decisions about child care don't need to be made for quite a while. However, it's time to start thinking about it if you plan to return to work after baby's birth.

Quality care is in high demand and short supply! Experts advise you to begin looking for a child-care situation *at least 6 months* before you need it. For some women, that may be the end of the second trimester!

During your third trimester, you may discover your nesting instinct—the overwhelming urge to clean and get organized. Experts believe this may be caused by an increase in oxytocin.

Dad Tip

Now is the time to think about changing your work schedule so you can be near home during the last part of the pregnancy and after baby is born. If you travel a lot, you may need to alter your schedule. Babies come on their own schedule. If you want to be present for the delivery, plan ahead!

Read the information in Appendix E, page 612, if you will need child care for your baby. Starting early is better than starting too late and not being able to find a good care situation for your baby.

Mad Cow Disease

We've all heard about mad cow disease, an illness in cattle. The type that affects humans is a variant of Creutzfeldt-Jacob disease, called *vCJD.* It is extremely hard to contract vCJD; only a few cases have occurred in the United States. It can take many years (even decades) for the disease to progress in a human.

You can put your mind to rest about eating beef in the United States. Our beef is tested extensively, so you have little cause for concern. If you travel outside the country, avoid eating beef in countries that are at risk.

Some Information May Scare You

In an effort to give you as much information as possible about pregnancy, we do include serious discussions throughout the book that some might find "scary." The information is not included to frighten you; it's there to provide facts about particular medical situations that may occur during pregnancy.

If a woman experiences a serious problem, she and her partner will probably want to know as much about it as possible. If a woman has a friend or knows someone who has problems during pregnancy, reading about it might relieve her fears. We also hope our discussions can help you start a dialogue with your doctor, if you have questions.

Nearly all pregnancies are uneventful, and serious situations don't arise. However, please know we have tried to cover as many aspects of pregnancy as we possible can so you'll have all the information at hand that you might need and want. Knowledge is power, so having various facts available can help you feel more in control of your own pregnancy. We hope reading information helps you relax and have a great pregnancy experience.

If you find serious discussions frighten you, don't read them! Or if the information doesn't apply to your pregnancy, just skip over it. But realize information is there if you want to know more about a particular situation.

Exercise for Week 30

Sit tall on a straight-backed side chair. Hold a towel above your head, with your hands shoulder-width apart. Slowly twist from your waist to the left side as far as is comfortable for you. Return to the center, then twist to the right. Do 8 times. *Stretches spine, and strengthens shoulders and upper-back muscles.*

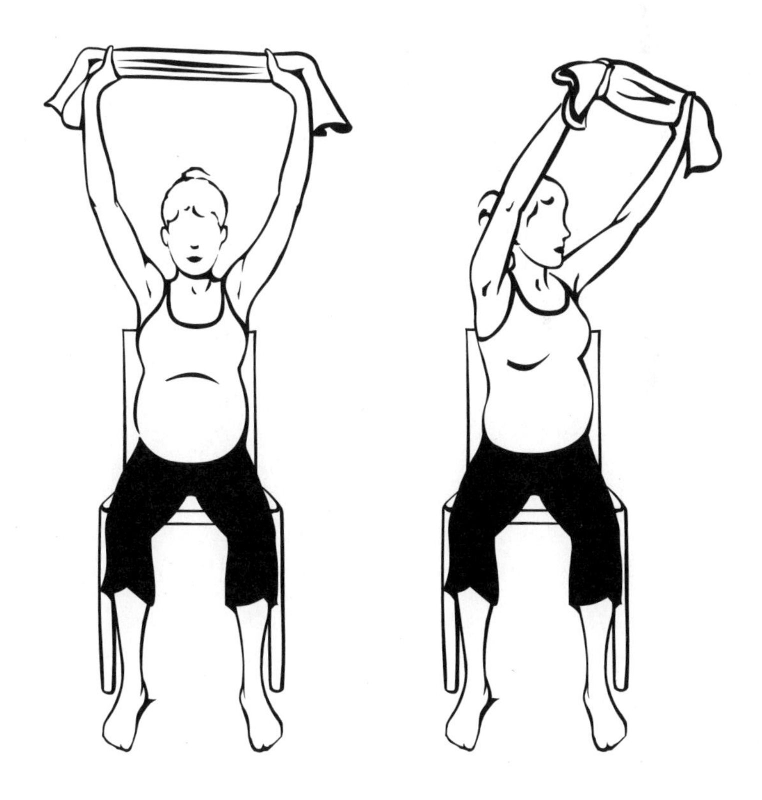

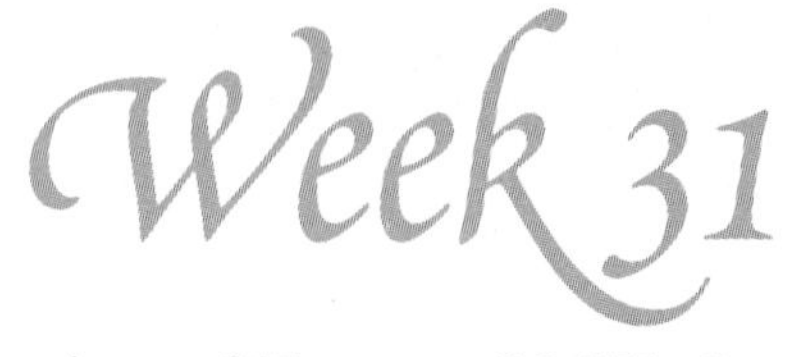

Week 31

Age of Fetus—29 Weeks

How Big Is Your Baby?

Your baby weighs about 3⅓ pounds (1.5kg), and crown-to-rump length is 11¾ inches (28cm). Its total length is nearly 16 inches (41cm).

How Big Are You?

It is now a little more than 12 inches (31cm) from the pubic symphysis to the top of the uterus. From your bellybutton, it is almost 4½ inches (11cm). Your total pregnancy weight gain should be between 21 and 27 pounds (9.45 and 12.15kg). As you can see in the illustration on page 440, your uterus now fills a large part of your abdomen.

How Your Baby Is Growing and Developing

Intrauterine-growth restriction (IUGR) indicates a fetus is small for its gestational age. Weight is below the 10th percentile (in the lowest 10%) for the baby's gestational age. This means 9 out of 10 babies of normal growth are larger.

When dates are correct and the pregnancy is as far along as expected and weight falls below the 10th percentile, it's cause for concern. Growth-restricted babies can have problems.

Your healthcare provider measures you at each visit to see how your uterus and baby are growing. A problem is usually found by measuring the uterus over a period of time and finding little or no change. If you measured 10¾ inches (27cm) at 27 weeks gestation and at 31 weeks you measure only 11 inches (28cm), there might be concern about IUGR, and tests may be ordered.

What causes IUGR? Many conditions can raise the risk of IUGR. We know a woman who has delivered a growth-restricted baby may be more likely to do so again.

Anything that results in baby receiving less nutrition can be a factor. Lifestyle choices can cause IUGR, such as smoking. The more cigarettes smoked, the smaller the baby. Alcohol and drug use can also restrict growth.

A woman who doesn't gain enough weight may have a growth-restricted baby. When you eat fewer than 1500 calories a day for an extended time, IUGR may result. So eat a healthful diet during pregnancy. Don't restrict normal weight gain.

Pre-eclampsia and high blood pressure can have an effect on baby's growth. Some infections in mom may restrict growth. Anemia may also be a cause.

Women who live at high altitudes are more likely to have babies who weigh less. Carrying more than one baby may also cause smaller-than-normal babies.

Other reasons for a small baby, unrelated to IUGR, include the fact a woman who is small might have a small baby. In addition, an overdue pregnancy can lead to a smaller baby. A baby with birth defects may be smaller.

Detecting IUGR is one important reason to keep all your prenatal appointments. You may not like being measured and weighed at every appointment, but it helps your healthcare provider see if your pregnancy is growing and baby is getting bigger.

IUGR can be diagnosed or confirmed by ultrasound. Ultrasound may also be used to assure baby is healthy and no malformations exist that must be dealt with at birth.

When IUGR is diagnosed, avoid doing anything that could make it worse. Bed rest is one treatment. Resting on your side allows the baby to

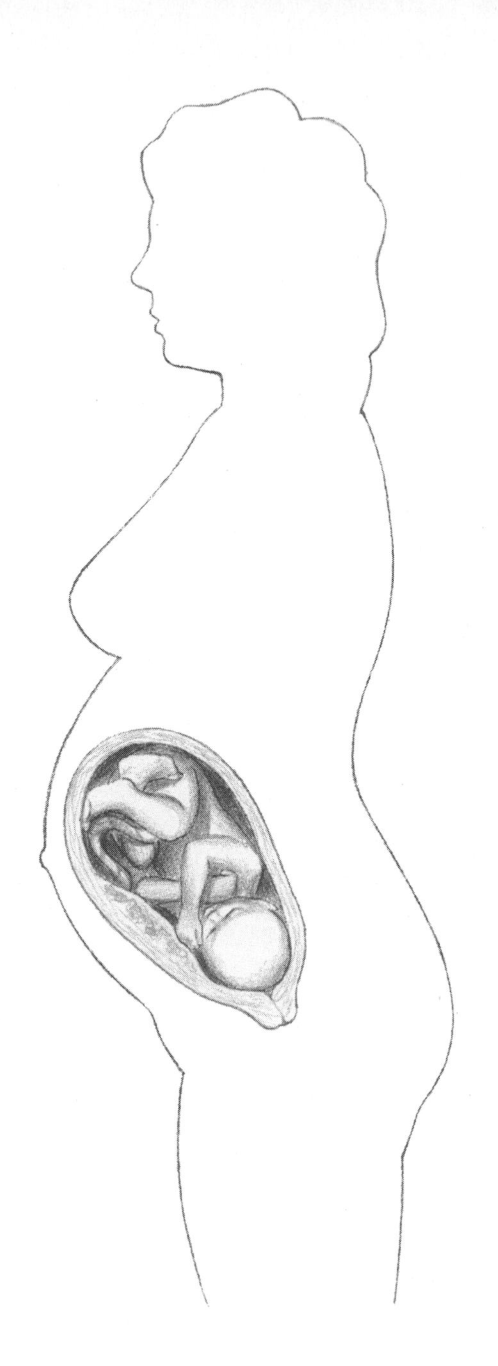

Comparative size of the uterus at 31 weeks of pregnancy (fetal age—29 weeks). The uterus can be felt about 4½ inches (11cm) above the bellybutton.

receive the best blood flow, and better blood flow is the best chance it has to improve growth. (For more on bed rest, see Week 29.) If maternal disease causes IUGR, you need to be treated to improve your health.

An infant with IUGR is at risk of dying before delivery. Baby may need to be delivered before it is full term. Infants with IUGR may not tolerate labor well; a Cesarean delivery may be necessary. The baby may be safer outside the uterus than inside of it.

Dad Tip

It's time to start looking for baby equipment, such as cribs, car seats and layette items. You'll need to make some of these purchases before baby's birth. Most hospitals or birthing centers won't let you take baby home without an approved car seat.

Changes in You

Too Much Saliva

Some women experience an increase in saliva during pregnancy. Hormones are the culprit. Too much saliva is called *ptyalism;* it occurs when estrogen levels increase. The condition often runs in families. Morning sickness may also contribute to the problem.

Often when you feel queasy, you don't swallow as much as you normally do, which results in buildup of saliva. The good news is saliva decreases the amount of tooth-decaying acid produced by bacteria.

To treat the condition, drink plenty of fluid to increase swallowing. Sucking on hard candies may also offer relief.

Swelling in Your Legs and Feet during Pregnancy

Your body produces as much as 50% more blood and body fluids during pregnancy. Some of this extra fluid leaks into your body tissues. When your growing uterus pushes on pelvic veins, blood flow in the lower part of your body is partially blocked. This pushes fluid into your legs and feet, causing swelling.

Tip for Week 31

Wearing rings and watches may cause circulation problems. Sometimes a ring becomes so tight on a pregnant woman's finger that the ring must be cut off by a jeweler. You might not want to wear rings if swelling occurs. Some pregnant women purchase inexpensive rings in larger sizes to wear during pregnancy. Or you could put your rings on a pretty chain and wear them around your neck or on a bracelet.

You may notice if you take your shoes off and leave them off for a while, you may not be able to put them back on. This is related to swelling. You may also notice wearing nylon stockings that are tight at the knee (or tight socks) leaves an indentation in your legs. It may look like you still have clothing on. Avoid tight, restrictive clothing.

The way you sit can also affect your circulation. Crossing your legs at the knee or ankle restricts blood flow to your legs. It's best not to cross your legs.

How Your Actions Affect Your Baby's Development

We've already described the importance of lying on your side when resting or sleeping in Week 15. Now's the time it will pay off. You may notice you begin to retain water if you don't lie on your side.

Visiting Your Healthcare Provider

It's important to go to all prenatal appointments. It may seem not much happens at these visits, especially when everything is normal and going well. But the information collected tells your healthcare provider a lot about your condition and your baby's.

Your healthcare provider is looking for signs of problems, such as changes in your blood pressure or weight, or inadequate growth of the baby. If problems aren't found early, they may have serious consequences for you and baby.

Childbirth Methods

It's time to start thinking about how you want to deliver your baby. It's not too early to do this because many of the methods used need a lot of time and practice to prepare you and your partner or labor coach to use them.

If you decide you want to use a particular method, such as Lamaze, you may have to sign up early to get a place in a class. In addition, you and your labor coach will want time to practice what you learn so you'll be able to use it during labor and delivery.

Some women decide before birth they are going to labor and deliver with *natural childbirth*. What does this mean? The description and/or definition of natural childbirth varies from one couple to another. Many people equate natural childbirth with a drug-free labor and delivery. Others equate natural childbirth with the use of mild or local pain medications. Most agree natural childbirth is birth with as few artificial procedures as possible. However, a woman who chooses natural childbirth usually needs some advance instruction to prepare for it.

Childbirth Philosophies and Methods. There are various philosophies of natural childbirth. Three of the most well-known are Lamaze, the Bradley Method and Grantly Dick-Read.

Lamaze is the oldest childbirth-preparation technique. Through training, it conditions women to replace unproductive laboring efforts with fruitful ones and emphasizes relaxation and breathing as ways to relax during labor and delivery.

The *Bradley Method* embraces a basic belief in the ability of all women to give birth naturally. Classes teach relaxation and inward focus; many types of relaxation are used. Emphasis is put on deep abdominal breathing to make labor more comfortable. Bradley includes a woman's partner in the birthing process. Classes teach expectant parents how to stay healthy and keep their risk of complications low through good nutrition, exercise and lifestyle choices. Classes begin when pregnancy is confirmed and continue until after birth.

In 1933, Dr. Grantly Dick-Read published the book *Childbirth without Fear* to put forth the belief that fear and tension cause pain in 95%

of women giving birth. (He did believe pain-relief medication was useful for women who had problems or a difficult birth.) The *Grantly Dick-Read* method tries to break the fear-tension-pain cycle of labor and delivery through relaxation techniques. The classes were the first to include fathers in the birth experience.

Other childbirth methods are also taught. Marie Mongan, a hypnotherapist, used the work of Dr. Grantly Dick-Read to develop *hypnobirthing*. She believes if you're not afraid, pain is reduced or eliminated, so anesthetics during labor are unnecessary.

Physical therapist Cathy Daub is the founder of *Birth Works Childbirth Education*. The goal of Birth Works is to help women have more trust and faith in their ability to give birth and to help build self-confidence. Classes are taught once a week for 10 weeks. They may be taken any time during pregnancy; it's best to take them before you become pregnant or during your first trimester.

Birthing from Within was developed by Pam England, a midwife. She believes birth is a rite of passage, not a medical event. Classes center on self-discovery. Pain-coping measures are intended to be integrated into daily life, not just used for labor.

ICEA, ALACE and *CAPPA* are three associations that share a similar philosophy. They believe in helping women trust their bodies and gain the knowledge necessary for making informed decisions about childbirth. The International Childbirth Education Association (ICEA) most commonly certifies hospital and physician educators. The Association of Labor Assistants & Childbirth Educators (ALACE) and the Childbirth and Postpartum Professional Association (CAPPA) usually offer independent classes.

Each of the above groups teach the stages of labor and coping techniques for each stage. Class series vary in length.

Should You Consider Natural Childbirth? Natural childbirth isn't for every woman. If you arrive at the hospital dilated 1cm, with strong contractions and in pain, natural childbirth may be hard for you. In this situation, an epidural might be appropriate.

On the other hand, if you arrive at the hospital dilated 4 or 5cm and contractions are OK, natural childbirth might be a reasonable choice. It's impossible to know what will happen ahead of time, but it helps to be aware of, and ready for, everything.

Keep an open mind during the unpredictable process of labor and delivery. Don't feel guilty or disappointed if you can't do all the things you planned. You may need an epidural. Or the birth may not be accomplished without an episiotomy. You should *never* feel guilty or feel you've failed if you need a Cesarean, an epidural or an episiotomy.

Beware of instructors in childbirth-education classes who tell you labor is free of pain, no one really needs a Cesarean delivery, I.V.s are unnecessary or an episiotomy is foolish. This can create unrealistic expectations for you. You may *need* some of these procedures.

The goal in labor and delivery is a healthy baby and a healthy mom. If this means you end up with a C-section, it's OK. Be grateful a Cesarean delivery can be done safely. Babies that would not have survived birth in the past can now be delivered safely. This is a wonderful accomplishment!

Your Nutrition

Salmonella poisoning can negatively impact a pregnancy. Salmonella bacteria can cause a lot of problems for you. Any could be serious.

Salmonella bacteria has many sources—there are over 1400 different strains! They're found in raw eggs and raw poultry. The bacteria is destroyed when a food is cooked, but it's wise to take additional precautions. Keep in mind the following measures to stay safe.

- Clean your counters, utensils, dishes and pans with hot water and soap or a disinfecting agent when you clean up.
- Cook poultry thoroughly.
- Don't eat products made with raw eggs, such as Caesar salad, hollandaise sauce, homemade eggnog, homemade ice cream and so on. Don't taste cake batter, cookie dough or anything else that contains raw eggs before it's cooked.

- When you eat eggs, be sure they're cooked thoroughly. Boil eggs for at least 7 minutes. Poach eggs for 5 minutes. Fry them on each side for 3 minutes—cook them so the yolk and white are firm. Don't eat "sunnyside up" eggs.

You Should Also Know

Carpal Tunnel Syndrome during Pregnancy

If you have carpal tunnel syndrome, you have pain in the hand and wrist, which can extend into the forearm and shoulder. It's caused when the median nerve in the wrist is squeezed by swelling in the wrist and arm area. Symptoms can be numbness, tingling or burning of the inner half of one or both hands. At the same time, fingers feel numb and useless. More than half of the time, both hands are involved.

> Pineapple contains bromelain, an enzyme that helps ease swelling, inflammation and bruising. Consider adding some to your meal plan.

Up to 25% of all pregnant women experience mild symptoms, but treatment is usually unnecessary. The full syndrome, in which treatment may be needed, is less frequent; it occurs in only 1 to 2% of pregnant women.

Treatment depends on symptoms. In pregnant women, splints are often used during sleep and rest to try to keep the wrist straight. Symptoms usually disappear after delivery.

Occurrence of carpal tunnel syndrome during pregnancy does *not* mean you'll suffer from it after baby's birth. In rare instances, symptoms may recur long after pregnancy. In these cases, surgery may be necessary.

Pregnancy-Induced Hypertension (PIH)

When high blood pressure occurs only during pregnancy, it is called *pregnancy-induced hypertension (PIH)* or *gestational hypertension.* The problem usually disappears after baby is born.

With PIH, the systolic pressure (the first number) increases to higher than 140ml of mercury or a rise of 30ml of mercury over your beginning blood pressure. A diastolic reading (the second number) of over 90ml or a rise of 15ml of mercury also indicates a problem. An example is a woman whose blood pressure at the beginning of pregnancy is 100/60. Later in pregnancy, it is 130/90. This signals she may be developing high blood pressure or pre-eclampsia.

If pizza has been left out on the counter for over 2 hours, throw it out. Bacteria can grow on the cheese and toppings, and cause food poisoning. If you want to keep leftover pizza, refrigerate it in an airtight plastic container immediately after you're finished eating.

We have seen some articles in magazines and newspapers that incorrectly equate high blood pressure with pre-eclampsia. They are *not* the same problem. High blood pressure is one common *sign* of pre-eclampsia, but it must be accompanied by other serious symptoms for you to be diagnosed with pre-eclampsia. See the discussion below. Be sure to follow your healthcare provider's advice about taking care of high blood pressure, but don't panic.

Your healthcare provider will be able to determine if your blood pressure is rising to a serious level by checking it at every prenatal appointment. That's one of the reasons it's so important to keep all your prenatal appointments.

What Is Pre-eclampsia?

Pre-eclampsia describes a group of symptoms that occur *only* during pregnancy or shortly after delivery. Pre-eclampsia seems to be on the rise; the condition affects 1 in 20 pregnancies and accounts for over 15% of all maternal deaths during pregnancy.

No one knows what causes pre-eclampsia (or eclampsia). It occurs most often during a woman's first pregnancy. Women over 35 years old who are having their first baby are more likely to develop high blood pressure and pre-eclampsia. Some experts believe *job stress* may be a contributing factor. If you're in a stressful job situation, discuss it with your healthcare provider.

Pre-eclampsia occurs more often in women who have had chronic high blood pressure and pre-eclampsia in a previous pregnancy. Keeping a close watch on you throughout pregnancy and checking your blood pressure and weight at every prenatal visit can alert your healthcare provider to a developing problem.

Pre-eclampsia problems are characterized by a collection of symptoms. The first four are the most common:

- **swelling (edema)**
- **protein in the urine (proteinuria)**
- **high blood pressure (hypertension)**
- **a change in reflexes (hyperreflexia)**
- swelling and pain in a foot may worsen
- rapid weight gain, such as 10 to 12 pounds in 5 days
- flulike aches and pain, without a runny nose or sore throat
- headaches
- vision changes or problems
- elevated level of uric acid
- pain under the ribs on the right side
- seeing spots

Report symptoms to your healthcare provider immediately, particularly if you've had blood-pressure problems during pregnancy!

Most pregnant women have some swelling during pregnancy. Swelling in the legs and/or hands does *not* mean you have pre-eclampsia.

Weight gain can be a sign of a developing problem. Pre-eclampsia increases water retention, which can increase your weight. If you notice an unusual, rapid weight gain, contact your healthcare provider.

Risk factors for developing pre-eclampsia include the following:

- history of high blood pressure before pregnancy
- kidney disease
- thrombophilia (blood-clotting disorders)
- some autoimmune disorders
- younger than 20 years old
- delaying childbirth until after age 35
- overweight or obesity
- multiple fetuses
- diabetes or kidney disease
- Black/African American ethnicity

Taking a multivitamin regularly before getting pregnant may help reduce your risk of pre-eclampsia. Eating high-fiber foods during the first trimester may also help reduce risks. Garlic has been shown to help reduce risks. Even eating five servings a week of *dark* chocolate may reduce your risk. Ask your healthcare provider his or her opinion, if you have questions.

Controlling asthma during pregnancy may help lower your risk of developing pre-eclampsia. Talk to your healthcare provider if you have questions.

A father-to-be's age may play a role in pre-eclampsia. One study showed the problem is 80% higher among women whose partners are 45 years or older.

There are ways to help lower your risk of developing pre-eclampsia. Get regular exercise. Take care of your teeth so you don't get gum disease. Take folic acid. Eat foods high in fiber.

Some researchers believe if a woman has pre-eclampsia, her blood vessels may never have properly dilated from the beginning of pregnancy.

Treating Pre-eclampsia. Pre-eclampsia can progress to *eclampsia*—seizures or convulsions in a woman with pre-eclampsia. The goal in treating pre-eclampsia is to avoid eclampsia. Seizures are not caused by a previous history of epilepsy or a seizure disorder.

Some experts believe low-dose-aspirin therapy may help prevent pre-eclampsia. The crucial time to begin taking it is around 12 weeks of pregnancy. Talk to your healthcare provider about it if you had pre-eclampsia with a previous pregnancy.

Treatment begins with bed rest at home. You may not be able to work or to spend much time on your feet. Bed rest provides the greatest blood flow to the uterus.

Lie on your side, not on your back. Drink lots of water. Avoid salt, salty foods and foods that contain sodium, which may make you retain fluid. Diuretics are not prescribed to treat pre-eclampsia and are not recommended. If a woman with pre-eclampsia has a systolic blood-pressure reading of 155 to 160ml, she should be treated with antihypertensive therapy to help prevent a stroke.

If you can't rest at home in bed or if symptoms don't improve, you may be admitted to the hospital or your baby may need to be delivered. A baby is delivered for its well-being and to avoid seizures in you.

During labor, pre-eclampsia may be treated with magnesium sulfate. It is given by I.V. to prevent seizures during and after delivery.

If you think you've had a seizure, call your healthcare provider immediately! Diagnosis may be difficult. If possible, someone who saw the possible seizure should describe it to your healthcare provider. Eclampsia is treated with medications similar to those prescribed for seizure disorders.

Exercise for Week 31

Sit up straight in a chair or on the floor. Lace your fingers together behind your head; keep your elbows apart. Inhale and push your hands, with your fingers still together, toward the ceiling. Exhale and return your hands to the position behind your head. Repeat 5 times. *Tones arms and shoulder muscles.*

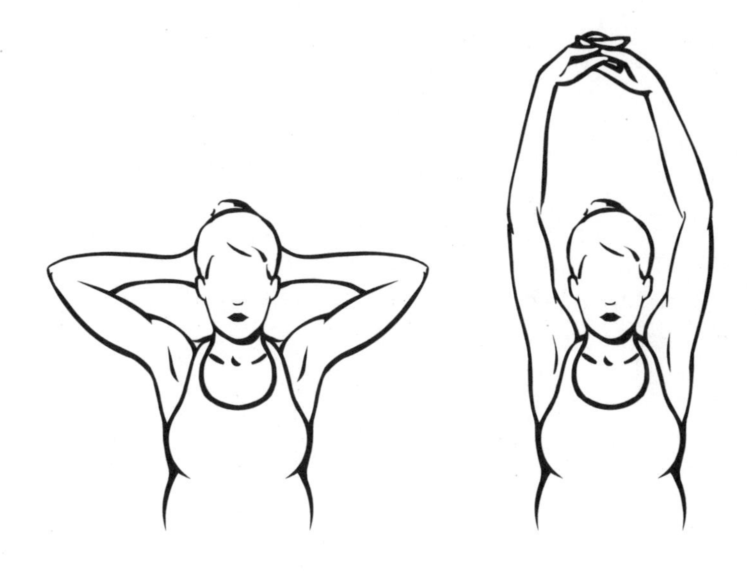

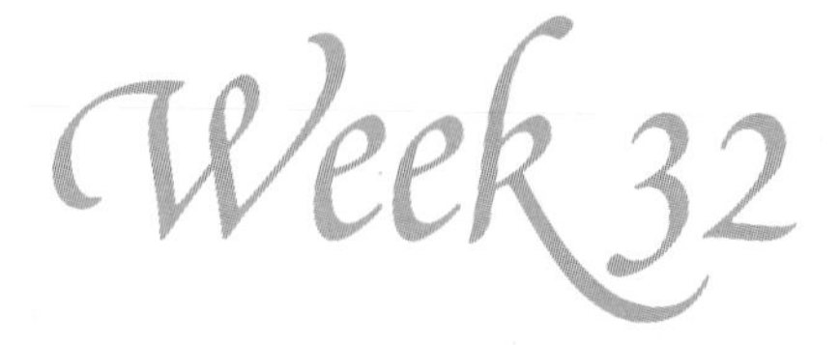

Age of Fetus—30 Weeks

How Big Is Your Baby?

By this week, your baby weighs almost 3¾ pounds (1.7kg). Crown-to-rump length is over 11½ inches (29cm), and total length is nearly 16¾ inches (42cm).

How Big Are You?

Measurement to the top of the uterus from the pubic symphysis is about 12¾ inches (32cm). Measuring from the bellybutton, it now measures almost 5 inches (12cm).

How Your Baby Is Growing and Developing

Twins? Triplets? More?

The rate of multiple births is going up—since 1980, the rate of twin births has increased 70%. Statistics show that close to 4% of all births in the United States are multiple births. If you're expecting more than one baby, you're not alone!

When talking about pregnancies of more than one baby, in most cases we refer to twins. The chance of a twin pregnancy is more likely than pregnancy with triplets, quadruplets or quintuplets (or even more!). However, we are seeing more triplet and higher-order births. A triplet birth is not very common; it happens about once in every 7000 deliveries. (Dr. Curtis has been fortunate to deliver two sets of triplets in his medical career.) Quadruplets are born once in every 725,000 births; quintuplets once in every 47 million births!

No matter how it happens, being pregnant with two or more babies can affect you in many ways. Your pregnancy will be different, and the adjustments you may need to make may be more wide-ranging. These changes may be necessary for your health and the health of your babies. Work closely with your healthcare provider to help make your pregnancy healthy and safe.

A multiple pregnancy occurs when a single egg divides after fertilization or when more than one egg is fertilized. Twin fetuses usually result (over 65% of the time) from the fertilization of two separate eggs; each baby has his or her own placenta and amniotic sac. These are called *fraternal twins* or *dizygotic* (two zygotes) *twins.* With fraternal twins, you can have a boy and a girl. Fraternal twins occur in 1 out of every 100 births. These rates vary for different races and areas of the world.

About 35% of the time, twins come from a single egg that divides into two similar structures. Each has the potential of developing into a separate individual. These are known as *identical twins* or *monozygotic* (one zygote) *twins.* Identical twins occur about once in every 250 births around the world.

Either or both processes may be involved when more than two fetuses are formed. What we mean by that is triplets may result from fertilization of one, two or three eggs, or quadruplets may result from fertilization of one, two, three or four eggs.

A twin pregnancy that results from fertility treatment most often results in fraternal twins. In some cases of higher-number fetuses, a pregnancy resulting from fertility treatment can result in fraternal *and* identical twins, when more than one egg is fertilized (fraternal twins) and, in addition, one or more of the eggs divides (identical twins).

The percentage of boys decreases slightly as the number of babies increases. In other words, as the number of babies a woman carries goes up, her chances of having more girls increases.

Special Issues for Identical Twins. With identical twins, division of the fertilized egg occurs between the first few days and about day 8. If division of the egg occurs after 8 days, the result can be twins that are connected, called *conjoined twins.* (Conjoined twins used to be called *Siamese twins.*) These babies may share important internal organs, such as the heart, lungs or liver. Fortunately this is a rare occurrence.

Identical twins may face some risks. There's a 15% chance they will develop a serious problem called *twin-to-twin transfusion syndrome.* There is one placenta, and the babies' blood vessels share the placenta. The problem occurs when one baby gets too much blood flow and the other too little. See the discussion in Week 23.

Dad Tip

Together with your partner, make a list of important telephone numbers and keep it with you. Include numbers for your work, your partner's work, the hospital, the healthcare provider's office, a back-up driver, baby-sitter or others. You may also want to make a list of numbers of people you want to call after the delivery of your baby. Take this list to the hospital with you.

There's a chance that several different types of diseases may occur in identical twins during their lifetimes. This is less likely to happen with fraternal twins.

It may be important later in life for your children to know whether they were identical or fraternal because of health concerns. Before delivery, tell your healthcare provider you would like to have the placenta(s) examined (with a pathology exam) so you'll know whether babies were identical or fraternal. It may be valuable information in the future. Even if there are two placentas, research shows it doesn't mean twins are fraternal; nearly 35% of all identical twins have two placentas.

The Frequency of Multiples. The frequency of twins depends on the type of twins. Identical twins occur about once in every 250 births around the world. It doesn't seem to be influenced by age, race, heredity, number of pregnancies or medications taken for infertility (fertility drugs).

The incidence of fraternal twins *is* influenced by race, heredity, mom's age, the number of previous pregnancies and the use of fertility drugs and assisted-reproductive techniques. Twins occur in 1 out of every 100 pregnancies in white women compared to 1 out of every 79 pregnancies in black women. Certain areas of Africa have an incredibly high frequency of twins. In some places, twins occur once in every 20 births. Hispanic women also have a slightly higher number of twin births. The occurrence of twins among Asians is less common—about 1 in every 150 births. In Japan, only 6 sets of twins are born per 1000 births while in Nigeria that rate is over 7 times greater. In Nigeria, fraternal twins are born at a rate of 45 per 1000 births.

Heredity also plays a part. The incidence of twin births can run in families, on the *mother's* side. In one study of fraternal twins, the chance of a female twin giving birth to a set of twins herself was about 1 in 58 births. The study also showed if a woman is the daughter of a twin, she has a higher chance of having twins. Another study reported 1 out of 24 (4%) of twins' mothers was a twin, but only 1 out of 60 (1.7%; about the national average) of twins' fathers was a twin.

If you've already given birth to a set of fraternal twins, your chance of having another set of twins quadruples! Other reasons for multiple fetuses include the use of fertility drugs, in-vitro fertilization, women having babies later in life, some women having more children, being very tall or obese, you recently discontinued oral contraception or taking large doses of folic acid.

Women having babies later in life accounts for nearly 35% of all multiple births. Age 30 seems to be the magic age beyond which the number of multiple births increases. Over 70% of all multiple births are to women over age 30. In the United States, the highest number of multiple births occurs in women over 40; the next highest group is women between the ages of 30 and 39.

The increase in multiple births among older women has been attributed to higher levels of gonadotropins. As a woman ages, gonadotropin increases, and she's more likely to produce two or more eggs during one menstrual cycle. Most twin births in older women are fraternal twins.

Having more children (or pregnancies) can also result in more than one baby. This is true in all populations and may be related to the mother's age and hormone changes.

Some families are just more "blessed" than others. In one case we know of personally, a woman had three single births. Her fourth pregnancy was twins, and her fifth pregnancy was triplets! She and her husband decided on another pregnancy; they were surprised (and probably relieved) when that pregnancy resulted in only one baby.

Discovering You're Carrying More than One Baby. Diagnosis of twins was more difficult before ultrasound was available. The illustration on page 457 shows an ultrasound of twins. You can see parts of both fetuses.

It is uncommon to discover twin pregnancies just by hearing two heartbeats. Many people believe when they hear only one heartbeat, there could be no possibility of twins. This may not be the case. Two rapid heartbeats may have a similar or almost identical rate, which could make it difficult to know there are two babies.

Measuring and examining your tummy during pregnancy is important. Usually a twin pregnancy is noted during the second trimester because you're too big and growth seems too fast for one baby. Ultrasound is the best way to diagnose a multiple pregnancy.

Do Multiple Pregnancies Have More Problems? With a multiple pregnancy, the possibility of problems goes up. Possible problems include the following:

- increased risk of miscarriage
- fetal death or mortality
- birth defects
- low birthweight or growth restriction
- pre-eclampsia
- problems with the placenta
- maternal anemia
- maternal bleeding or hemorrhage
- problems with the umbilical cord, including entwinement or tangling of the babies' umbilical cords
- too much or too little amniotic fluid
- abnormal fetal presentations, such as breech or transverse lie
- premature labor
- difficult delivery and Cesarean delivery

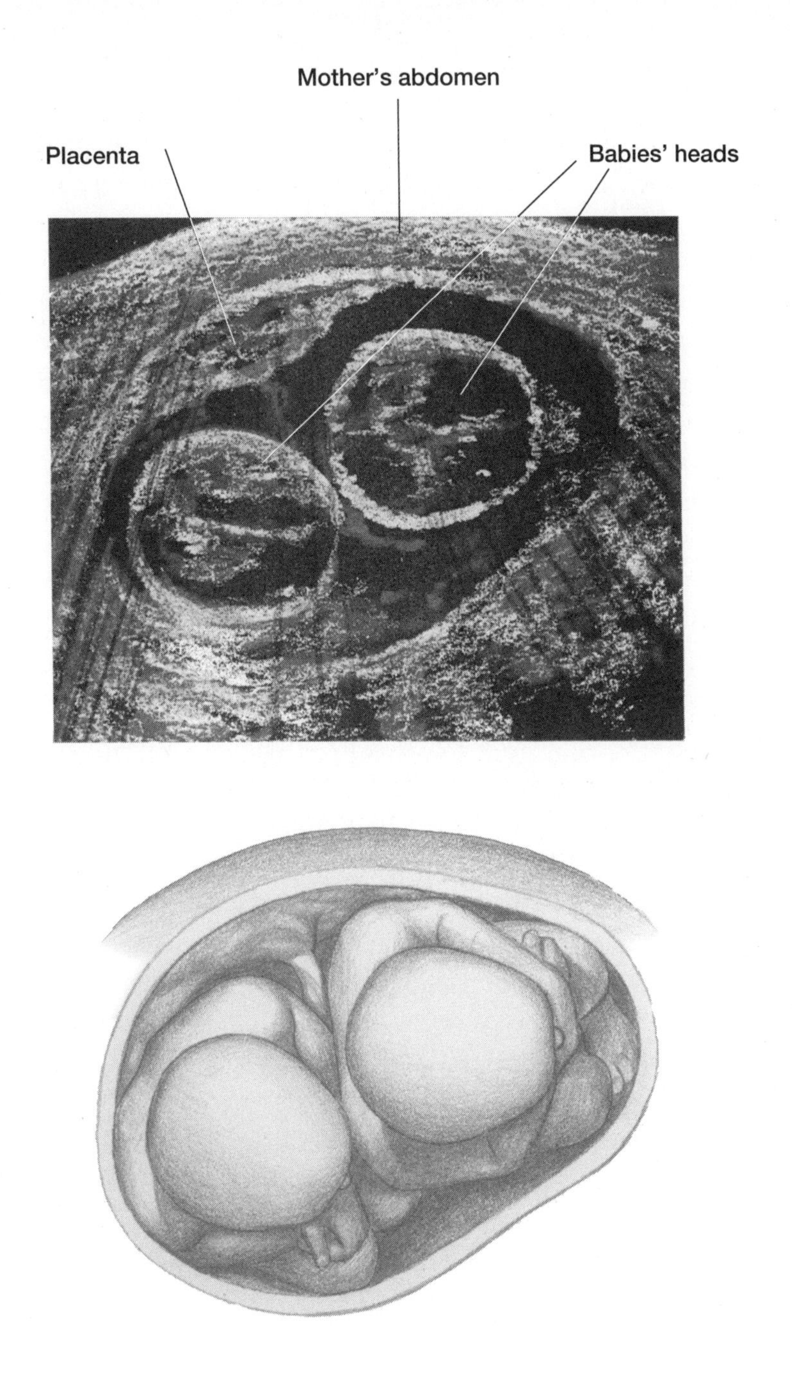

Ultrasound of twins shows two babies in the uterus. If you look closely, you can see the two heads. The interpretive illustration shows how the babies are lying.

Birth defects are more common among identical twins than fraternal twins. The incidence of minor problems is twice as high as it is in a single pregnancy, and major defects are also more common.

One of the biggest problems with multiple pregnancies is premature delivery. As the number of babies increases, the length of gestation and the birthweight of each baby decreases, although this is not true in every case.

The average length of pregnancy for twins is about 37 weeks. For triplets it's about 35 weeks. For every week the babies stay inside the uterus, their birth weights increase, along with the maturity of organs and systems.

It's important to continue your pregnancy as long as possible; this may be achieved by bed rest. You may not be able to carry on with regular activities for the entire pregnancy. If your healthcare provider recommends bed rest, follow his or her advice.

Weight gain is important. You may be advised to gain more than the normal 25 to 35 pounds, depending on the number of babies you carry. With twins, if you were normal weight before pregnancy, you may be advised to gain 40 to 54 pounds. For overweight women, a weight gain between 31 and 50 pounds may be recommended; for obese women, a gain between 25 and 42 pounds may be recommended. If you're expecting triplets, your weight gain may be between 50 and 60 pounds.

Some researchers believe use of a *tocolytic agent* (medication to stop labor), such as ritodrine, is critical in preventing premature delivery. These medicines are used to relax the uterus to keep you from going into premature labor.

Follow your healthcare provider's instructions closely. Every day and every week you can keep the babies inside you are days or weeks you won't have to visit them in an intensive-care nursery while they grow, develop and finish maturing.

Delivering More Than One Baby

How multiple fetuses are delivered often depends on how babies are lying in your uterus. Possible complications include abnormal presentation of one or more of the babies, the umbilical cord coming out ahead of the babies, placental abruption, fetal stress or bleeding after delivery.

Because risk is higher, safeguards are taken during labor and before delivery. These include an I.V., the presence of an anesthesiologist, the ability to perform an emergency Cesarean delivery and the availability and/or presence of pediatricians or other medical personnel to take care of the babies.

With twins, all possible combinations of fetal positions can occur. Both babies may come head first (vertex). They may come *breech,* meaning bottom or feet first. They may be lying sideways or *oblique,* meaning at an angle that is neither breech nor vertex. Or they may come in any combination of the above.

When both twins are head first, a vaginal delivery may be tried and may be accomplished safely. It may be possible for one baby to deliver vaginally. But the second one could need a Cesarean delivery if there are problems. Some healthcare providers believe delivery of multiples is more safely accomplished with a Cesarean delivery.

After delivery, healthcare providers pay close attention to bleeding in you because of the rapid change in the size of the uterus. It is overdistended with more than one baby. Medicine, usually oxytocin (Pitocin), is given by I.V. to contract the uterus to stop bleeding so you don't lose too much blood. Heavy blood loss could produce anemia and make a blood transfusion or long-term treatment with iron supplementation necessary.

Changes in You

Until this week, your visits to the healthcare provider have probably been on a monthly basis. At week 32, most healthcare providers begin seeing a pregnant woman every 2 weeks. This continues until the last month of pregnancy, then you'll probably switch to weekly visits.

By this time, you probably know your healthcare provider fairly well and feel comfortable talking about your concerns. Now is a good time to ask questions and to discuss concerns about labor and delivery. If there are complications or problems later in pregnancy or at delivery, you'll be able to communicate better and know what's going on. You'll feel comfortable with the care you're receiving.

Your healthcare provider may plan on talking to you about many things in the weeks to come, but you can't always assume this. You may be taking prenatal classes and hearing different things about labor and delivery. Don't be afraid to ask questions. Most healthcare providers are receptive to your queries. They want you to discuss things you're concerned about instead of worrying about them unnecessarily.

How Your Actions Affect Your Baby's Development

Do you wear contacts? You may want to wait until after baby is born to refill your contact-lens prescription. You may experience eye discomfort and irritation during pregnancy because of hormonal changes that change the curvature of the cornea. Hormones can also alter your vision slightly and dry your eyes. Don't use any products for dry eyes until you talk to your healthcare provider about it at a prenatal visit.

Tip for Week 32

Your requirements for calories, protein, vitamins and minerals increase if you carry more than one baby. You'll need to eat about 300 calories a day more *per baby* than for a normal pregnancy.

If you have problems, one solution is disposable contacts that correct for the changes. You might also try your old glasses if your contacts don't seem to work. Wait until after baby's birth to make any permanent changes. It can take up to 6 weeks before your vision returns to normal.

Your Nutrition

If you're expecting more than one baby, your nutrition and weight gain are very important during pregnancy. Food is your best source for nutrients, but keep taking your prenatal vitamin every day. The vitamins and iron in prenatal vitamins are still essential to your well-being and the well-being of your baby or babies.

Iron supplementation may be necessary. If you're anemic at the time of delivery, a low blood count could have a negative effect. You might need a blood transfusion.

> If you're on the go and want a salad, buy a prepackaged bowl that contains dressing and toppings. It's a healthy choice on days you may be tempted to buy fast food.

If you don't gain weight early in pregnancy, you have a higher chance of developing pre-eclampsia. Your babies may also be tiny.

Don't be alarmed when your healthcare provider discusses the amount of weight he or she wants you to gain. Studies show if you gain the targeted amount of weight with a multiple pregnancy, your babies are often healthier. In addition, gaining half of your weight by week 20 can help your babies, especially if they're born early.

How can you gain the amount of weight you need to gain? Just adding extra calories won't help you or growing babies. Avoid junk food because of empty calories.

Get your calories from specific sources. Eat an extra serving of a dairy product and an extra serving of protein each day. These will provide you with the extra calcium, protein and iron you require to meet the needs of your growing babies. Discuss the situation with your healthcare provider; he or she may suggest you see a nutritionist.

You Should Also Know

Bird Flu

To date, few people in the world have been infected with avian influenza H5N1, also called *bird flu*. Research shows most of these people worked closely with birds infected with the disease; they caught it from the birds themselves, not from other people.

At this time, the average American doesn't have to be concerned with catching bird flu. No special precautions are called for. Health authorities keep a close watch on the disease in birds and humans. Researchers continue to work on a vaccine.

If you want to be cautious, wash your hands with soap and hot water, or use a hand sanitizer, after handling any birds. This is sound advice to help prevent the spread of any type of germs from the bird to you.

Laparoscopy during Pregnancy

As many as 2% of all pregnancies are complicated by a surgical problem. The most common surgical condition during pregnancy is appendicitis. Other surgical emergencies include cholecystitis, intestinal obstruction, ovarian cysts and ovarian torsion.

The second trimester is generally the safest time to perform surgery. Advantages of laparoscopic surgery include small incisions resulting in faster recovery, early return of bowel and gastrointestinal activity, smaller scars, less pain (requiring less pain medicine) and shorter hospitalization.

Laparoscopy may not always be the best choice. As the uterus gets bigger, it may not be possible. However, we can't give you an exact time or week of pregnancy when laparoscopy can no longer be done. It's an individual decision in each case.

Cancer and Pregnancy

Pregnancy is a happy time for most women. Occasionally, however, serious problems can occur. Cancer in pregnancy is one serious complication that occurs rarely.

This discussion is included not to scare you but to provide you with information. It is not a pleasant subject to discuss, especially at this time. However, every woman should have this information available. Its inclusion in this book is twofold:

- to inform you of a serious problem that can occur during pregnancy
- to provide you with a resource to help you form questions for a dialogue with your healthcare provider, if you wish to discuss it

If you're now pregnant and you have had cancer in the past, tell your healthcare provider as soon as you find out you're pregnant. He or she may need to make decisions about individualized care for you during pregnancy.

Cancer during Pregnancy. Tremendous changes affect your body during pregnancy. Some researchers believe cancers influenced by increased hormones may increase in frequency during pregnancy. Increased blood flow may increase cancer to other parts of the body. Body changes during pregnancy can make it difficult to find or to diagnose an early cancer.

When cancer occurs during pregnancy, it can be very stressful. The healthcare provider must consider how to treat the cancer, but he or she is also concerned about the developing baby.

How these issues are handled depends on when cancer is discovered. A woman's concerns may include the following.

- Will the pregnancy have to be terminated so the cancer can be treated?
- Will treatment or medications harm the baby?
- Will the malignancy affect the baby or be passed to the baby?
- Should therapy be delayed until after delivery or after termination of the pregnancy?

Cancer during pregnancy is a rare occurrence; it must be treated on an individual basis. Some cancers found during pregnancy include breast tumors, leukemia, lymphomas, melanomas, bone tumors and cancer of female organs, such as the cervix, uterus and ovaries.

Anticancer drugs stop cell division to help fight the cancer. If taken during the first part of pregnancy, they can affect cell division of the embryo.

Breast Cancer. Breast cancer is uncommon in women younger than 35. Fortunately, it's a rare complication of pregnancy. However, breast cancer is the most common type of cancer diagnosed during pregnancy. Of all women who have breast cancer, about 2% are pregnant at the time of diagnosis.

During pregnancy, it may be harder to discover breast cancer because of changes in the breasts. Most evidence indicates pregnancy does *not* increase the rate of growth or spread of a breast cancer.

Studies indicate pregnancy is safe in women with a history of breast cancer if the cancer has been successfully treated. Treatment of breast cancer during pregnancy varies. It may require surgery, chemotherapy and/or radiation. Recent studies indicate chemotherapy for breast cancer during pregnancy may be safe.

A form of breast cancer you should be aware of is *inflammatory breast cancer* (IBC). Although rare, it can occur during and after pregnancy, and may be mistaken for mastitis, which is inflammation of the breast. Symptoms of inflammatory breast cancer include swelling or pain in the breast, redness, nipple discharge and/or swollen lymph nodes above the collarbone or under the arm. You may feel a lump, although one is not always present.

If you experience any of these symptoms, *do not panic!* Nearly all of the time it will be a breast infection related to breastfeeding. However, if you're concerned, contact your healthcare provider. A biopsy is used to diagnose the problem. To learn more about IBC, visit www.ibcsupport.org.

Other Cancers. Cervical cancer is believed to occur about once in every 10,000 pregnancies. However, about 1% of the women who have cancer of the cervix are pregnant when it's diagnosed. Cancer of the cervix is curable, particularly when found and treated in its early stages.

Malignancies of the vulva, the tissue surrounding the vaginal opening, have also been reported during pregnancy. It is a rare complication.

Hodgkin's disease (a form of cancer) commonly affects young people. It is now being controlled for long periods with radiation and chemotherapy. The disease occurs in about 1 of every 6000 pregnancies. Pregnancy does not appear to have a negative effect on the course of Hodgkin's disease.

Pregnant women who have *leukemia* have demonstrated an increased chance of premature labor or increased bleeding after pregnancy. Leukemia is usually treated with chemotherapy or radiation therapy.

Melanoma is a cancer derived from skin cells that produce *melanin* (pigment). A malignant melanoma can spread through the body. Pregnancy may cause symptoms or problems to worsen. A melanoma can spread to the placenta and baby.

Bone tumors are rare during pregnancy. However, two types of noncancerous bone tumors can affect pregnancy and delivery. These tumors, *endochondromas* and *benign exostosis,* can involve the pelvis; tumors may interfere with labor. The possibility of having a Cesarean delivery is more likely with these tumors.

It may be harder to lose your pregnancy weight after having twins, so stick to the weight goal your healthcare provider gives you. In addition, carrying two babies causes more changes in your body, which may cause you to hold onto the weight you gain during pregnancy.

Exercise for Week 32

One exercise you can do during pregnancy may help during labor. Using your diaphragm to breathe is beneficial to you. These are the muscles you will use during labor and delivery. Breath training decreases the amount of energy you need to breathe, and it improves the function of your respiratory muscles. Practice the different breathing exercises below for benefits in the near future (labor and delivery!).

- Breathe in through your nose, and exhale through pursed lips. Making a little whistling sound is OK. Breathe in for 4 seconds, and breathe out for 6 seconds.
- Lie back, propped on some pillows, in a comfortable position. Place your hand on your tummy while breathing. If you breathe using your diaphragm muscles, your hand will move up when you inhale and down when you exhale. If it doesn't, try using different muscles until you can do it correctly.
- Bend forward to breathe. If you bend slightly forward, you'll find it's easier to breathe. If you feel pressure as your baby gets bigger, try this technique. It may offer some relief.

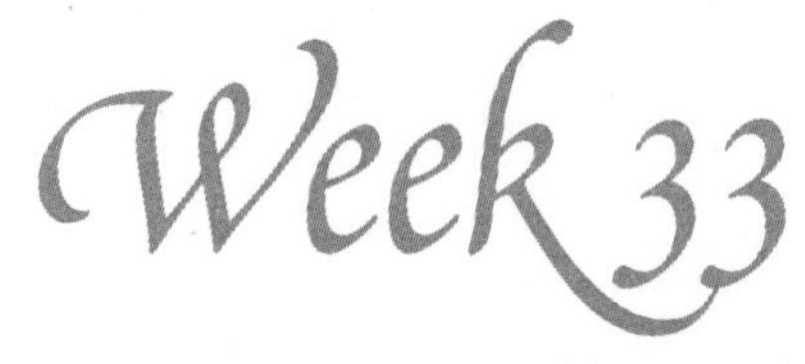

Age of Fetus—31 Weeks

How Big Is Your Baby?

Your baby weighs about 4¼ pounds (1.9kg) by this week. Its crown-to-rump length is about 12 inches (30cm), and total length is nearly 17¼ inches (44cm).

How Big Are You?

Measuring from the pubic symphysis, it's about 13¼ inches (33cm) to the top of the uterus. Measurement from your bellybutton to the top of your uterus is about 5¼ inches (13cm). Total weight gain should be between 22 and 28 pounds (9.9 and 12.6kg).

How Your Baby Is Growing and Developing

Placental Abruption

The illustration on page 468 shows placental abruption—premature separation of the placenta from the uterine wall. Normally, the placenta doesn't separate from the uterus until after baby is delivered. Separation before delivery can be very serious.

Placental abruption occurs in about 1 in every 80 pregnancies. The time of separation can vary. If it separates at the time of delivery and the infant is delivered without incident, it's not as significant as a placenta separating during pregnancy.

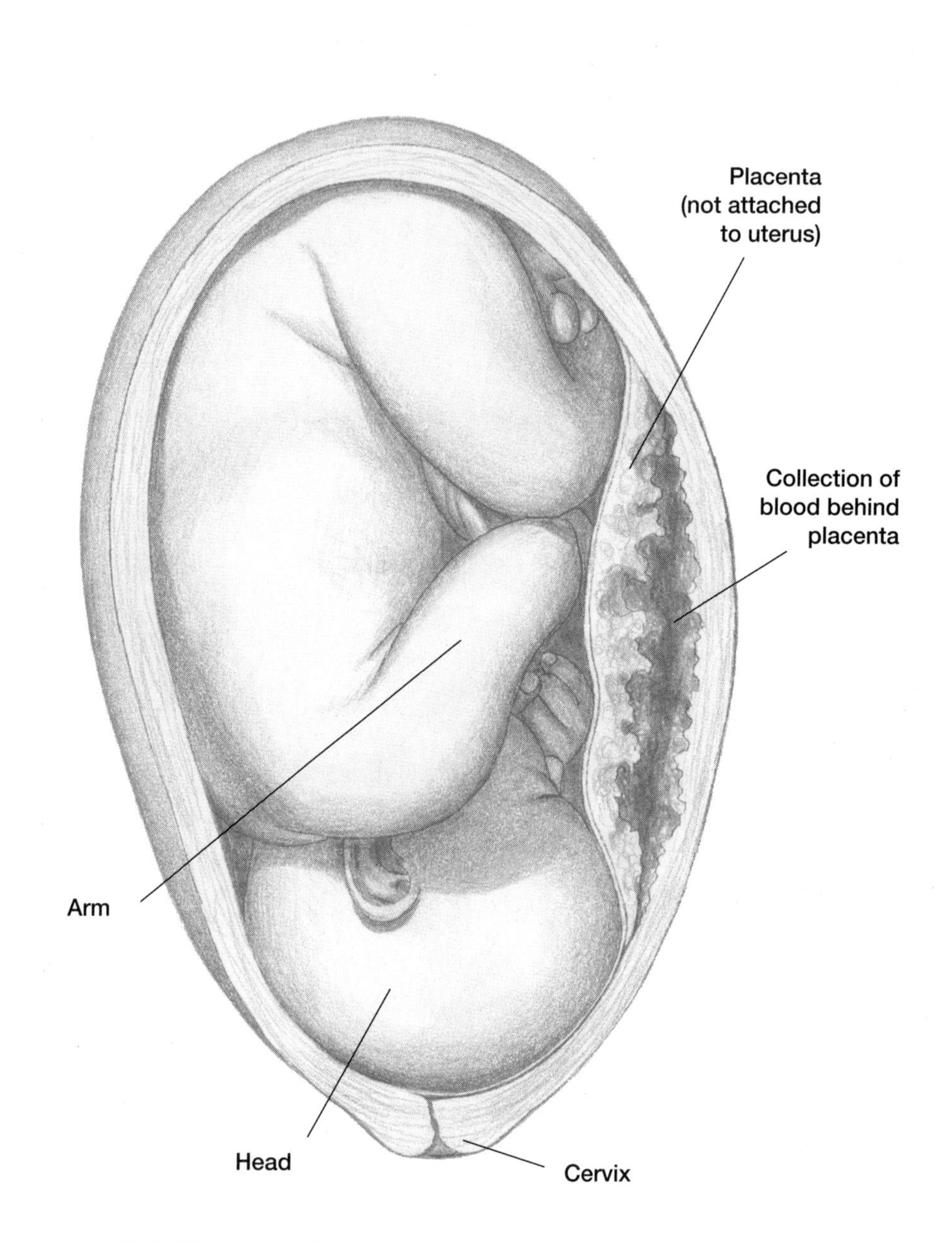

This illustration of placental abruption shows that the placenta has separated from the wall of the uterus.

The cause of placental abruption is unknown. Certain conditions may increase the chance of it happening, including:

- physical injury to the mother, as from a car accident or a bad fall
- a short umbilical cord
- sudden change in the size of the uterus from water breaking
- high blood pressure
- dietary deficiency
- a uterine abnormality
- previous surgery on the uterus or D&C for abortion or miscarriage

Studies indicate a folic-acid deficiency may play a role. Other researchers suggest smoking and alcohol use may make a woman more likely to have placental abruption.

A woman who has had placental abruption in the past is at increased risk of having it recur. Rate of recurrence has been estimated to be as high as 10%. This can make a subsequent pregnancy a high-risk pregnancy.

The situation is most severe when the placenta totally separates from the uterine wall. The fetus relies entirely on the placenta for its circulation. When it separates, the fetus doesn't receive blood from the umbilical cord, which is attached to the placenta.

Symptoms of placental abruption can vary. There may be heavy bleeding from the vagina, or you may experience no bleeding at all. Vaginal bleeding occurs in about 75% of all cases. Other symptoms can include lower-back pain, tenderness of the uterus or abdomen, and contractions or tightening of the uterus.

Serious problems, such as shock, may occur with rapid loss of large quantities of blood. A large blood clot can also be a problem. Factors that clot the blood may be used up, which can make bleeding a problem.

Ultrasound may help diagnose the problem, but it doesn't always provide an exact diagnosis. This is particularly true if the placenta is located at the back of the uterus where it can't be seen easily with ultrasound examination.

Can Placental Abruption Be Treated? Treatment of placental abruption varies, based on the ability to diagnose the problem and the status of the mother and baby. With heavy bleeding, delivery of the baby may be necessary.

When bleeding is not heavy, the problem may be treated more conservatively. This depends on whether the fetus is stressed or if it appears to be in immediate danger.

Placental abruption is one of the most serious problems related to the second and third trimesters of pregnancy. If you have any symptoms, call your healthcare provider immediately!

Changes in You

Fibroid Tumors

Fibroid tumors are growths that develop in the uterine wall or on the outside of the uterus; most are noncancerous (benign). Most women with fibroids don't have problems during pregnancy, but pregnancy hormones can make fibroids grow larger. However, they often shrink after baby is born.

Research shows if you have fibroids, you may have a higher chance of having problems during pregnancy. Fibroids can also slightly increase the chance of miscarriage, especially if growths are large. Placental abruption may occur more readily if the placenta embeds itself over a large fibroid. Fibroids have also been known to block the opening to the cervix. Discuss the situation with your healthcare provider if you're concerned.

Obstructive Sleep Apnea

About 2% of all pregnant women develop obstructive sleep apnea during pregnancy; the condition seems to be more common in pregnant women than in the general population. If you have obstructive sleep apnea, airways narrow and you stop breathing briefly, then resume normal breathing. This can occur up to 100 times a night, which can greatly disturb your sleep!

Lack of oxygen causes your body to release adrenaline and cortisol, which raises blood pressure and releases sugar into the bloodstream.

Over time, this release of sugar into your blood may increase your risk of developing diabetes.

When it occurs during pregnancy, sleep apnea has been linked to high blood pressure, gestational diabetes, fatigue and cardiovascular problems in a mom-to-be. Some women with sleep apnea are at higher risk for developing pre-eclampsia. It can also negatively affect your baby's growth and development.

Some women need a CPAP (continuous positive-airway pressure) machine to breathe more healthfully during sleep. A mask is placed over your nose and mouth, and delivers continuous air to you during sleep so you keep breathing. The good news is that obstructive sleep apnea often disappears after baby is born.

When Your Water Breaks

The membranes around the baby that contain the amniotic fluid are called the *bag of waters.* These membranes help protect baby from infection. They usually don't break until just before labor begins, when labor begins or during labor.

Sometimes membranes break earlier in pregnancy. See the discussion that begins on page 472. After your water breaks, your risk of infection increases, so you need to take precautions. An infection could be harmful to your baby.

Call your healthcare provider immediately when your water breaks. Avoid sexual intercourse because it can increase the possibility of introducing an infection into your uterus and thus to your baby.

When your water breaks, there is often a gush of amniotic fluid, usually followed by a leakage of small amounts of fluid. Amniotic fluid is usually clear and watery, but it may have a bloody appearance or it may be yellow or green. Women describe their water breaking as a constant wetness or water running down their leg when they stand. *Continuous* leakage of water is a good clue membranes have ruptured.

Tests can be done to see if your water has broken. One is a *nitrazine test* based on the acidity of the amniotic fluid. When amniotic fluid is placed on a small strip of paper, it changes color. However, blood can change the color of nitrazine paper, even if your water hasn't broken.

Another test is a *ferning test.* Amniotic fluid or fluid from the back of the vagina is taken with a swab and placed on a slide for examination under a microscope. Dried amniotic fluid looks like a fern or branches of a pine tree. Ferning may be more helpful in diagnosing ruptured membranes than looking at color changes on nitrazine paper.

Premature Rupture of Membranes (PROM). When membranes rupture earlier in pregnancy, it is called *premature rupture of membranes (PROM).* There are two categories of premature rupture. *Premature rupture of membranes (PROM)* refers to rupture of fetal membranes before the onset of labor and occurs in 8 to 12% of all pregnancies. PPROM is the *preterm-premature rupture of membranes* and refers to rupture of fetal membranes before 37 weeks of pregnancy. It occurs in 1% of all pregnancies. In the United States, about 30% of all pregnant women are checked for PROM.

The exact cause is unknown. Black/African-American women appear to have a higher incidence of PPROM than white women. Smoking is strongly correlated with PPROM. Vitamin and mineral deficiencies have also been considered causes. Uterine bleeding has been strongly tied to PPROM; infection also plays an important role in many cases. If you had PPROM with a previous pregnancy, you have a 35% chance it will occur again.

If ruptured membranes are not detected and treated within 24 hours, infection and other serious complications may occur. A test is available to diagnose whether membranes have ruptured prematurely; it is called *Amnisure.*

The test detects a protein found in amniotic fluid that isn't normally present in the vagina unless membranes have ruptured. It's a vaginal test but does not require use of a speculum or a vaginal exam. A sterile

Dad Tip

Is your home safe for your new baby? Things to consider when thinking about safety include pets, furniture, second-hand and third-hand smoke, window coverings or other things in your home that could pose a danger to your little one. Start now to check for problems so you'll have time to take care of them before baby's birth.

swab is inserted about 2 to 3 inches (5 to 7cm) into the vagina, and a sample is taken. Results are ready in about 10 minutes.

How Your Actions Affect Your Baby's Development

You may be gaining weight faster than at any other time during pregnancy. However, *you* are not putting on most of this weight—the baby is! Your baby is growing and may be gaining as much as 8 ounces (½ pound) or more every week.

Heartburn may become more of a problem as baby crowds your stomach. Eating several small meals a day, rather than three large meals, may make you more comfortable.

Hepatitis

Hepatitis is a viral infection of the liver. It's near the top of the list of serious infections that affect a large percentage of our population every year. That's one reason all pregnant women are screened for hepatitis B at the beginning of pregnancy.

When people talk about hepatitis, it can be confusing. Six different forms of hepatitis have been identified—hepatitis A, hepatitis B, hepatitis C, hepatitis D, hepatitis E and hepatitis G. The most serious type of hepatitis during pregnancy is hepatitis B. See the discussions below.

Hepatitis A (HAV). Hepatitis A (HAV) accounts for 50% of all hepatitis cases in the United States. It is transmitted by the oral-fecal path, such as drinking contaminated water or eating contaminated food or touching something contaminated with feces, like a dirty diaper, then touching your mouth with your hands. You're more likely to contract this type of hepatitis if you travel to developing countries.

Fortunately, the occurrence of HAV during pregnancy is less than 1 in 1000. In our country, pregnant women most likely to be infected are those who have recently emigrated from, or traveled to, various places, such as Southeast Asia, China, Africa, Central America, Mexico and the Middle East.

Symptoms of HAV include fever, malaise, anorexia, nausea, abdominal pain and jaundice. Hepatitis A is diagnosed with a blood test. A pregnant woman will *not* pass hepatitis A to her developing baby. If a woman is exposed during pregnancy, she may be given hepatitis immune gamma globulin to help protect her from getting the disease.

Serious complications from HAV are rare. Treatment is rest and a healthful diet. Usually a woman with hepatitis A recovers within a few months.

Hepatitis B (HBV). Hepatitis B (HBV) is one of the most contagious forms of hepatitis and accounts for over 40% of all cases of hepatitis in the United States. More than 1 million Americans are chronic carriers of HBV and over 15,000 pregnant women have HBV.

During pregnancy, HBV can be passed from mother to baby, especially if the mother becomes infected late in pregnancy. Nearly all cases occur from exposure to the mother's blood or to secretions in the birth canal.

People at risk for contracting hepatitis B include those with a history of sexually transmitted diseases, intravenous drug use or exposure to people with HBV or to blood products that contain HBV. Sexual transmission accounts for most cases. The risk of contracting HBV is higher if a person was born in Southeast Asia or the Pacific Islands; hepatitis B is 25 to 75 times more common in these populations.

We are not completely certain of the safety of the hepatitis-A vaccine. However, it's made from dead viruses, so risks may be low. Hepatitis-B vaccine is safe to receive during pregnancy but is suggested only for women who are at high risk.

HBV symptoms include nausea, flu-like symptoms, jaundice, dark urine and pain in or around the liver or upper-right abdomen. Some symptoms of HBV, such as nausea and vomiting, are common in normal pregnancies so testing is important.

Nearly half of all cases of HBV in adults have no symptoms. Those without symptoms can pass the disease to other people, even though they're not actively infected. That's one reason all blood donors are screened for HBV.

Between 10 and 20% of all babies born to moms who test positive for hepatitis B get the disease. An infant can also get it through close contact with its mother and by breastfeeding. An infected baby can be very sick.

If a woman is exposed and blood tests show she doesn't have HBV antibodies, she should be vaccinated as soon as possible after exposure. The vaccine stimulates her body to make antibodies. If she is exposed in the future, she won't get hepatitis B. She may also need to receive immune globulin. The HBV vaccine is safe during pregnancy. A woman at risk can be vaccinated while she's pregnant.

It is now recommended that all babies be vaccinated against HBV at birth, then again at 1 week, 1 month and 6 months after birth. Ask your pediatrician about it.

Hepatitis C (HCV). In the past, hepatitis C was called *non-A, non-B hepatitis.* Hepatitis C (HCV) may be contracted by those who have blood transfusions or use contaminated needles. The current risk of contracting HCV through a blood transfusion is less than 1 in a million. It's estimated that 2.7 million people in the United States are infected with HCV. Most are between the ages of 40 and 59.

There is no vaccine or preventive treatment available at this time. Immune globulin doesn't work for HCV. If you have hepatitis C, you may see a liver specialist so your liver function can be checked throughout pregnancy.

The transmission rate to a baby from an infected mom is low. Breastfeeding does not appear to transmit the hepatitis-C virus to the newborn. However, discuss this situation with your healthcare provider before the baby's birth.

Other Types of Hepatitis. Hepatitis D (HDV) does not occur unless you're already infected with hepatitis B. It occurs as a *co-infection* with acute HBV. Transmission to a baby from an infected mom is rare. Treatments to protect the baby are effective.

Another type of hepatitis—hepatitis E (HEV)—is not well known. It results from fecal-oral transmission, similar to HAV. While HEV is rare in the United States, it's common in Asia, Africa, the Middle East, Central America and Mexico.

HEV is not transmitted to baby from mom. If a woman has hepatitis E, it can worsen during pregnancy, especially if contracted in the third trimester. About 65% of all women with acute HEV deliver their babies early.

Hepatitis G (HGV) occurs more often in people already infected with HBV or HCV, or in those with a history of intravenous drug use.

Your Nutrition

Eating a well-balanced diet of fresh fruits and vegetables, dairy products, whole-grain products and protein contributes to the healthy development of baby. You may be concerned about what foods to avoid. Some foods may be OK to eat when you're not pregnant but should be avoided now.

When possible, avoid food additives. We aren't certain how they can affect a developing baby, but if you can avoid them, do so.

Fresh produce can carry lots of germs; fruits and vegetables can also carry pesticides. Use soap and water to wash all produce to remove any contaminants. Even if you don't eat the peel, contaminants could get on your hands if the item isn't washed. After washing, peel the fruit or vegetable, if that's the way you normally eat it. If you're not going to peel it but just cut through it, rinse the skin well.

If it's a root vegetable or one with grooves, like some melons, clean it with a brush, soak in a bowl of water then rinse under running water. Don't eat alfalfa sprouts, radish sprouts and mung beans; they often have germs.

Below are some facts about fruits and vegetables and how eating them can impact your pregnancy.

- Cook carrots whole; they retain more of a chemical that helps fight cancer.

- To increase your intake of some veggies, purée them and add them to sauces. For example, cook and purée carrots and add them to a spaghetti sauce.
- Butternut squash is low in calories, high in beta-carotene, folate and potassium, and full of fiber and vitamin A. It may help protect you against high blood pressure and increase your immunity to illnesses.
- Asparagus is high in folate.
- Black beans are high in potassium and fiber; potassium may help control your blood pressure.
- A medium artichoke is low in calories and full of folate, potassium, iron, magnesium and vitamins A, C and K. Use artichoke hearts in an omelet or casserole, or top some with Parmesan cheese and bread crumbs, and bake.
- Blueberries help protect the collagen in your skin.
- Many fruits and vegetables are over 75% water, so eating them increases your fluid intake.

Tip for Week 33

Don't stop eating or start skipping meals as your weight increases. You and your baby need the calories and nutrition you receive from a healthy diet.

You Should Also Know

Whooping Cough (Pertussis)

In the last 10 years, the cases of whooping cough, also called *pertussis,* have tripled. The disease we see today is a milder form of whooping cough than in the past, but it still produces a nagging cough that can last a long time.

Nearly everyone has been vaccinated with the DPT vaccine (diphtheria, pertussis and tetanus). But immunity decreases over time, leaving many people at risk, including young people, healthcare workers and childcare providers. If it's been 2 years since your last tetanus/diphtheria booster, talk to your healthcare provider about getting another one.

The disease begins as a cold with a mild cough, then intense coughing begins. A person coughs until no air is left in the lungs, then takes a deep breath that produces a heaving, whooping sound when air passes the larynx. The person eventually coughs up phlegm, which may be followed by vomiting. Coughing attacks may occur up to 40 times a day. The disease can last up to 8 weeks, and you may cough for months afterward. If whooping cough is diagnosed early enough, antibiotics can treat the disease and keep it from being passed to other people.

The FDA has approved two booster vaccines. Talk to your healthcare provider about them if you believe you may be at risk. If you have any symptoms of whooping cough, call your healthcare provider immediately! The faster the infection is treated, the sooner you'll feel better.

Will Your Healthcare Provider Perform an Episiotomy?

An episiotomy has been one of the most commonly performed procedures in obstetrics and has almost become routine in some places. In 2000, about 33% of women giving birth vaginally had an episiotomy. However, many experts believe it's being used less frequently now than in the past. Today, many healthcare providers let the tissue between the vagina and rectum tear naturally during childbirth. Some studies show torn tissue may heal more easily.

An episiotomy is a controlled, straight, clean cut, made from the vagina toward the rectum during delivery. It's done to help avoid tearing as baby's head passes through the birth canal. An incision may be better than a tear or rip that could go in many directions. The cut may be made directly in the midline toward the rectum, or it may be a cut to the side. After delivery, layers are closed with absorbable sutures that don't require removal. A surgical episiotomy may heal better than a ragged tear.

Benefits of an episiotomy for a woman include a lower risk of trauma to the area between the thighs, from the tailbone to the pubic bone, less relaxation of pelvic organs with prolapse, less chance of stool and/or urine incontinence, and lower likelihood of sexual dysfunction. Benefits to a baby may include more rapid delivery. However, there are disadvantages to an episiotomy. Research shows it may lead to a more-difficult recovery, sexual problems and an increased chance of incontinence.

The American College of Obstetricians and Gynecologists (ACOG) recommends restricted use of episiotomy, rather than routine use. Research shows women who have an episiotomy may feel more pain, take longer to heal and be more likely to suffer serious lacerations near, or through, the rectum than women with vaginal tearing. If you have questions, bring them up at a prenatal visit. Ask your healthcare provider why an episiotomy might be done and whether you will have any say in this procedure.

According to one study, prenatal perineal massage started after 34 weeks of pregnancy may reduce a woman's chances of tearing during birth and/or reduce the need for an episiotomy. It may also reduce pain after childbirth. It's most helpful for first-time moms. If you're interested, discuss it with your healthcare provider. It may work for some women, but it doesn't work for everyone.

The need for an episiotomy usually becomes evident when baby's head is in the vagina. An episiotomy is also necessary if baby is stressed or if a vacuum extractor or forceps will be used during the birth.

The description of an episiotomy includes a description of the depth of the incision. There are four different depths of the incision:

- A *first-degree* episiotomy cuts only the skin.
- A *second-degree* episiotomy cuts the skin and underlying tissue.
- A *third-degree* episiotomy cuts the skin, underlying tissue and rectal sphincter, which is the muscle that goes around the anus.
- A *fourth-degree* episiotomy goes through the three layers and the rectal mucosa.

After baby's birth, epifoam may be prescribed. It is useful in treating pain and itching if you have an episitomy. Epifoam comes in an applicator that provides a measured amount for each application. You may want to ask your healthcare provider about it. Other medications are also safe to use, even if you breastfeed your baby. Acetaminophen with codeine or other medications may be prescribed for pain.

Exercise for Week 33

Stand with your feet slightly apart and your knees soft, with arms by your side. Hold your tummy in. Using light weights (2 to 3 pounds each to start; if you don't have weights, use a 16-ounce can), raise your left arm to the front and your right arm to the rear; stop just below shoulder height. Don't swing your arms; control the movement. Lower your arms to the starting position. Repeat 16 times, alternating the arm to the front. *Strengthens upper body.*

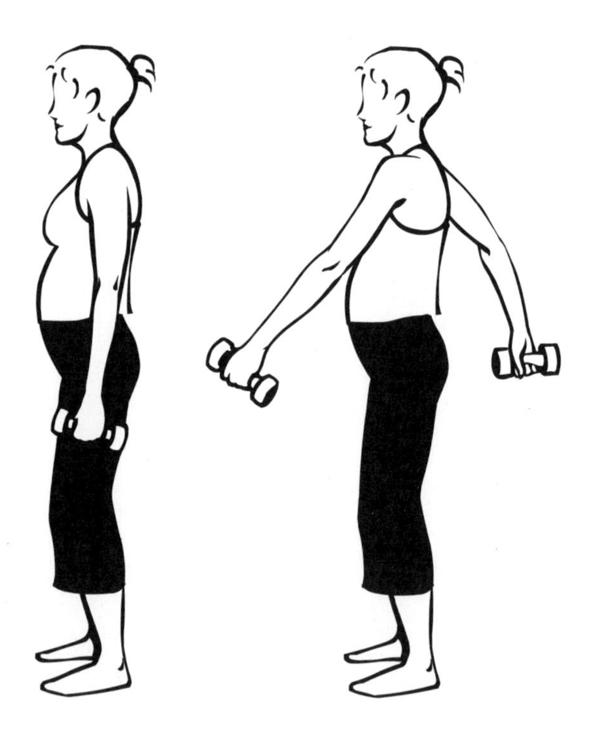

Week 34

Age of Fetus—32 Weeks

How Big Is Your Baby?

Your baby weighs almost 4¾ pounds (2.15kg) by this week. Its crown-to-rump length is about 12¾ inches (32cm). Total length is 17¾ inches (45cm).

How Big Are You?

Measuring from your bellybutton, it's about 5½ inches (14cm) to the top of your uterus. From the pubic symphysis, it measures about 13½ inches (34cm). When your uterus grows larger at an appropriate rate, it's a sign of normal growth of your baby.

It's not important that your measurements match anyone else's at similar points in their pregnancies. What's important is that you're growing appropriately and that your uterus grows and gets larger at an appropriate rate.

How Your Baby Is Growing and Developing

An ideal test to do before delivery would determine if the fetus is healthy. It would be able to detect fetal stress, which could indicate a problem.

Ultrasound accomplishes some of these goals by enabling healthcare providers to see the baby inside the uterus, as well as to evaluate the brain, heart and other organs. Along with ultrasound, a nonstress test and a contraction stress test can indicate well-being and/or problems.

Changes in You

Stress Incontinence

During the last trimester, you may leak a little urine when you cough, sneeze, exercise or lift something. Don't panic! This is called *stress incontinence;* it's normal as your uterus grows and puts pressure on your bladder.

You can control the problem by doing the Kegel exercise; see Week 14. Practice it now, and continue after baby arrives. It can also help you with incontinence that sometimes occurs after a baby's birth.

One in three women experiences light bladder leakage during pregnancy.

Bring up any incontinence you have at one of your prenatal visits. It will give your healthcare provider the opportunity to rule out a urinary-tract infection, which may also cause incontinence.

Feelings You May Be Having

A few weeks before labor begins or at the beginning of labor, you may notice a change in your abdomen. Measurement from your bellybutton or pubic symphysis to the top of the uterus may be smaller than on a previous prenatal visit. This phenomenon occurs as the head of the baby enters the birth canal and is called *lightening.*

With lightening, there may be advantages and disadvantages. You may have more room in your upper abdomen, giving you more room to breathe. However, you may have more pressure in your pelvis, bladder and rectum, which can make you uncomfortable. Some women have the uncomfortable feeling the baby is "falling out," which is also related to pressure baby exerts as it moves down in the birth canal.

Another feeling may occur around this time. Some pregnant women describe it as a "pins-and-needles" sensation. It's tingling, pressure or numbness in the pelvis or pelvic region from the pressure of the baby. It's common and shouldn't overly concern you.

The feelings described above may not be relieved until after delivery. Lying on your side may help lessen pressure on the nerves, vessels and

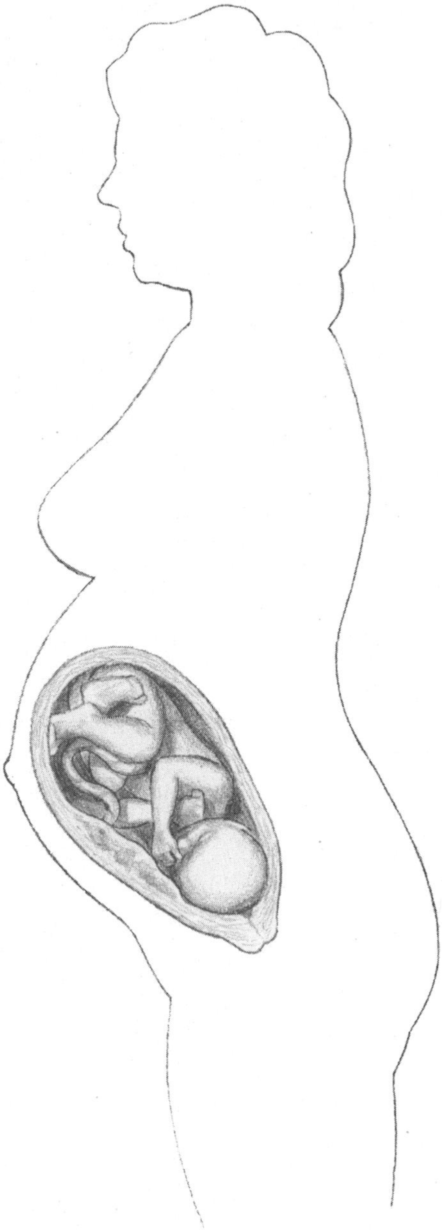

Comparative size of the uterus at 34 weeks of pregnancy (fetal age—32 weeks). The uterus can be felt about 5½ inches (14cm) above your bellybutton.

arteries in the pelvic area. If the problem is severe, talk to your healthcare provider about it.

Your healthcare provider may examine you and tell you your baby is "not in the pelvis" or "is high up." He or she is saying the baby has not yet come into the birth canal. If your healthcare provider says your baby is "floating" or "ballotable," it means part of the baby is felt high in the birth canal. But the baby is not fixed in the birth canal. Baby may even move away from your healthcare provider's fingers when you're examined.

If you're concerned or worried, call the office. It may be a reason to perform a pelvic exam to see how low the baby's head is.

Don't be concerned if you don't notice the baby drop. It doesn't occur with every woman or with every pregnancy. It's common for baby to drop as labor begins or during labor.

Braxton-Hicks Contractions and False Labor

Ask your healthcare provider to describe the signs of labor contractions. They are usually regular. They increase in length and strength over time. You'll notice a regular rhythm to real labor contractions. Time them to know how often they occur and how long they last. When you go to the hospital depends in part on your contractions.

> By this time, baby's hearing is much more refined—inside the uterus, it may turn its head in the direction of a noise.

Braxton-Hicks contractions are painless contractions you may be able to feel when you place your hand on your tummy. They often begin early in pregnancy and are felt at irregular intervals. They may increase in number and strength when the uterus is massaged. They are not positive signs of true labor.

False labor may occur before true labor begins. False-labor contractions can be painful and may feel like real labor to you. See the box on page 485. In most instances, they are irregular and short (less than 45 seconds). You may feel discomfort in the groin, lower abdomen or back. With true labor, contractions produce pain that starts at the top of the uterus and spreads over the entire uterus, through the lower back into the pelvis.

True Labor or False Labor?

Considerations	True Labor	False Labor
Contractions	Regular	Irregular
Time between contractions	Comes closer together	Does not get closer together
Contraction intensity	Increases	Doesn't change
Location of contractions	Entire abdomen	Various locations or back
Effect of anesthetic or pain relievers	Will not stop labor	Sedation may stop or alter frequency of contractions
Cervical change	Progressive cervical change	No cervical change

False labor seems to occur more often in women who have been pregnant before and delivered more babies. It usually stops as quickly as it begins. There doesn't appear to be any danger to your baby.

How Your Actions Affect Your Baby's Development

The end of your pregnancy begins with labor. Some women are concerned (or hope!) their actions can cause labor to begin. The old wives' tales about going for a ride over a bumpy road or taking a long walk to start labor aren't true. Going about your daily activities (unless your healthcare provider has advised bed rest) will not cause labor to start before baby is ready to be born.

Sex during late pregnancy may bring on labor. Semen contains prostaglandins that can cause contractions. Orgasm and nipple stimulation can also touch off uterine contractions.

Your Nutrition

It's a waste of time to have your cholesterol level checked during pregnancy. The level of cholesterol in your blood rises during pregnancy due to hormonal changes. Wait until after baby's birth or you stop breastfeeding to check your cholesterol.

A Vitamin-Rich Snack

When you're looking for something to snack on, you might not think of a baked potato, but it's an excellent snack! You get protein, fiber, calcium, iron, B vitamins and vitamin C when you eat one. Bake up a few, and store them in the refrigerator. Heat one up when you're hungry. Broccoli is another food filled with vitamins. Add it to your baked potato, and top both with some plain yogurt, cottage cheese or nonfat sour cream for a delicious treat!

You Should Also Know

Getting Ready for Baby

Your baby will need many things when it comes home from the hospital. You might want to start thinking about things baby will need now so you don't get caught short if baby comes a little early.

Items to consider for the nursery include some sort of bed (crib, bassinet), a changing table, a rocking chair, chest of drawers, diaper pail, baby monitor, small lamp, mobile, vaporizer or humidifier, and a smoke detector. Another item to consider is the paint in baby's room. Use nontoxic paint; if you're unsure, repaint the walls.

A word of caution: Be careful about buying secondhand nursery equipment or borrowing someone else's. Some items might not meet current safety standards.

Your baby needs a comfortable, safe place to sleep. A *bassinet* is a small, portable bed for baby to sleep in until she gets too big, then she can be moved to a crib. A *crib* is more permanent; buy a new crib if you can afford it. Before you make a purchase, check out various safety features, as established by the Juvenile Product Manufacturers' Association (JMPA), the Consumer Product Safety Commission (CPSC) and the American Academy of Pediatrics (AAP); they help ensure baby's safety.

Some parents believe baby should sleep with them in a "family bed." Discuss this practice with your pediatrician; safety is important. Many experts do not believe family bed sharing is safe.

> *Dad Tip*
>
> **Preregister at the hospital to save time when you finally get there for baby's birth. Ask your partner to ask at your healthcare provider's office, or ask about preregistering in your prenatal classes. If office personnel or prenatal instructors don't know, call the hospital and ask.**

It's fun to dress baby in the cutest outfits, but in reality, most babies don't need many clothes. They can get by just fine with some basic styles for the first year. A few cute outfits are OK, but don't spend your money on them if you don't need to. (You may receive many different clothing items as shower and baby gifts.)

A baby's needs are easy to meet. Diapers, T-shirts, gowns that open at the bottom, footed sleepers, socks, bibs, a hat, a warm cover-up, one-piece short- or long-legged "onesies," blankets and towels are the most basic items you'll need to stock up on. How many of each you need depends on your personal situation, but have about 8 dozen diapers on hand (order 100 a week for a newborn if you have a diaper service). They can be a combination of cloth and disposable diapers; both are good in various situations.

Car Seats. The most important piece of baby equipment you can buy is a *car seat;* choose one soon so you'll have it when baby is born. Once you've selected a car seat, go to your local police or fire station and ask them to show you how to install it correctly.

When choosing a car seat for baby, purchase a new one. This is one piece of equipment you don't want to borrow or to buy secondhand. The car seat could be damaged by previous wear and use, or it might be missing important parts. Technological advances may also make an older car seat outdated.

Your baby needs to ride in a car seat *every* time he rides in a car—it's the law in all 50 states. The safest place for baby is the middle of the back seat.

A car seat is the best protection your baby has in case of an accident. Don't take him out of the car seat for feeding, changing or comforting while the car is moving. From the time your baby goes home from the hospital, he should ride in a car seat.

There are different types of car seats available. When choosing one, be certain it meets the safety standards of the JMPA, the CPSC and the AAP.

Caution: Never put a car seat in the front passenger seat, especially if it has an air bag! If your car has side-impact air bags in the back seat, be sure baby's car seat is placed in the middle of the back seat or ask your dealer to disable those air bags.

The final word is: Keep your baby safe; never let her ride in any vehicle without being buckled up and belted in. One report found an average of 35 babies a year die in auto accidents on the way home from the hospital. Don't let your baby become a statistic.

Pets in the Home

You may have a pet that is your "baby," but now you're expecting a real baby. As soon as you learn you're pregnant, start thinking about how your pet may handle having a new baby in the house. You need to prepare your pet because baby's safety must always come first.

Be sure your pet is up to date on vaccinations. Have your vet check your pet for parasites. If your pet isn't neutered, now may be the time to do it—it can help reduce aggression.

When you bring baby home from the hospital, it means a lifestyle change for your pet. An animal is sensitive to a routine, so making changes before baby is born may be easier on your pet. During your pregnancy, try the following.

- Before baby's birth, begin reducing the time you spend with your pet. It can help prepare it for the future, when you'll have less time because of baby.

- Make any necessary changes in your pet's feeding, exercise or play schedule in the weeks before baby's birth.
- Make changes in where your pet will be kept. If baby will be in your room and your pet has slept there, move your pet's bed to another location so it'll be familiar.
- Evaluate your dog's obedience training. He should react to basic commands.
- Expose your pet to other children when possible. It can be a shock to an animal to be confronted with a small baby. A baby's crying can startle or frighten an animal.
- Put out baby's things, such as the bassinet, crib and changing table. Let your pet smell everything.
- Keep pets off baby furniture and out of baby's room.
- Keep pets and cages out of the kitchen and children's play areas.
- Give your pet an area that's all its own and off-limits to baby.

Nearly all pets are territorial. They like a routine they can follow. If you plan to rearrange furniture or change the functions of a room, do it early in your pregnancy. This allows the animal to become familiar with the new organization.

There are some general precautions with pets. Some pets can carry a bacteria that causes UTIs in humans. Washing hands for at least 10 seconds after patting or caring for a pet can help you lower your risk. Pet foods that aren't well-processed may be contaminated with salmonella. Always be sure to wash hands well after handling any pet food.

If you have a puppy or kitten, it may have a lot of energy. It could be a challenge handling it, especially when you have a baby to care for. You may have to spend extra time with a young pet.

If your animal is fairly old, a change in routine could cause problems. If your pet has had the run of the house, it may take some time to train it to stay out of certain areas. An older pet may be less flexible about adding baby to the household. It may sulk, ignore you or beg for your attention. Your pet may also be jealous of the time and attention you give baby. You may have to set aside some time alone with an older pet.

Introducing Your Dog to Baby. Give your dog a chance to meet and interact with children while you're pregnant. Ask friends or family members to bring their children over to expose your pet. You can get an idea of how your pet may respond to the expected baby. Pay attention to your dog's response to a baby crying. If you find your dog gets distressed, you may have to leave him with a friend or board him for a while. If you discover your dog has a tendency to bite, you may need to consider getting rid of him.

You might also want to consider training classes for your dog. Obedience classes can teach a dog to follow simple commands.

Introducing Your Cat to Baby. If you have a cat, you know how unpredictable it can be. It's best to keep a cat away from baby when possible. Let the cat watch from a distance. If she shows any signs of aggression, remove the cat from the area. If the cat slinks toward baby, it's a sign of aggression. Reward your cat for any positive actions, such as staying off furniture.

Cats usually run away from children and hide, if they're bothered by them. Cats usually adjust to a new baby more easily than dogs because they aren't as attached to humans. However, cats *are* curious, so set up any new furniture early, so kitty has a chance to check it out before baby's arrival.

Don't let your cat sleep on baby furniture. Cover the crib with a mesh cover sold exclusively for this purpose. Or fill the crib with balloons—cats don't like them, especially when they pop!

Other Household Pets. Birdcages need to be cleaned every day. Wear rubber gloves; wash the gloves in bleach water and your hands thoroughly when you have finished. Bird waste is highly toxic and may harbor bacteria that can cause disease. Keep your birds in the cage.

Pocket pets are hamsters, mice, gerbils and guinea pigs. Keep these pets in their cages, away from baby. Hamsters, mice, gerbils, guinea pigs, chicks, frogs and turtles can all carry salmonella. If you have a ferret, keep it away from your baby. They have been known to attack children.

If you have a reptile as a pet, you may want to consider getting rid of it. The Centers for Disease Control and Prevention (CDC) advises keeping children younger than 5 years old away from all pet reptiles. They can be a source of life-threatening salmonella infections.

> **Tip for Week 34**
> A strip of paper, tape or a bandage can help cover a bellybutton that is sensitive or poking through your clothing.

A child can become infected from handling a reptile or by handling objects contaminated with a reptile's feces. Some cases have been reported in infants who never touched the reptiles. Researchers believe infants were infected when they were held by those who handled the reptiles!

Vasa Previa

Vasa previa is a condition in which blood vessels of the umbilical cord cross the interior opening of the cervix, lying close to it or covering it. It occurs once in about every 2000 to 3000 pregnancies.

When the cervix dilates or membranes rupture, unprotected vessels can tear. Or they can become squeezed together, which shuts off blood and oxygen to the baby. It can also occur when baby drops into position for delivery and presses on the vessels, which limits or shuts off blood supply to the baby. Danger may also occur when membranes rupture. Fetal vessels may rupture at the same time, causing loss of blood from the fetus.

Detecting the problem can be achieved with a 5-second scan with color ultrasound. The test shows vessels lying across the cervical opening and measures the speed of the blood flow. Different rates of blood flow have distinct colors and reveal the location of the fetal blood vessels. However, this screening is not routine.

Diagnosis is difficult because there are no symptoms. Risks include placenta previa, painless bleeding, previous uterine surgery or D&C, pregnancy with multiples and in-vitro fertilization. If you have any of these risk factors, discuss having the color ultrasound with your healthcare provider.

When a woman is diagnosed with vasa previa, she may be put on bed rest the third trimester to help prevent labor. A Cesarean delivery is done after 35 weeks of pregnancy, with a success rate of over 95%.

"Bloody Show" and Mucus Plug

After a vaginal exam or at the beginning of early labor and early contractions, you may bleed a small amount. This is called a *bloody show;* it may occur as the cervix stretches and dilates. You should not lose a lot of blood. If it causes you concern or appears to be a large amount of blood, call your healthcare provider immediately.

Along with a bloody show, you may pass a mucus plug. A *mucus plug* is a buildup of cervical mucus found at the opening of the cervix to protect the uterus and baby by creating a barrier between the vagina and uterus. It keeps bacteria from entering the uterus. However, losing the mucus plug poses no danger to you or to baby.

A mucus plug may be clear, pink, brownish or reddish in color. It may be dislodged in small pieces, or it may come out in one large piece. Losing the mucus plug can be a sign your body is preparing for labor, but it doesn't mean labor is at hand.

Timing Contractions

Most women learn in prenatal classes or from their healthcare provider how to time contractions during labor. To time how long a contraction lasts, begin timing when the contraction starts and end timing when the contraction lets up and goes away.

It's also important to know how often contractions occur. There may be some confusion about this. You can choose from two methods. Ask your healthcare provider which method he or she prefers.

1. Note the time period from when a contraction starts to the time the next contraction starts. This is the most commonly used method and the most reliable.
2. Note the time period from when a contraction ends to the time the next contraction starts.

You'll know it's time to head for the hospital when contractions are 4 to 5 minutes apart for at least an hour. They'll also be increasing in intensity and length, and coming closer together.

It may be helpful for you and your partner or labor coach to time contractions before calling your healthcare provider or the hospital. Your healthcare provider will probably want to know how often contractions occur and how long each one lasts. With this information, he or she can decide when you should go to the hospital.

Exercise for Week 34

Sit on the edge of a chair. Using light weights (2 to 3 pounds each to start; if you don't have weights, use a 16-ounce can), raise your arms to shoulder level, and bend your elbows so you can point your hands toward the ceiling. Slowly bring your elbows and arms together in front of your face. Hold for 4 seconds, then slowly open to shoulder-width. Repeat 8 times; work up to 20 times. *Tightens breast muscles to help keep breasts from sagging.*

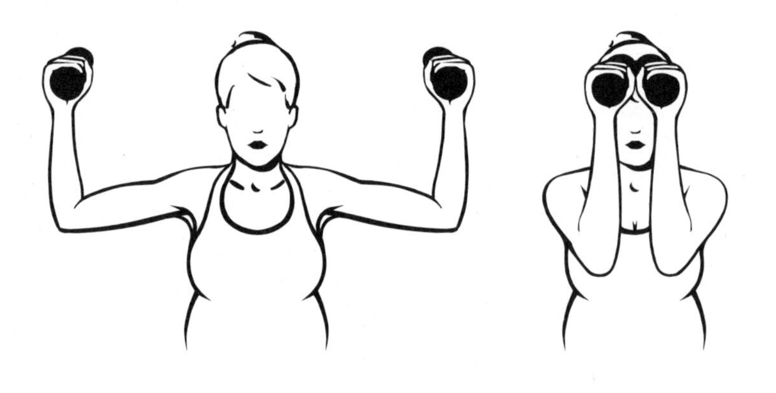

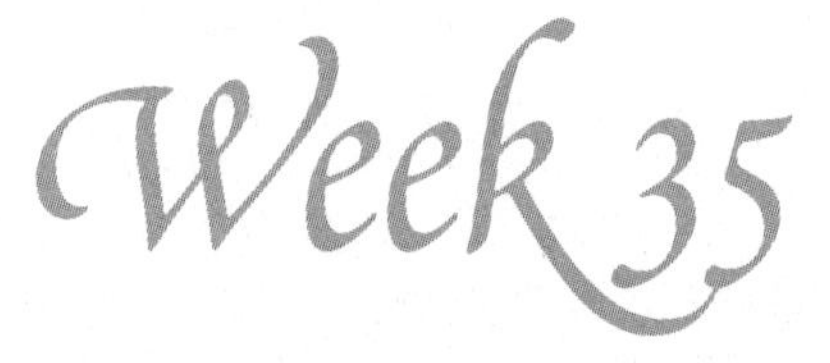

Week 35

Age of Fetus—33 Weeks

How Big Is Your Baby?

Your baby now weighs over 5¼ pounds (2.4kg). Crown-to-rump length is about 13¼ inches (33cm), and total length is 18¼ inches (46cm).

How Big Are You?

It's about 6 inches (15cm) to the top of your uterus from your belly-button. From the pubic symphysis, the distance is about 14 inches (35cm). By this week, your total weight gain should be between 24 and 29 pounds (10.8 and 13kg).

How Your Baby Is Growing and Changing

How Much Does Your Baby Weigh?

You've probably asked your healthcare provider several times how big your baby is or how much baby might weigh when it's born. This is one of the most frequently asked questions.

Ultrasound can be used to estimate baby's weight. Several measurements are used in a formula. Many believe ultrasound is the best way to estimate weight. However, estimates may vary as much as half a pound (225g) or more in either direction.

Even with a weight estimate, we can't tell if baby will fit through the birth canal. It's usually necessary for you to labor to see how baby fits into your pelvis and if there is room for it to pass through the birth canal.

Although this book is designed to take you through pregnancy by examining one week at a time, you may want specific information. Because the book can't include *everything* you need *before* you know you're looking for it, check the index, beginning on page 655, for a particular topic. We may not cover the subject until a later week.

In some women who appear to be average or better-than-average size, a 6- or 6½-pound (2.7 to 2.9kg) baby won't fit through the pelvis. Experience also shows women who are petite are sometimes able to deliver 7½-pound (3.4kg) or larger babies without much difficulty. The best test or method of assessing whether baby will deliver through your pelvis is labor.

Umbilical-Cord Prolapse

With umbilical-cord prolapse, the umbilical cord is pushed out of the uterus too soon. It's rare and is a life-threatening emergency for the baby. It happens when the cord passes alongside or past part of baby, which compresses the umbilical vessels and shuts off the supply of blood and oxygen to the baby.

The situation may occur when there's a poor fit between the part of the baby entering the birth canal and the mother's bony pelvis, and the cord passes baby. Abnormal fetal presentations, including breech, transverse lie and oblique lie, can increase the risk.

Prolapse is twice as likely to occur when a baby weighs less than 5½ pounds or when the mother-to-be has given birth at least twice before. Excessive amounts of amniotic fluid also increases the risk—when membranes rupture, the large amount of fluid released can cause the cord to pass beyond baby.

Tip for Week 35

Maternity bras provide extra support to your growing breasts. You may feel more comfortable wearing one during the day and at night while you sleep.

When the situation occurs, the healthcare provider may have to keep his or her hand inside the woman's vagina to lift the presenting part of the baby off the cord until baby can be delivered by Cesarean delivery. Lowering a woman's head or changing her position may help. Filling the woman's bladder to elevate the fetal head a little may be done until a Cesarean can be performed. If steps are taken promptly to deal with the situation and deliver the baby, there is usually a good outcome.

Changes in You

Shoes and Feet

Your feet may change and/or grow during pregnancy. This can happen as your baby grows and you add pregnancy pounds. If it does (and it happens to many women!), keep the following in mind.

- Give up your tie-on and strap-on shoes for slip-ons. They're much easier to get in and out of.
- Opt for flats—high heels and platform shoes can be dangerous.
- Sandals are great when they offer support. Buy a good pair.
- Consider adding foot treatments to your list of "must dos"—foot massages and pedicures can help make your feet and legs feel great. A pedicure can also help you keep your toenails trimmed—a tough job when you can't even see your feet!

Grandma's Remedy

If you want to avoid using medication, try a folk remedy. If you have a lot of gas, try taking 1 teaspoon of olive oil on an empty stomach.

Emotional Changes in Late Pregnancy

As you get closer to delivery, you and your partner may become more anxious about the events to come. You may have more mood swings, which seem to occur for no reason. You may become more irritable, which can strain your relationship. You may be concerned about insignificant or unimportant things.

While these emotions rage inside you, you'll notice you're getting bigger and aren't able to do things you used to do. You may feel uncomfortable, and you may not be sleeping well. These things can all work together to make your emotions swing wildly from highs to lows.

Emotional changes are normal; be ready for them. Talk with your partner, and tell him how you feel and what you're thinking about. You may be surprised to discover he has concerns about you, the baby and his role during labor and delivery. By talking, you both may find it easier to understand what the other is experiencing.

Your concern about baby's health and well-being may increase during the last weeks of pregnancy. You may also fret about how well you'll tolerate labor and how you'll get through delivery. You may be concerned about whether you'll be a good mother or be able to raise a baby properly.

Discuss emotional problems with your healthcare provider. He or she may be able to reassure you that what you're going through is normal. Take advantage of prenatal classes and information available about pregnancy and delivery.

Lactation Consultants

If you want to breastfeed, it may help to consult with a lactation specialist before baby's birth. A lactation consultant is a qualified professional who works in many settings, including hospitals, home-care services, health agencies and private practice. A consultant can help with basic breastfeeding issues, assess and observe both you and your baby, develop a care plan, inform healthcare providers of the situation and follow up with you as needed. You can even contact a lactation consultant before baby's birth. Ask your healthcare provider at one of your prenatal appointments for more information. Or check at the hospital where you plan to deliver to see if they have lactation consultants on staff. For more information on lactation consultants and breastfeeding, see Appendix B, page 596.

How Your Actions Affect Your Baby's Development

Preparing for Baby's Birth

You may be feeling a little nervous about knowing when it's time to call your healthcare provider or go to the hospital. Ask about signs to watch for at one of your prenatal visits. In prenatal classes, you should also learn how to recognize the signs of labor and when you should call your healthcare provider or go to the hospital.

Your bag of waters may break before you go into labor. In most cases, you'll notice this as a gush of water followed by a steady leaking.

During the last few weeks of pregnancy, have your suitcase packed and ready to go. See the list in Week 36 for some helpful suggestions for things you might want or need when you get to the hospital.

If possible, tour the hospital facilities with your partner a few weeks before your scheduled due date. Find out where to go and what to do when you get there.

Talk with your partner about the best ways to reach him if you think you're in labor. Cell phones are a good way to stay in touch. You might have him check with you periodically. Or he can wear a pager if he is often away from a phone, especially during the last few weeks of pregnancy.

Plan your route to the hospital. Have your partner drive it a few times. Plan an alternate route in case of bad weather or traffic tie-ups.

> **Dad Tip**
>
> At a prenatal visit, ask the healthcare provider about your part in the delivery. There may be some things you'd like to do, such as cutting the cord or videotaping your baby's birth. It's easier to talk about these things ahead of time. Not every new father wants an active role in the delivery. That's OK, too.

Ask your healthcare provider what you should do if you think you're in labor. Is it best to call the office? Should you go directly to the hospital? By knowing what to do, and when, you can relax a little and not worry about the beginning of labor and delivery.

Preregistering at the Hospital

It may be helpful and save you time if you register at the hospital a few weeks before your due date. You'll be able to do this with forms you get at the office or by getting forms from the hospital. It's smart to do this early because when you go to the hospital, you may be in a hurry or concerned with other things.

You should know certain facts that may not be included in your chart, such as:

- your blood type and Rh-factor
- when your last period was and what your due date is
- details of any past pregnancies
- your healthcare provider's name
- your pediatrician's name

Your healthcare provider has recorded various things that have occurred during your pregnancy. A copy of this record is usually kept in the labor-and-delivery area.

Certified Nurse-Midwives, Nurse Practitioners and Physician Assistants

In today's obstetric-and-gynecology medical practices, you may find many types of highly qualified people helping to take care of you. These people—mostly women, but not all!—are on the forefront in guiding women through pregnancy to delivery. They may even help deliver their babies!

A *certified nurse-midwife* (CNM) is an advance-practice registered nurse (RN). He or she has received additional training delivering babies and providing prenatal and postpartum care to women. A CNM works closely with a doctor or team of doctors to address specifics about a particular pregnancy, and labor and delivery. Often a CNM delivers babies.

A certified nurse midwife can provide many types of information to a pregnant woman, such as guidance with nutrition and exercise, ways to deal with pregnancy discomforts, tips for managing weight gain, dealing with various pregnancy problems and discussions of different methods of pain relief for labor and delivery. A CNM can also address issues of family planning and birth control and other gynecological care, including breast exams, Pap smears and other screenings. A CNM can prescribe medications; each state has their own specific requirements.

A *nurse practitioner* is also an advanced-practice registered nurse (RN). He or she has received additional training providing prenatal and postpartum care to women. A nurse practitioner may work with a doctor or work independently to address specifics about a woman's pregnancy, and labor and delivery.

(continues)

A nurse practitioner can provide many types of information to a pregnant woman, such as guidance with nutrition and exercise, ways to deal with pregnancy discomforts, tips for managing weight gain, dealing with various pregnancy problems and discussions of different methods of pain relief for labor and delivery. He or she can also address issues of family planning and birth control and other gynecological care, including breast exams, Pap smears and other screenings. In some cases, a nurse practitioner may prescribe medications or provide pain relief during labor and delivery (as a certified registered nurse anesthetist [CRNA]).

A *physician assistant (PA)* is a qualified healthcare professional who may take care of you during pregnancy. He or she is licensed to practice medicine in association with a licensed doctor. In a normal, uncomplicated pregnancy, many or most of your prenatal visits may be with a PA, not the doctor. This may include labor and delivery. Most women find this is a good thing—often these healthcare providers have more time to spend with you answering questions and addressing your concerns.

A PA's focus is to provide many health-care services traditionally done by a doctor. They care for people who have conditions (pregnancy is a condition they see women for), diagnose and treat illnesses, order and interpret tests, counsel on preventive health care, perform some procedures, assist in surgery, write prescriptions and do physical exams. A PA is *not* a medical assistant, who performs administrative or simple clinical tasks.

We are fortunate to have these dedicated professionals working in OB/GYN practices and clinics. The care they provide is crucial to the medical community and makes quality medical care for women something every woman can look forward to.

Your Nutrition

Your body continues to need lots of vitamins and minerals for baby. You'll need even more of them if you breastfeed! On page 502 is a chart showing your daily vitamin-and-mineral requirements during pregnancy and breastfeeding. It's important to realize how necessary your continued good nutrition is for you and your baby.

Nutrient Requirements during Pregnancy and Breastfeeding

Vitamins & Minerals	During Pregnancy	During Breastfeeding
A	800mcg	1300mcg
B_1 (thiamine)	1.5mg	1.6mg
B_2 (riboflavin)	1.6mg	1.8mg
B_3 (niacin)	17mg	20mg
B_6	2.2mg	2.2mg
B_{12}	2.2mcg	2.6mcg
C	70mg	95mg
Calcium	1200mg	1200mg
D	10mcg	10mcg
E	10mg	12mg
Folic acid (B_9)	400mcg	280mcg
Iron	30mg	15mg
Magnesium	320mg	355mg
Phosphorous	1200mg	1200mg
Zinc	15mg	19mg

You Should Also Know

Ultrasound in the Third Trimester

If you have an ultrasound exam in the third trimester, your healthcare provider is looking for particular information. Performed later in pregnancy, this test can:

- evaluate baby's size and growth
- determine the cause of vaginal bleeding
- check for IUGR
- determine the cause of vaginal or abdominal pain
- evaluate a baby after an accident or injury to the mother-to-be
- detect some birth defects
- monitor the growth of multiples
- monitor a high-risk pregnancy
- measure the amount of amniotic fluid
- check whether baby is head first or breech

- determine which delivery method to use
- find out the maturity of the placenta
- be used with amniocentesis, to determine fetal lung maturity
- be used as part of a biophysical profile

Shingles during Pregnancy

Shingles occurs when a type of herpes virus becomes active after having been dormant in nerve root ganglia. This can happen long after the primary infection has gone away. The condition is also called *herpes zoster.* It occurs more often in people who are older, although it can occur in younger people as well.

Baby's sucking reflex develops before birth.

A time of great concern for a pregnant woman is during the first trimester because of concern about viral infections affecting a fetus. Around the time of delivery concern is for the baby coming through the birth canal and contracting the virus from mom. Pain from shingles occurs in specific areas of nerve distribution. Treatment centers around pain control with pain medications. If you think you have shingles, contact your healthcare provider, who can decide on treatment for you.

What Is Placenta Previa?

With *placenta previa*, the placenta attaches to the lower part of the uterus instead of the upper wall; it lies close to the cervix or covers it. The problem occurs about once in every 170 pregnancies. The illustration on page 504 shows placenta previa.

Placenta previa is serious because of the chance of heavy bleeding. Bleeding may occur during pregnancy or during labor. There are three main types of placenta previa:

- placenta touches the cervix (low-lying placenta)
- the placenta partially covers the cervix (partial placenta previa)
- the placenta completely covers the cervix (total placenta previa)

The cause of placenta previa is not completely understood. Risk factors include previous Cesarean delivery, over age 30, smoking and delivery of several babies.

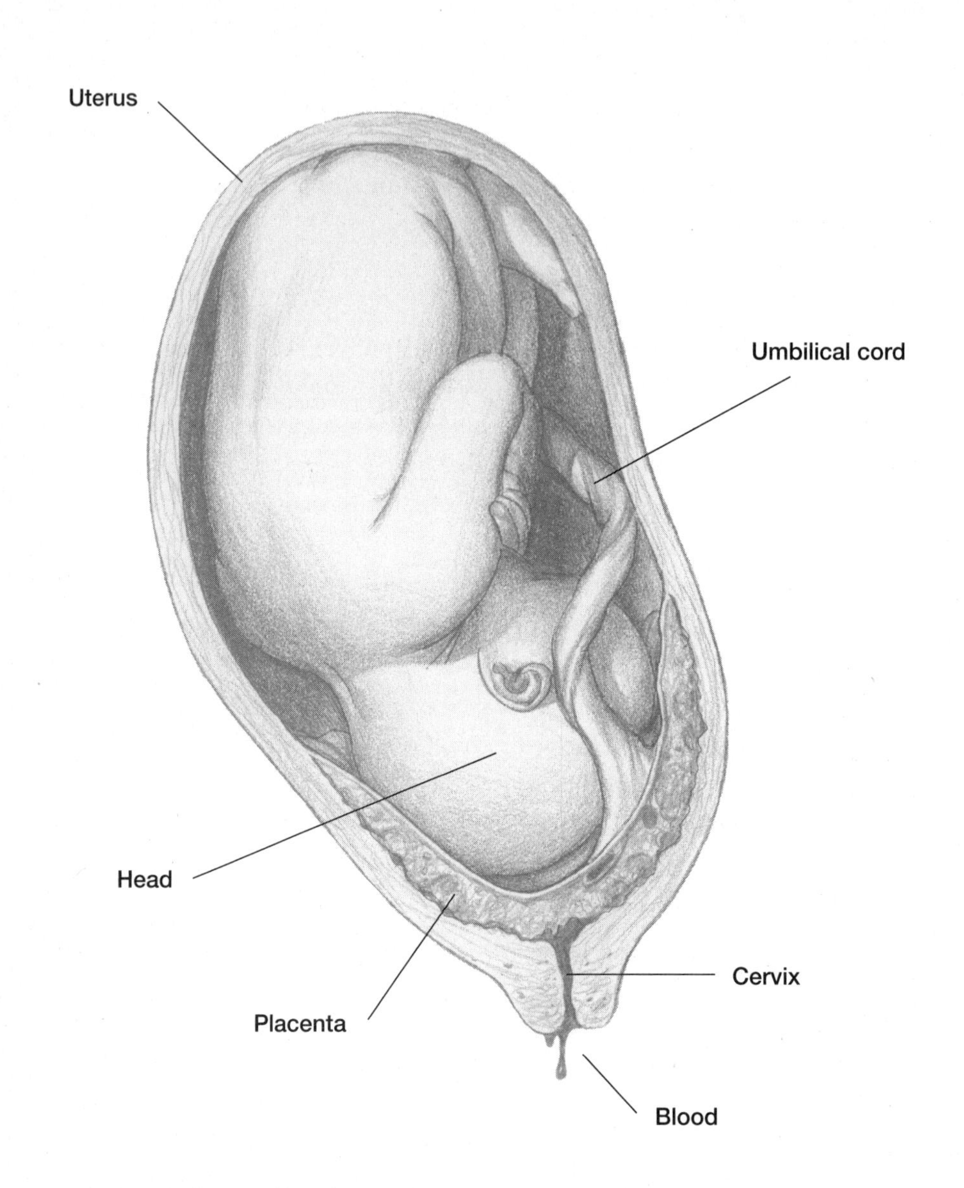

In this illustration of total placenta previa, note how the placenta completely covers the cervical opening to the uterus.

A woman who conceives with in-vitro fertilization has a greater chance of developing placenta previa. Experts believe insertion of the embryo into the uterus may cause contractions, which could cause the embryo to implant low in the uterus, raising the risk of placenta previa. In addition, embryos may intentionally be implanted low in the uterus because research shows this placement may improve the chance of pregnancy.

The most characteristic symptom of placenta previa is painless bleeding without contractions. This doesn't usually occur until close to the end of your second trimester or later when the cervix thins out, stretches and tears the placenta loose.

Bleeding may occur without warning and may be extremely heavy. It occurs when the cervix begins to dilate with early labor, and blood escapes.

Placenta previa should be considered when a woman has vaginal bleeding during the second half of pregnancy. The problem can't be diagnosed with a physical exam because a pelvic examination may cause heavier bleeding. Healthcare providers use ultrasound to identify the problem. Ultrasound is particularly accurate in the second half of pregnancy because the uterus and placenta are bigger, and things are easier to see.

Your healthcare provider may advise you not to have a pelvic exam if you have placenta previa. This is important to remember if you see another healthcare provider or when you go to the hospital.

It's not possible to deliver the placenta first, followed by the baby. The baby may also be in a breech presentation. Babies are usually delivered by Cesarean delivery. The baby is delivered first, then the placenta is delivered so the uterus can contract. Bleeding can be kept to a minimum.

Some Information May Scare You

In an effort to give you as much information as possible about pregnancy, we do include serious discussions throughout the book that some might find "scary." The information is not included to frighten you; it's there to provide facts about particular medical situations that may occur during pregnancy.

If a woman experiences a serious problem, she and her partner will probably want to know as much about it as possible. If a woman has a friend or knows someone who has problems during pregnancy, reading about it might relieve her fears. We also hope our discussions can help you start a dialogue with your doctor, if you have questions.

Nearly all pregnancies are uneventful, and serious situations don't arise. However, please know we have tried to cover as many aspects of pregnancy as we possibly can so you'll have all the information at hand that you might need and want. Knowledge is power, so having various facts available can help you feel more in control of your own pregnancy. We hope reading it helps you relax and have a great pregnancy experience.

If you find serious discussions frighten you, don't read them! Or if the information doesn't apply to your pregnancy, just skip over it. But realize information is there if you want to know more about a particular situation.

Exercise for Week 35

Stand with your feet apart, knees softly bent. Raise your arms so your upper arms are parallel to the floor and your hands point up into the air. Squeeze your shoulder blades together, hold for 3 seconds, then release. Do 10 times. *Improves posture and relieves upper-back stress.*

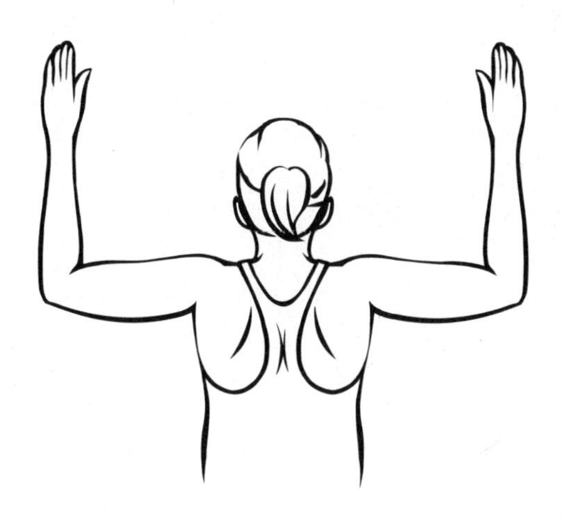

Week 36

Age of Fetus—34 Weeks

How Big Is Your Baby?

By this week, your baby weighs about 5¾ pounds (2.6kg). Its crown-to-rump length is over 13½ inches (34cm), and total length is 18⅔ inches (47cm).

How Big Are You?

From the pubic symphysis, it's about 14½ inches (36cm) to the top of the uterus. From your bellybutton, it's more than 5½ inches (14cm) to the top of the uterus.

How Your Baby Is Growing and Developing

An important part of your baby's development is maturing of its lungs and respiratory system. The respiratory system is the last system to mature. Knowing how mature a baby's lungs are helps in deciding about early delivery, if it must be considered. Tests can predict whether baby will be able to breathe without assistance.

Respiratory-distress syndrome (RDS) or *hyaline membrane disease* occurs when lungs aren't completely mature, and baby can't breathe on its own after birth. The baby may require a machine to breathe for it.

Several fetal-lung-maturity tests can be done. The test done depends on availability of the test in your area and the experience of your healthcare team. Your healthcare provider will determine if a test is necessary and which one to do.

Two methods for evaluating fetal-lung maturity require amniocentesis. They are discussed below.

The *L/S ratio* is done around 34 weeks of pregnancy. The ratio in amniotic fluid changes between lecithin and sphingomyelin at this time. Levels of lecithin increase, while levels of sphingomyelin stay the same. The ratio between the two levels indicates if a baby's lungs are mature.

The *phosphatidyl glycerol (PG)* test is the second way to evaluate lungs. The test is positive or negative. If phosphatidyl glycerol is present in amniotic fluid (positive), the infant will probably not have respiratory distress at birth.

Changes in You

You have only 4 to 5 weeks until your due date. You may have gained 25 to 30 pounds (11.25 to 13.5kg), and you still have a month to go. It isn't unusual for your weight to stay the same or change very little at your weekly visits after this point.

The maximum amount of amniotic fluid surrounds the baby now. In the weeks to come, the baby continues to grow, but some amniotic fluid is reabsorbed by your body. This reduces the amount of room in which the baby has to move. You may notice a difference in baby's movements. For some women, it feels as if baby isn't moving as much as it has been.

Restless-Leg Syndrome (RLS)

You may have *restless-leg syndrome (RLS)* for the first time during pregnancy; it can rob you of sleep. If you develop RLS, you will feel a sensation in your legs that makes you feel as if you must move your lower limbs. Experts suggest RLS may be linked to anemia and could be caused by an iron or folic-acid deficiency.

Treatment includes increasing your iron intake and taking folic acid. Talk to your doctor *before* you do either. Applying a heating pad for 15

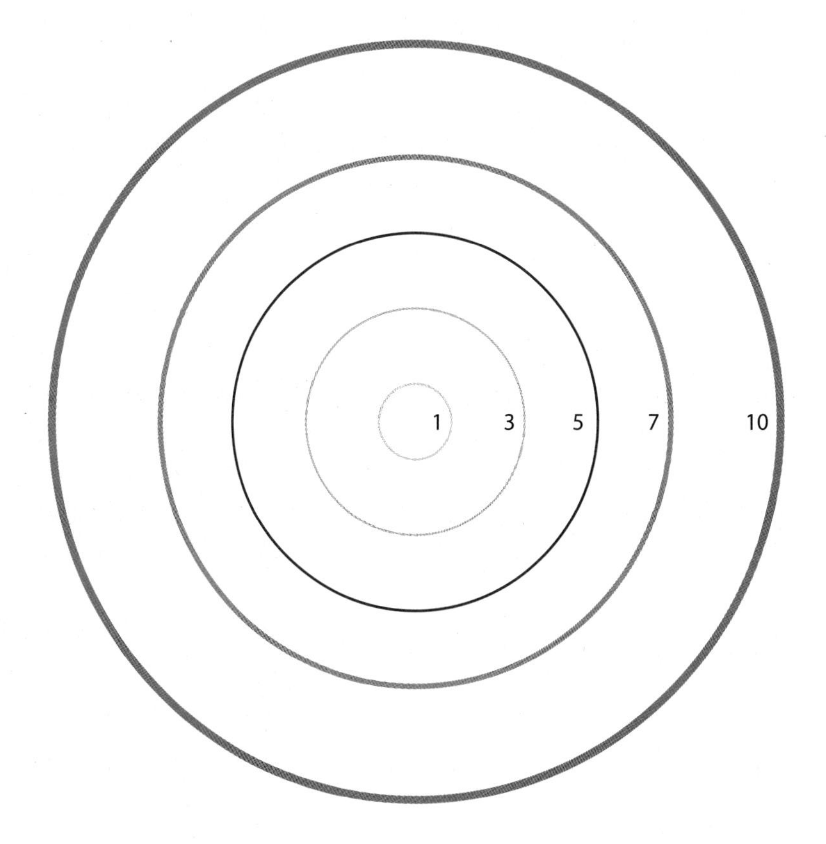

Cervical dilatation in centimeters (shown actual size).

to 20 minutes may help. The good news is RLS often disappears completely after baby's birth.

What Is Labor?

It's important to understand the labor process. You'll be more informed when labor occurs, and you'll know what to do. *Labor* is defined as the stretching and thinning (dilatation) of your cervix. This happens when the uterus, which is a muscle, tightens and relaxes to squeeze out the baby. As the baby is pushed out, the cervix stretches. Your cervix must open to 10cm (about 4 inches) for your baby to pass through it. (See the cervical dilation chart on the opposite page.)

We don't know what causes labor to begin, but there are many theories. One is that hormones made by the mother and baby together trigger labor. It's believed both release the hormone oxytocin, which triggers labor. Or it could be the baby produces some hormone that causes the uterus to contract.

The cervix must also soften and thin out (become effaced). To put it in more understandable terms, before pregnancy, your cervix is about as hard as the end of your nose. Close to delivery, it is about as soft as your ear lobe.

At various times, you may feel tightening, contractions or cramps, but it isn't actually labor until there is a *change in the cervix*. As you can see from the discussion below, there are many aspects to labor. You'll go through them all to deliver your baby.

Three Stages of Labor. There are three distinct stages of labor.

- **Stage one**—The first stage of labor begins with uterine contractions of great enough intensity, duration and frequency to soften and dilate the cervix. The first stage ends when the cervix is fully dilated (10cm) and open enough to allow baby's head to come through it.
- **Stage two**—The second stage of labor begins when the cervix is completely dilated at 10cm. This stage ends with the delivery of baby.

- **Stage three**—The third stage of labor begins after baby's birth. It ends with delivery of the placenta and the membranes that have surrounded the fetus.

Some doctors have described a fourth stage of labor, referring to a time after delivery of the placenta during which the uterus contracts. Contraction of the uterus is important in controlling bleeding after delivery.

How Long Will Labor Last? The length of the first and second stages of labor can last 14 to 15 hours or more in a first pregnancy. The average length of *active* labor is between 6 and 12 hours. When you hear about a *long labor,* most of the time is spent in early labor. Contractions may start and stop or be weaker or farther apart, then get regular and strong.

Every labor is different, in great part because of the level of pain you experience. Be aware that contractions *can* hurt.

A woman who has already had one or two children will probably have a shorter labor, but don't count on that either! The average time for labor usually decreases by a few hours for a second or third delivery.

Everyone's heard of women who barely made it to the hospital or had a 1-hour labor. For every one of those women, there are others who have labored 18, 20, 24 hours or longer. It's impossible to predict the amount of time that will be required for labor. You may ask your healthcare provider, but his or her answer is only a guess.

How Your Actions Affect Your Baby's Development

Choosing Your Baby's Doctor

It's time to choose a doctor for your baby. You might choose a pediatrician—a doctor who specializes in treating children. Or you might choose a family practitioner. If the doctor you are seeing during pregnancy is a family practitioner, and you want him or her to care for your baby, you probably don't need to consider this at all.

It's good to meet the person who will care for baby *before* the birth—many pediatricians welcome it. It gives you an opportunity to discuss important matters with this new doctor.

The first visit is important, so ask your partner to go with you. It's a good time for the two of you to discuss any concerns or questions about the care of your baby and to receive helpful suggestions. You can also discuss the doctor's philosophy and learn his or her schedule and "on-call" coverage.

Tip for Week 36

To find a pediatrician for baby, ask for referrals. Your pregnancy doctor might be able to give you one. Or ask family, friends or people in your childbirth-education classes for names of doctors they like.

When baby is born, the pediatrician will come to the hospital to check him or her. Selecting a pediatrician before the birth ensures your baby will see the same doctor for follow-up visits at the hospital and at the doctor's office.

If you belong to an HMO, and there are a group of pediatricians, arrange a meeting with one physician. If you have a conflict or don't see eye to eye with this person, you may be able to choose another doctor. Ask your patient advocate for information and advice.

Questions to Ask a Pediatrician. The questions below may help you when you talk with your pediatrician. You will probably also have other questions.

- What are your qualifications and training?
- Are you board certified? If not, will you be soon?
- What hospital(s) are you affiliated with?
- Do you have privileges at the hospital where I will deliver?
- Will you do the newborn exam?
- If I have a boy, will you perform the circumcision (if we want to have it done)?
- What is your availability for regular office visits and emergencies?
- How long is a typical office visit?

- Are your office hours compatible with our work schedules?
- Can an acutely ill child be seen the same day?
- How can we reach you in case of an emergency or after office hours?
- Who responds if you are not available?
- Do you return phone calls the same day?
- Do you have advance-practice nurses or physician assistants in your office?
- Can we contact you by email if we have routine questions? How soon do you respond?
- What sort of advice do you give parents who both work outside the home?
- Are you interested in preventive, developmental and behavioral issues?
- Do you provide written instructions for well-baby and sick-baby care?
- Do you support women in their efforts to breastfeed?
- What are your fees?
- Do your fees comply with our insurance?
- What is the nearest (to our home) emergency room or urgent-care center you would send us to?

Analyzing Your Visit. Some issues can be resolved only by analyzing your feelings *after* your visit. Below are some things you and your partner might want to discuss after your visit.

- Are the doctor's philosophies and attitudes acceptable to us, such as use of antibiotics and other medications, child-rearing practices or related religious beliefs?
- Did the doctor listen to us?
- Did he or she seem genuinely interested in our concerns?
- Is the office comfortable, clean and bright?
- Did the office staff seem cordial, open and easy to talk to?

By choosing someone to care for your baby before it's born, you have a chance to take part in deciding who will have that important task. If you don't, the healthcare provider who delivers your baby or hospital personnel will select someone. Another good reason for choosing someone ahead of time is if your baby has complications, you'll at least have met the person who will be treating him or her.

Your Nutrition

You may be having a harder time with your food plan than you had earlier in pregnancy. You may be bored with the food you've been eating. Baby is getting bigger, and you don't seem to have much room for food. Heartburn or indigestion may be more challenging now.

Don't give up on good nutrition! Continue to pay attention to what you eat. Continue to give your baby the best nutrition you can before its birth.

Every day, try to eat one serving of a dark-green leafy vegetable, a serving of food or juice rich in vitamin C, and one serving of a food rich in vitamin A. Many yellow foods, such as yams, carrots and cantaloupes, are good sources of vitamin A. Remember to keep up your fluid intake.

Eat high-fiber foods for good nutrition and to help with constipation. High-fiber foods can also deal with heartburn. And keep the peel on your potatoes! They add fiber, potassium, calcium, vitamin C and vitamin B_6 to your diet. You can even mash cooked potatoes that still have the peel—they're very tasty.

You Should Also Know

How Is Your Baby Presenting?

You probably want to know at what point in your pregnancy your doctor can tell how baby is presenting for delivery. Is the baby's head down, or is the baby breech? At what point will the baby stay in the position it's in?

Usually between 32 and 34 weeks of pregnancy, you can feel baby's head in the lower abdomen below your umbilicus. Some women can feel different parts of the baby earlier than this, but baby's head may not have been hard enough until now to identify it.

Baby's head has a distinct feeling. It's different from the feeling your doctor gets with a breech presentation. A breech baby has a soft, round feeling.

Beginning at 32 to 34 weeks, your doctor may feel your abdomen to determine how baby is lying inside you. This position may change many times during pregnancy.

At 34 to 36 weeks of pregnancy, the baby usually gets into the position it's going to stay in. If you have a breech at 37 weeks, it's possible the baby can still turn to be head-down. But it becomes less likely the closer you get to the end of your pregnancy. (See Week 38 for further discussion.)

Dad Tip

You should also pack for the hospital. Some essential items you might need include magazines, a list of phone numbers, a change of clothes, something to sleep in, a camera, a charged battery, your cell phones and charger, a telephone calling card or lots of change, nonperishable snacks, insurance information, a comfortable pillow and extra cash.

Packing for the Hospital

Packing for the hospital can be unnerving. You don't want to pack too early and have your suitcase staring at you. But you don't want to wait till the last minute, throw your things together and take the chance of forgetting something important.

It's probably a good idea to pack about 3 or 4 weeks before your due date. Pack things you'll need during labor for you and your labor coach, items you and the baby will need after delivery and personal articles for your hospital stay. There are a lot of things to consider, but the list below should cover nearly all of what you might need:

- completed insurance or preregistration forms and insurance card
- heavy socks to wear in the delivery room
- an item to use as a focal point
- 1 cotton nightgown or T-shirt for labor

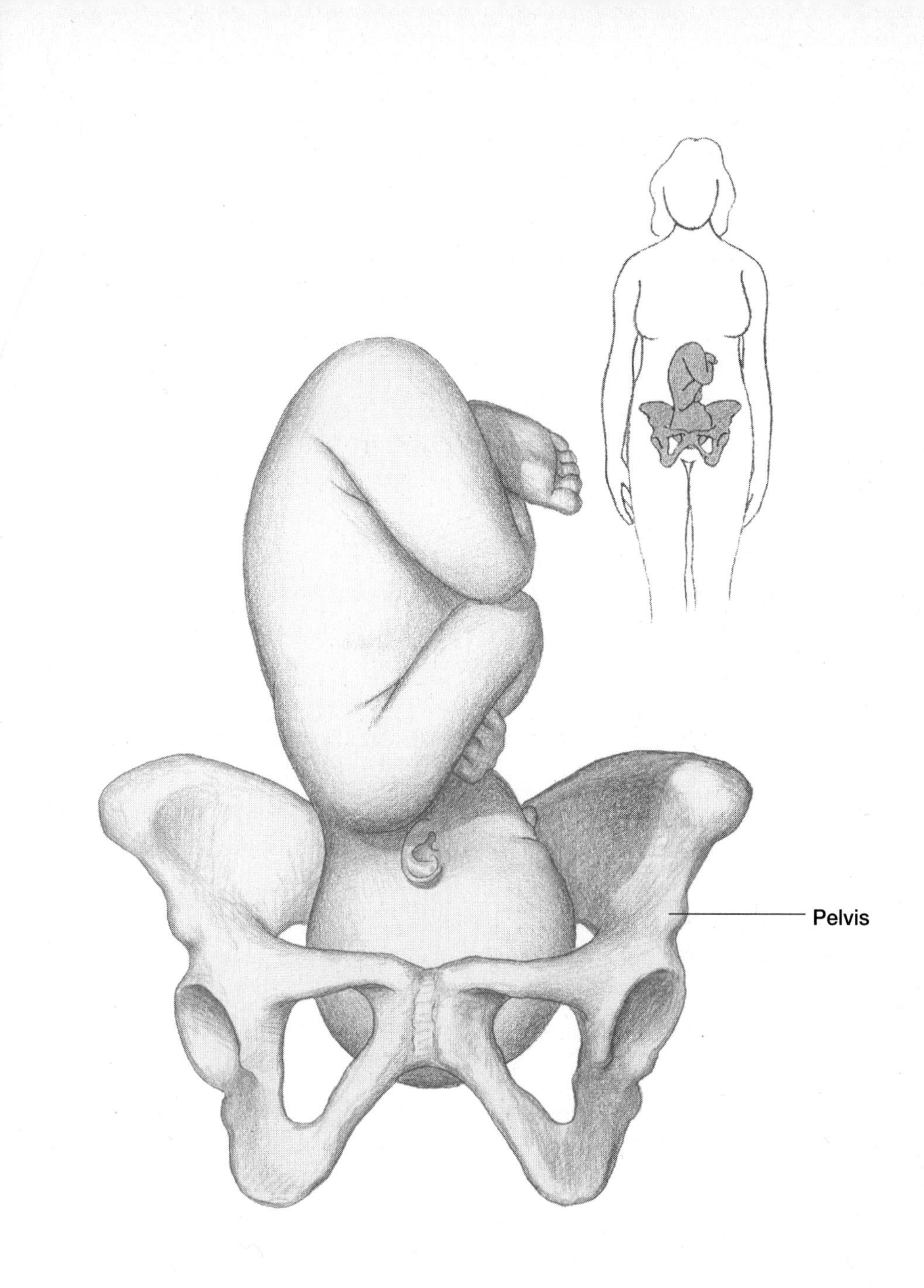

Alignment of baby with head in pelvis before delivery.
This is the preferable presentation.

- lip balm, lollipops or fruit drops, to use during labor
- light diversion, such as books or magazines, to use during labor
- breath spray
- 1 or 2 nightgowns for after labor (bring a nursing gown if you're going to breastfeed)
- slippers with rubber soles
- 1 long robe for walking in the halls
- 2 bras (nursing bras if you breastfeed)
- breast pads for leaking breasts
- 3 pairs of panties
- toiletries you use, including brush, comb, toothbrush, toothpaste, soap, shampoo, conditioner
- hairband or ponytail holder, if you have long hair
- loose-fitting clothes for going home
- sanitary pads, if the hospital doesn't supply them
- glasses, if you wear contacts (you can't wear contacts during labor)

You may also want to bring one or two pieces of fruit to eat after the delivery. Don't pack them too early!

It's a good idea to include some things in your hospital kit for your partner or labor coach to help you both during the birth. You might bring the following:

- a watch with a second hand
- talc or cornstarch for massaging you during labor
- a paint roller or tennis ball for giving you a low-back massage during labor
- tapes or CDs and a player, or a radio to play during labor
- a camera
- list of telephone numbers and a long-distance calling card
- change for vending machines
- snacks for your partner or labor coach

The hospital will probably supply most of what you need for baby, but you should have a few things:

- clothes for the trip home, including an undershirt, sleeper, outer clothes (a hat if it's cold outside)

- a couple of baby blankets
- diapers, if your hospital doesn't supply them

Be sure you have an approved infant car seat for baby's first ride. It's important to put your baby in a car seat the very first time he or she rides in a car! Many hospitals won't let you take your baby home without one.

What You May See in the Delivery Room

You'll see lots of equipment when you enter the labor and/or delivery room. You won't recognize most of it, so we include descriptions of equipment you may encounter.

An electronic vital-signs monitor measures your heart rate and blood pressure with a cuff. It tells doctor how well you and baby are doing. I.V. infusion pumps deliver fluids into your veins if the doctor orders them.

There are many types of birthing beds. In many, the bottom section can be removed, converting the bed into a delivery table. Some beds can also accommodate alternate birthing positions.

An epidural pump delivers pain-relief medication after the epidural catheter is put in place by an anesthesiologist. A vacuum extractor helps baby through the birth canal in some cases. An amniohook looks like a crochet hook; it's used to rupture membranes.

Suction bulbs are used to draw blood and mucus from baby's nose and mouth after birth and in the days after delivery. An infant warmer helps stabilize baby's temperature. An infant scale weighs him or her.

> Women who listen to lyric-free, instrumental music (synthesizer, harp, piano, orchestra or jazz) for 3 hours during early phases of active labor experience less pain and distress. We believe the slow music helps a woman relax and distracts her from her pain.

Fetal Monitoring

A fetal monitor detects baby's heart rate and contractions, and can be used to track baby's response to them. It shows contractions and baby's heartbeat; the readout is seen in the labor room, nurses' station and possibly on your doctor's computer.

Each baby needs to be evaluated individually using fetal monitor tracing and other information about your pregnancy. ACOG recommends the use of three categories to describe the results of fetal monitoring.

- *Category I*—Tracings are normal.
- *Category II*—Tracings are indeterminate; this means they aren't normal, but they aren't absolutely abnormal. They require evaluation, continued surveillance and re-evaluation. Eighty percent of all tracings fall into this category.
- *Category III*—Tracings are abnormal and require prompt evaluation. Elements used to categorize them include fetal heart rate, variability, decelerations and reaction to contractions.

Exercise for Week 36

To help improve your posture, stand or sit on the floor, and clasp your hands behind you. Lift your arms until you feel a good stretch in your upper-chest area and upper arms. Hold for a count of 5, then lower your arms. Repeat 8 times. *Stretches arm and back muscles, and opens upper chest.*

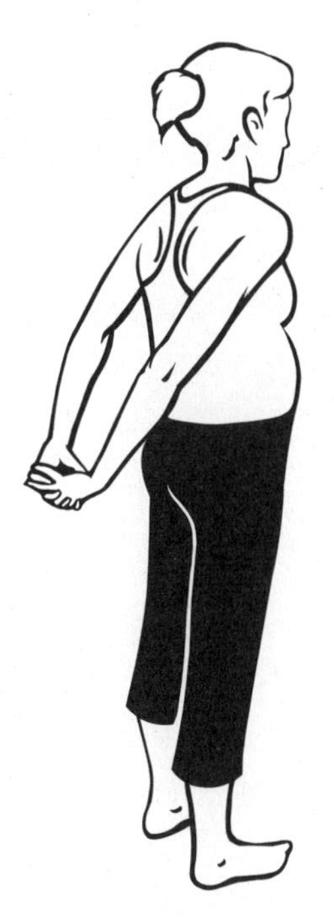

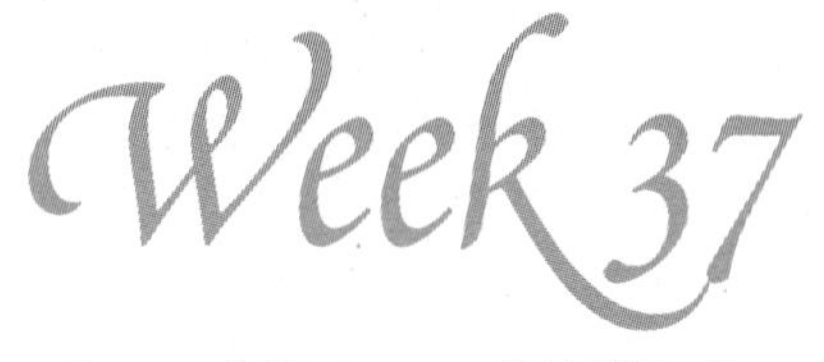

Week 37

Age of Fetus—35 Weeks

How Big Is Your Baby?

Your baby weighs almost 6⅓ pounds (2.8kg). Crown-to-rump length is 14 inches (35cm). Its total length is around 19 inches (48cm).

How Big Are You?

The size of your uterus may not have changed much since your last visit. Measuring from the pubic symphysis, the top of the uterus is about 14¾ inches (37cm). From the bellybutton, it is 6½ to 6¾ inches (16 to 17cm). Your total weight gain by this time should be about as high as it will go at 25 to 35 pounds (11.3 to 15.9kg).

How Your Baby Is Growing and Developing

Your baby continues to grow and to gain weight, even during these last few weeks. A change in pressure on your tummy, such as laying a book there, may cause baby to react by kicking vigorously.

Baby's head is usually directed down into the pelvis around this time. But in about 3% of all pregnancies, the baby's bottom or legs enter the pelvis first, called a *breech presentation,* which we discuss in Week 38.

Changes in You

Pelvic Exam in Late Pregnancy

Your healthcare provider may do a pelvic exam to help evaluate your pregnancy. One of the first things he or she will look for is whether you're leaking amniotic fluid. If you think you are, it's important to tell your healthcare provider.

He or she will examine your birth canal and cervix during the pelvic exam. Think of the birth canal as a tube going from the pelvic girdle down through the pelvis and out the vagina. The baby travels through this tube from the uterus. During labor, the cervix usually becomes softer and thins out. Your cervix may be evaluated for its softness or firmness and the amount of thinning.

Before labor begins, the cervix is thick. When you're in active labor, the cervix thins out; when it is half-thinned, it is "50% effaced." Immediately before delivery, the cervix is "100% effaced" or completely thinned out.

The amount the cervix is open is also important. This is measured in centimeters. The cervix is fully open when the diameter of the cervical opening measures 10cm. The goal is to be a 10! Before labor begins, the cervix may be closed or open a little way, such as 1cm (nearly ½ inch).

You will be checked to see if baby's head, bottom or legs are coming first; this may be referred to as the "presenting part." The shape of your pelvic bones is also noted.

The station is then determined. Station describes the degree to which the presenting part of the baby has descended into the birth canal. If the baby's head is at a -2 station, it means the head is higher inside you than if it were at a +2 station. The 0 point is a bony landmark in the pelvis, the starting place of the birth canal.

Your healthcare provider may describe your situation in medical terms. You might hear you are "2cm, 50% and a -2 station." This means the cervix is open 2cm (about 1 inch), it is halfway thinned out (50% effaced) and the presenting part (baby's head, feet or buttocks) is at a -2 station.

Write down this important information. It's helpful to know when you go to the hospital and are checked there. You can tell the medical personnel what your dilatation and effacement were at your last checkup so they can know if your situation has changed.

How Your Actions Affect Your Baby's Development

Cesarean Delivery

Most women plan on a vaginal birth, but a Cesarean delivery is always a possibility. With a Cesarean, the baby is delivered through an incision made in the mother's abdominal wall and uterus. An *emergency Cesarean delivery* is one that is unplanned. An *elective Cesarean delivery* is planned and done without a medical reason.

The illustration on page 525 shows a Cesarean delivery. Common names for this type of surgery are *C-section, Cesarean section* and *Cesarean delivery.*

The main advantage to having a Cesarean delivery is delivery of a healthy infant. A Cesarean may be the safest way for your baby to be born. The disadvantage is Cesarean delivery is a major operation and carries with it all the risks of surgery.

It would be nice to know you're going to need a Cesarean so you wouldn't have to go through labor. Unfortunately, you don't know ahead of time if you will have problems.

Some women believe if they have a Cesarean, "it won't be like having a baby." They falsely believe they won't experience the birth process. That's not true. If you have a Cesarean delivery, try not to feel this way. You haven't failed in any way!

It may be difficult at times to tell the exact location of different parts of the baby. You may have a good idea according to where you feel kicks and punches. Ask your doctor to show you on your tummy how the baby is lying. Some doctors will take a marking pen and draw on your stomach to show you how baby is lying. You can leave it so you can later show your partner how baby was lying when you were seen in the office that day.

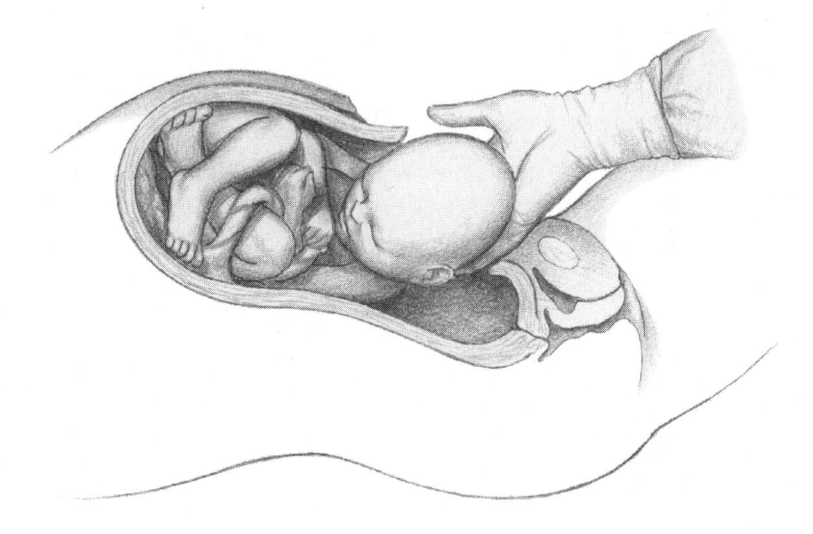

Delivery of a baby by Cesarean section.

Remember, having a baby has taken 9 long months. Even with a Cesarean delivery, you have accomplished an amazing feat.

Reasons for Cesareans. Cesareans are done for many reasons. They are often performed when there's a problem during labor. The most common reason for having one is a previous Cesarean delivery. Nine out of 10 women who have had a previous Cesarean delivery choose a repeat Cesarean for the next birth.

Some women who have had Cesareans may be able to have a vaginal delivery with later pregnancies; this is called *vaginal birth after Cesarean* (VBAC). See the discussion that begins on page 530. Doctors are doing fewer VBACs because of concerns for the safety of the mother and baby when a woman labors after a previous Cesarean.

Nonmedical factors for having a Cesarean include maternal choice, more conservative practice guidelines and legal pressures. If you're exhausted when you begin labor, you may also be at a higher risk for a Cesarean section. Pre-eclampsia or an active herpes sore may require a Cesarean delivery.

A Cesarean may be necessary if your baby is too big to fit through the birth canal, called *cephalo-pelvic disproportion (CPD).* CPD may be suspected during pregnancy, but usually labor must begin before it can be confirmed. A Cesarean may be recommended if an ultrasound shows your baby is very large—9½ pounds or larger—and may not be easily delivered vaginally.

It's possible for you to dilate during labor without the baby moving down through the pelvis. When baby's head is too large to fit through the birth canal, it results in *failure to progress.* This situation is one of the most common reasons for a Cesarean delivery.

Fetal stress is an important reason a Cesarean delivery may be performed. The fetal heartbeat and its response to labor is often monitored. If the heartbeat indicates baby is having trouble with labor contractions, a Cesarean may be necessary.

If the umbilical cord is compressed, a Cesarean may be necessary. The cord may come into the vagina ahead of the baby's head or the baby can press on part of the cord. This is a dangerous because a compressed cord can cut off baby's blood supply.

A Cesarean may be needed if you're older. The Cesarean-delivery rate for mothers between 40 and 54 years old is more than double the rate for women younger than age 20.

A Cesarean is often necessary if baby is in a breech presentation, which means baby's feet or buttocks enter the birth canal first. Delivering the shoulders and the head after baby's body may damage the baby's head or neck, especially with a first baby.

> If complications arise during pregnancy or while you're in labor, your CNM, NP or PA will consult a physician specializing in pregnancy.

Placental abruption or placenta previa are also reasons for a Cesarean delivery. If the placenta separates from the uterus before delivery (placental abruption), the baby loses its supply of oxygen and nutrients. This is usually diagnosed when a woman has heavy vaginal bleeding. If the placenta blocks the birth canal (placenta previa), the baby can't be delivered any other way.

A Cesarean delivery for a first baby increases a woman's chances for placenta previa or placental abruption in her next pregnancies. A repeat Cesarean increases a woman's risk of placenta accreta in subsequent pregnancies if the placenta implants low in the uterus and grows into the area of the previous Cesarean-delivery incision.

Rising Rate of Cesarean Deliveries. In 1965, only 4% of all deliveries were by C-section. Between 1996 and 2007, there was a 71% increase in Cesarean births. In 2007, 32% of all live births in the United States were Cesarean deliveries (more than 1.2 million); in 2008 that number rose to 32.3%. Today in the United States, Cesarean deliveries account for over 30% of all deliveries. In some areas, this percentage is even higher.

The rising rate is related in part to closer monitoring during labor and safer procedures for Cesarean deliveries. Part of the increase can also be attributed to the increase in multiple births, but the Cesarean rate actually increased more for singletons than for multiples.

Babies delivered by a scheduled Cesarean delivery between 37 and 39 weeks have more respiratory problems than babies born vaginally or by emergency Cesarean at the same point in pregnancy. It's believed hormones released during labor help baby deal with fluid in the lungs. The compressions of the baby's chest from labor are also believed to help clear amniotic fluid from baby's lungs.

Elective Cesarean Deliveries. Part of the increase in Cesarean deliveries in the United States is due to *Cesarean delivery on maternal request (CDMR).* It is also called *patient-requested Cesarean.*

There are many reasons for choosing a Cesarean delivery, including fear of labor, concern over vaginal tearing and worry about incontinence later. Some women believe a Cesarean will help them retain their prepregnancy figure; however it's pregnancy, not giving birth, that stretches the waistline. Other women believe a Cesarean is safer for baby.

In some parts of the world, elective Cesarean delivery is not a big issue. In many Latin American countries, the rate of elective Cesareans is 40 to 50%. One survey conducted in Brazil showed private hospitals, where the wealthiest patients go, had an 80 to 90% rate of elective Cesareans.

U.S. doctors are split on the question of elective Cesarean delivery. There's evidence supporting both sides. Some believe with improved anesthesia, antibiotics, infection control and pain management, a Cesarean is no riskier than vaginal delivery. However, ACOG, the federal government, the American College of Nurse-Midwives and Lamaze International believe we should look more closely at the present Cesarean-delivery rate.

The point in pregnancy when a Cesarean is scheduled is also important. It's amazing how much difference a few days can make to the health of your baby. The latest recommendations are that a woman *not* schedule a Cesarean delivery any earlier than 39 weeks, unless tests show the baby's lungs are mature. Research shows a baby will do better if he or she is born within 7 days of its due date. If a baby is delivered earlier than this, he or she may have more problems. When compared with babies delivered at 37 or 38 weeks, those born at 39 weeks or more had significantly *lower* rates of problems.

How Is a Cesarean Delivery Performed? If problems arise during pregnancy and/or labor, if your care has been provided by a CNM, PA or NP, he or she may consult a physician. In most areas, an obstetrician performs a Cesarean. In small communities, a general surgeon or a family practitioner may perform Cesarean deliveries.

If you're scheduled to have a Cesarean, follow directions for eating before surgery. You are often awake when a Cesarean is done. If you are, you may be able to see your baby immediately after delivery!

You're first visited by the anesthesiologist to discuss pain-relief methods. Up to 90% of all elective Cesarean deliveries are done with spinal anesthesia.

After you receive anesthesia, your doctor begins by making a 5- to 6-inch incision in the area above your pubic bone. A cut is made through tissue down to the uterus, where a horizontal incision is made into the lower part of the uterus. After all the incisions are made, the doctor reaches into the uterus and removes the baby, then the placenta. Each layer is sewn together with absorbable sutures; the entire procedure takes 30 minutes to an hour.

In the past, a Cesarean was often done with a classical incision, in which the uterus was cut down the midline. This incision doesn't heal as well because it is made in the muscular part of the uterus. It's more likely to pull apart with contractions (as in a vaginal birth after Cesarean). This can cause heavy bleeding and injure the baby. If you have had a classical Cesarean section in the past, you *must* have a Cesarean delivery every time you have a baby.

Today, most Cesarean deliveries are *low-cervical* Cesareans or *low-transverse* Cesareans. This means the incision is made low in the uterus. Or a T-incision may be used. It goes across and up the uterus in the shape of an inverted T. It provides more room to get baby out. If you have a T-incision, you may need a Cesarean delivery with all subsequent pregnancies because it may be more likely to rupture.

After Your Cesarean Delivery. If you're awake for baby's birth, you may be able to hold him or her immediately. You may also have a chance to begin nursing.

You may need pain relief for the incision. One device to help deal with the pain after a Cesarean is *ON-Q*. A small catheter is inserted underneath the skin, which sends a local painkiller to the *incision* area of the Cesarean so very little, if any, medication gets to baby through your breast milk. Studies show moms who receive ON-Q after a Cesarean are able to get out of bed and walk around more quickly, and their hospital stays are shorter. Ask your doctor about it at one of your prenatal visits.

You'll probably stay in the hospital 2 to 4 days. Recovery at home from a Cesarean delivery takes longer than recovery from a vaginal delivery. The normal time for full recovery is usually 4 to 6 weeks.

Vaginal Birth after Cesarean (VBAC)

Should you attempt a vaginal delivery after having had a Cesarean delivery? Medically speaking, the method of delivery isn't as important as the well-being of you and your baby. Before any final decision is made, weigh the risks and benefits. In some cases, there may not be any choice in the matter. In other cases, you and your doctor may decide to let you labor for a while to see if you can deliver vaginally.

> If a woman has a Cesarean delivery, she is at increased risk for postpartum depression.

Some women like having a repeat Cesarean delivery because they don't want to go through labor only to end up with a Cesarean delivery. You may need another Cesarean if you have had problems with this pregnancy. Discuss it with your doctor if you have questions.

If you are small and the baby is large, you may need another Cesarean. Multiple fetuses may make vaginal delivery difficult or impossible without danger to the babies.

Inducing labor with a VBAC may be necessary; however, there's an increased risk of the uterine scar from an earlier Cesarean stretching and pulling apart with induction. This is especially true if hormones are used to ripen the cervix and/or induce labor. It is believed that contractions may be too strong for a uterus scarred by previous surgery. A repeat Cesarean may be advised to avoid rupturing the uterus.

Risk also increases for a woman who gets pregnant within 9 months of having a previous Cesarean. In this case, the uterus is more likely to rupture during a vaginal delivery. Researchers believe this might occur because it can take from 6 to 9 months for the uterine scar to heal (this is the scar on the uterus—not your abdomen). Until enough healing time has passed, the uterus may not be strong enough to stand up to the stress of a vaginal delivery. VBACs are safest when at least 18 months have passed between the previous Cesarean and the attempted vaginal delivery.

Advantages of VBAC include a decreased risk of problems associated with surgery, which a Cesarean is. Recovery after a vaginal delivery is shorter. You can be up and about in the hospital and at home in a much shorter amount of time.

If you want to try VBAC, discuss it with your doctor in advance so plans can be made. Not all hospitals are equipped for VBAC. During labor, you will probably be monitored more closely. You may be attached to I.V.s, in case a Cesarean delivery becomes necessary.

Tip for Week 37

Be prepared for delivery with bags packed, insurance papers filled out and available, and other important details taken care of.

Consider the benefits and risks in deciding whether to attempt a vaginal delivery after a previous Cesarean delivery. Discuss them at length with your doctor and your partner before making a final decision. Don't be afraid to ask your doctor his or her opinion of your chances for a successful vaginal delivery. He or she knows your health and pregnancy history.

Your Nutrition

You and your partner have been invited to a big party. You've been careful about your nutrition, and your pregnancy is almost over. Should you let yourself go, and eat and drink whatever you want? Probably not.

Maintain your good eating habits. You *can* party healthfully. Before you go, eat or drink something to take the edge off your appetite. It may be easier to avoid high-fat, high-calorie foods if you're not ravenous.

At the party, eat food when it's fresh or hot—at the beginning of the party. As the party goes on, the food may not be chilled or heated enough to prevent bacteria from growing. So eat early or when dishes are refilled.

Avoid alcohol. Drink fruit juice "spiked" with ginger ale or lemon-lime soda. If it's the holiday season and they're serving eggnog, have a glass if it's pasteurized and alcohol-free.

Raw fruits and vegetables can be satisfying. Avoid raw seafood, raw meat and soft cheeses, such as Brie, Camembert and feta. They may contain listeriosis.

Stay away from the refreshment table if you can't resist the goodies. It may feel better to sit down (away from food), relax and talk with friends.

You Should Also Know

Will You Have an Enema?

Will you be required to have an enema when you arrive at labor and delivery? An *enema* is a procedure in which fluid is injected into the rectum to clear out the bowel. An enema before labor can make the birth of your baby more pleasant for you. When the baby's head comes out through the birth canal, anything in the rectum also comes out. An enema decreases the amount of contamination from feces during labor and at the time of delivery, which may also help prevent infection.

Most hospitals offer an enema at the beginning of labor, but it's not always mandatory. There are certain advantages to having one early in labor. You may not want to have a bowel movement soon after your

Dad Tip

You may not understand how nervous your partner may be about getting in touch with you when she needs you. Be sure to let her know how she can reach you at work or when you're out. Keep your cell phone or a beeper with you all the time. This can comfort her and provide her with peace of mind.

baby's birth because of discomfort. Having an enema before labor can prevent this discomfort.

For a discussion of depression after pregnancy—Postpartum Distress Syndrome—see Appendix F, page 616.

Ask your doctor if an enema is routine or considered helpful. Tell him or her you'd like to know about the benefits of an enema and the reasons for giving one. It isn't required by all doctors or all hospitals.

What Is Back Labor?

Some women experience back labor. *Back labor* refers to a baby coming through the birth canal looking straight up. With this type of labor, you will probably experience lower-back pain. Back labor can also last longer.

The mechanics of labor work better if baby is looking down at the ground so it can extend its head as it comes out through the birth canal. If the baby can't extend its head, its chin points toward its chest, which may cause pain in your lower back during labor. Your doctor may need to rotate the baby so it comes out looking down at the ground rather than up at the sky.

Will Your Doctor Use a Vacuum Extractor or Forceps?

The goal with every birth is to deliver a baby as safely as possible. Sometimes baby needs a little help. Your doctor may use a vacuum extractor or forceps to help safely deliver baby. Vacuum and forceps delivery methods each have about the same risks. Use of either is associated with a more frequent need for mechanical ventilation in infants and with more 3rd- and 4th-degree perineal tears.

Vacuum extractors are used more today than forceps. There are several types of vacuum extractors. Some have a plastic cup that fits on baby's head by suction. Another type has a metal cup that fits on baby's head. The doctor attaches the cup to baby's head and gently pulls on it to deliver baby's head and body.

Forceps is a metal instrument used to deliver babies; it looks like two large metal hands. Use of forceps has decreased in recent years. If a lot of traction with forceps is needed to deliver baby, a Cesarean may be a better choice. Cesarean deliveries are also used more often to deliver a baby that is high up in the pelvis.

If the possible use of a vacuum extractor or forceps causes you concern, discuss it with your healthcare provider. It's important to discuss issues that may come up during labor and delivery so you can communicate your concerns.

If your baby is born this week, you may not finish reading this book. However, you may be interested in reading an excerpt from our baby book, *Your Baby's First Year, Week by Week*, which begins on page 637.

The book covers your baby's first year of life in a weekly format, similar to *Your Pregnancy Week by Week*. Information in the excerpt relates to the first week of your baby's life–we hope you find it helpful.

Exercise for Week 37

Sit on a chair or on the floor in a crossed-leg position. Inhale, and slowly tilt your head to the right until you feel a stretch in your neck. Breathe deeply 3 times while holding the stretch. Slowly bring your head to the center, then tilt your head to the left. Hold while you breathe deeply 3 times. Do 4 times on each side. *Helps stretch the neck, and relieves neck and shoulder tension.*

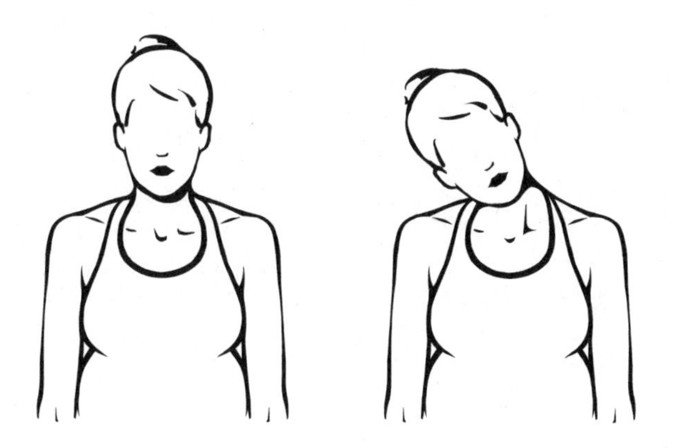

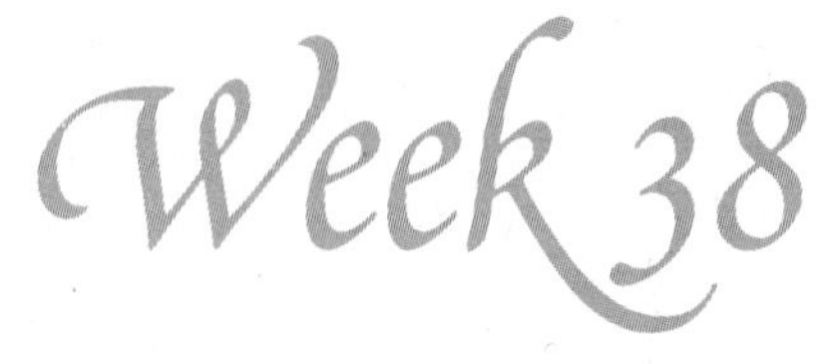

Week 38

Age of Fetus—36 Weeks

How Big Is Your Baby?

At this time, your baby weighs about 6¾ pounds (3.1kg). Crown-to-rump length is still about 14 inches (35cm). Total length is around 19⅔ inches (49.5cm).

How Big Are You?

Many women feel uncomfortable during the last weeks of pregnancy because their uterus is so large. It's about 14½ to 15¼ inches (36 to 38cm) between your uterus and the pubic symphysis. From your bellybutton to the top of your uterus is about 6½ to 7¼ inches (16 to 18cm).

How Your Baby Is Growing and Developing

Specific cells in the lungs produce chemicals needed for breathing immediately after birth. An important factor is the chemical *surfactant.* A baby born before its lungs are mature may not have surfactant in its lungs. It can be introduced directly into a newborn's lungs and baby can use it immediately. Many premature babies who receive surfactant do not have to be put on respirators—they can breathe on their own!

Changes in You

Tests You May Have during Labor

If you think you may be in labor and go to the hospital, you will have a *labor check*. Vital signs will be taken, a monitor will be placed on your abdomen and a pelvic exam will be done. Tests are done to find out if you're in labor and if your pregnancy is doing OK. If you're not in labor, you'll be given advice and sent home. Instructions may include precautions and warning signs. No one wants to be sent home, but don't fret. You'll be back soon.

Fetal blood sampling is one way to measure how well a baby can stand the stress of labor. Before the test can be performed, your water must have broken, and the cervix must be dilated at least 2cm (about an inch). An instrument is placed into the vagina, through the dilated cervix, to the top of the baby's head and makes a small nick in baby's scalp. Baby's blood is collected in a small tube, and acidity is checked. This signals whether baby is having any trouble or is under stress and helps your healthcare team decide whether labor can continue or if a Cesarean delivery is needed.

In many hospitals, a baby's heartbeat is monitored with *external fetal monitoring* or *internal fetal monitoring*. External fetal monitoring can be done before your water breaks. A pair of belts is strapped to your tummy. One strap holds a device that monitors baby's heart rate, the other holds a device to measure the length of contractions and how often they occur.

Internal fetal monitoring monitors the baby more precisely. An electrode, called a *scalp electrode,* is placed through the vagina and attached to baby's scalp to measure its heart rate. A thin tube is used inside the uterus to monitor the strength of the contractions. This is done only after membranes have ruptured. It may be a little uncomfortable, but it's not painful.

Information is recorded on a strip of paper; results can usually be seen in your room and at the nurses' station. In some places, your healthcare provider can check results on his or her computer.

In most cases, while you're being monitored, you must stay in bed. In some places, wireless monitors are available so you can move around.

How Your Actions Affect Your Baby's Development

Breech and Other Abnormal Presentations

It's common for a baby to be in the breech presentation early in pregnancy. However, when labor starts, only 3 to 5% of all babies, not including multiple pregnancies, are a breech or other abnormal presentation.

Certain factors can make a breech presentation more likely. One of the main causes is a baby's prematurity. Near the end of the second trimester, a baby may be in a breech presentation. By taking care of yourself, you may avoid going into premature labor, which gives baby the best opportunity to change its position naturally.

Although we don't always know why a baby is in the breech presentation, we know breech births occur more often when:

- you have had more than one pregnancy
- you're carrying twins, triplets or more
- there is too much or too little amniotic fluid
- the uterus is abnormally shaped
- you have abnormal uterine growths, such as fibroids
- you have placenta previa
- your baby has hydrocephalus

New research shows a breech position may be inherited from either the mom-to-be *or* the dad-to-be. Both men and women who were delivered in a breech presentation have more than twice the risk of having their firstborn child in a breech presentation at the time of birth.

There are different kinds of breech presentations. A *frank breech* occurs when the legs are flexed at the hips and extended at the knees. This is the

Tip for Week 38

If baby may be in a breech presentation, your healthcare provider may order an ultrasound to confirm it. It helps determine how baby is lying in your uterus.

most common type of breech found at term or the end of pregnancy; feet are up by the face or head. With a *complete breech presentation*, one or both knees are flexed, not extended. See the illustration on page 541.

Other unusual presentations are also possible. One is a *face presentation*. The baby's head is hyperextended so the face comes into the birth canal first. This type of presentation may need to be delivered by Cesarean delivery.

In a *shoulder presentation*, the shoulder presents first. In a *transverse lie*, the baby is lying almost as if in a cradle in the pelvis. The baby's head is on one side of your abdomen, and its bottom is on the other side. The only way to deliver these types of presentation is by Cesarean delivery.

Studies show 30% of all abnormal presentations aren't detected before labor begins; your risk increases if you're overweight. Your healthcare provider may order a fetal ultrasound to check your baby's position toward the end of pregnancy if you're overweight.

Delivering a Breech Baby. If your baby is breech when labor begins, the chance of problems increases. This has led to debate over the best way of delivering a breech baby. For many years, breech deliveries were done vaginally. Then it was believed the safest method was by Cesarean, especially with a first baby. Today, experts believe a baby in the breech position can probably be delivered more safely by Cesarean delivery before labor begins or during early labor.

Some experts believe a woman can deliver a breech presentation if the situation is right. This usually includes a frank breech in a mature baby if the woman has had previous normal deliveries. Most agree a *footling breech presentation* (one leg extended, one knee flexed) should be delivered by Cesarean delivery.

If your baby is in an abnormal presentation, your healthcare provider may suggest you get on your hands and knees, with your hips above your heart, then lower yourself onto your forearms. This position may help baby turn into a head-down position.

If you know baby is breech, tell them when you get to the hospital. If you call with a question about labor and have a breech presentation, mention it to the person you talk with.

If your baby is born this week, you may not finish reading this book. However, you may be interested in reading an excerpt from our baby book, *Your Baby's First Year, Week by Week*, which begins on page 637.

The book covers your baby's first year of life in a weekly format, similar to *Your Pregnancy Week by Week*. Information in the excerpt relates to the first week of your baby's life–we hope you find it helpful.

Turning a Breech Baby. Attempts may be made to turn the baby from a breech to a head-down (vertex) position before your water breaks, before labor begins or in early labor. Using his or her hands, the healthcare provider turns baby into the head-down birth position. This is called *external cephalic version (ECV)* or just *version*.

Problems can occur with ECV; it's important to know about them. Talk with your physician about whether this procedure is an option for you. Possible risks include:

- rupture of membranes
- placental abruption
- affect on baby's heart rate
- onset of labor

More than 50% of the time, turning baby is successful. However, some stubborn babies shift again into a breech presentation. ECV may be tried again, but version is harder to perform as your delivery date draws closer.

Your Nutrition

You may not feel much like eating now, but it's important to eat healthfully. Snacks might be the answer—eat small snacks throughout the day to keep your energy levels up and to help avoid heartburn. You may also be tired of the foods you've been eating. The list below offers some smart snacks for your healthy nutrition:

- bananas, raisins, dried fruit and mangoes to satisfy your sweet tooth and to provide you with iron, potassium and magnesium
- string cheese; it's high in calcium and protein
- fruit shakes made with skim milk and yogurt, ice milk or ice cream for calcium, vitamins and minerals

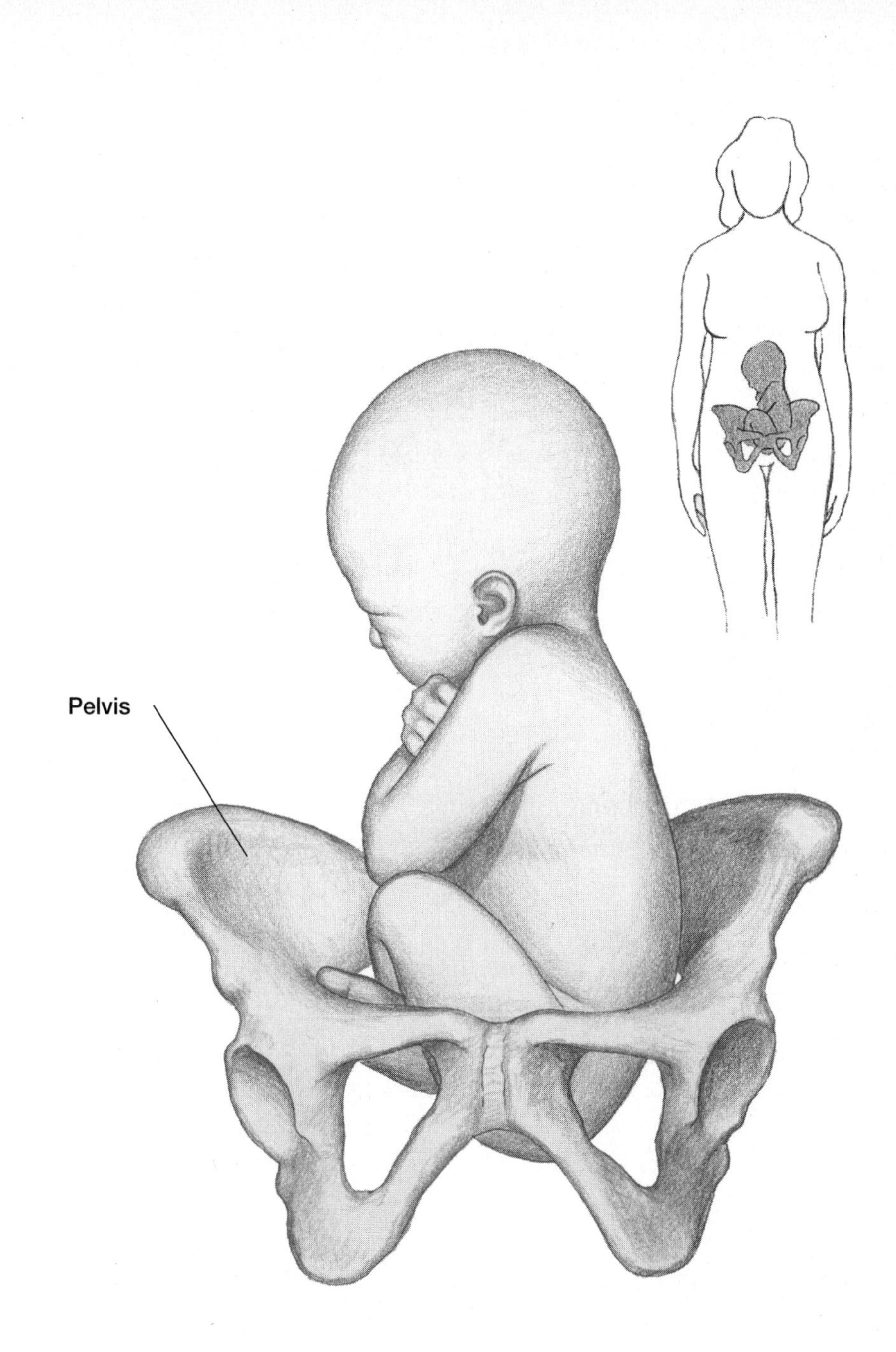

Baby aligned in the pelvis bottom first, with knees flexed, is called a *complete breech presentation.*

- high-fiber crackers, spread with a little peanut butter for taste and protein
- cottage cheese and fruit, flavored with a little sugar and some cinnamon, for tasty milk and fruit servings
- salt-free chips or tortillas with salsa or bean dip for fiber and good taste
- hummus and pita slices for fiber and good taste
- fresh tomatoes, flavored with some olive oil and fresh basil; eat with a few thin slices of Parmesan cheese for a vegetable serving and dairy serving
- chicken or tuna salad (made from fresh chicken or tuna packed in water) and crackers or tortilla pieces for protein and fiber

You Should Also Know

What Is a Retained Placenta?

The placenta is usually delivered within 30 minutes after baby's birth; it's a routine part of delivery. In some cases, a piece of placenta remains inside the uterus and doesn't deliver on its own. This is called a *retained placenta.* When it occurs, the uterus can't contract enough, resulting in vaginal bleeding that can be heavy.

A retained placenta can occur for many reasons. A placenta may attach over a previous Cesarean-section scar or other scars on the uterus. Some experts are concerned the increasing Cesarean-delivery rate may result in more placental problems. The placenta may also attach over an area that was scraped or over an area of the uterus that was infected at one time.

When the placenta doesn't separate from the uterine wall, it

Grandma's Remedy

If you want to avoid using medication, try a folk remedy. If you have a stomachache, drink a 4-ounce glass of warm water to which you've added 1 teaspoon of baking soda.

can be serious. However, it's rare. Bleeding is usually severe after delivery, and surgery may be necessary to stop it. An attempt may be made to remove the placenta by D&C.

The medical term *abnormal placentation* is used to describe placenta accreta, percreta and increta, in which the placenta grows through the uterine wall, resulting in a retained placenta. Serious bleeding can result.

Your healthcare provider will pay attention to the delivery of your placenta while you're paying attention to your baby. Some people ask to see the placenta after delivery; you may wish to have your healthcare provider show it to you.

Will You Need to Be Shaved?

Many women want to know if they have to have their pubic hair shaved before birth. It's not a requirement; many women are not shaved today. However, some women who chose not to have their pubic hair shaved later said it hurt a lot when their pubic hair became tangled in their underwear due to the normal vaginal discharge after birth. You might want to think about this and discuss it with your healthcare provider.

Dad Tip

Ask your partner if there are things she'd like you to bring to the hospital for her, such as an iPod or special CDs and a CD player. Have things ready. If you take a tour of the hospital or birthing center, you might get other ideas. Discuss your role in labor and delivery with her; learn what you can do to help her. You may be able to help maintain privacy. When people visit during labor or after baby's birth, be sure they don't get too loud or it doesn't get crowded. Let your partner rest and recover; be her knight in shining armor.

Exercise for Week 38

Stand with your feet shoulder-width apart and your knees soft, with your arms by your side. Hold your tummy in. Using light weights (2 to 3 pounds each to start; if you don't have weights, use a 16-ounce can), keep your hands by your hips, your head up and back straight. Inhale as you squat about 6 inches; hold for 5 seconds. Exhale as you squeeze your buttocks muscles and return to the standing position. Repeat 8 times. *Strengthens quadriceps.*

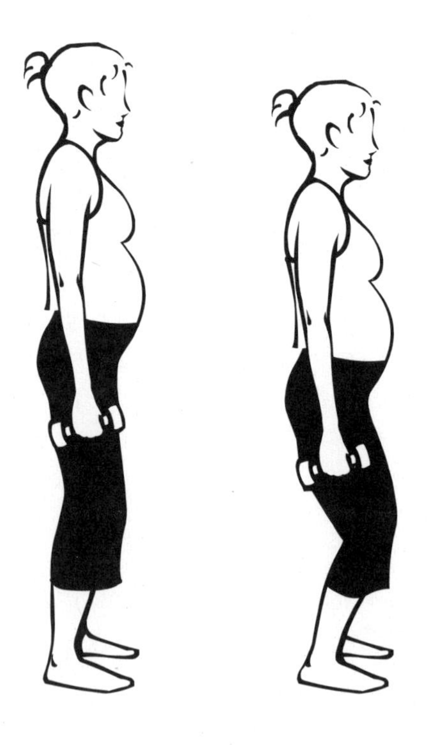

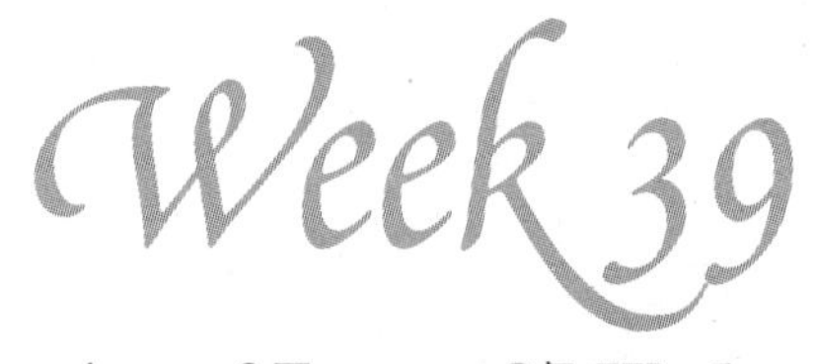

Week 39

Age of Fetus—37 Weeks

How Big Is Your Baby?

Your baby weighs about 7¼ pounds (3.3kg). Crown-to-rump length is about 14½ inches (36cm). The baby's total length is close to 20 inches (50.5cm).

How Big Are You?

The illustration on page 547 shows a side view of a woman's uterus with baby inside it. She's about as big as she can get. You probably are, too! Your weight should remain between 25 and 35 pounds (11.4 and 15.9kg) gained until delivery.

If you measure from the pubic symphysis to the top of the uterus, the distance is 14½ to 16 inches (36 to 40cm). Measuring from the belly-button, the distance is about 6½ to 8 inches (16 to 20cm).

How Your Baby Is Growing and Developing

Your baby continues to gain weight. It doesn't have much room to move. All the organ systems are developed. The last organ to mature is the lungs.

Can Your Baby Get Tangled in the Cord?

You may have been told by friends not to raise your arms over your head or to reach high to get things because it may cause the cord to wrap around the baby's neck. There doesn't seem to be much truth to this old wives' tale.

The term *nuchal cord* refers to an umbilical cord wrapped around a baby's neck. It occurs in nearly 25% of all births. Nothing you do during pregnancy causes or prevents this from happening. A tangled umbilical cord isn't necessarily a problem during labor. It only becomes a problem if the cord is stretched tight around the baby's neck or is in a knot. The good news is this situation is not always dangerous for baby.

Changes in You

It would be unusual for you *not* to be uncomfortable and feel huge at this time. Your uterus fills your pelvis and most of your abdomen. It has pushed everything else out of the way. By this time, you may want baby to be born because you're so uncomfortable.

How Your Actions Affect Your Baby's Development

Feeding Your Baby

Feeding your baby is one of the most important tasks you will perform. The nutrition you give your baby *now* will have an effect on the rest of his life. You want to give your baby the best start nutritionally that you can. If you any have questions, discuss them with your healthcare provider.

ACOG discourages elective delivery of a baby before the 39th week of pregnancy. The best time to deliver is between 39 weeks and one day before you reach 41 weeks.

You may decide to breastfeed baby; it may be the best nutrition you can give him. The baby receives more than just breast milk from you. He will also receive important nutrients, antibodies to help prevent infections and other important substances for growth and development. However, you may choose not to breastfeed—if you bottle-feed, you can still provide good nutrition for your baby.

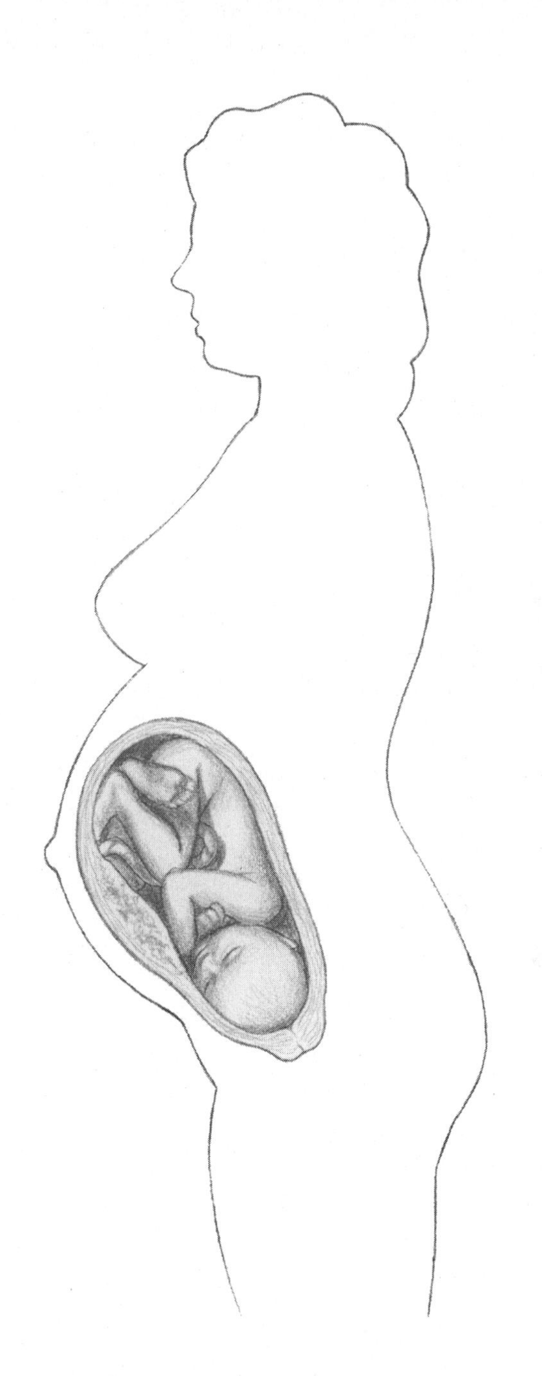

Comparative size of the uterus at 39 weeks of pregnancy (fetal age—37 weeks) with a baby that is close to full term.

In Appendix B, page 596, and Appendix C, page 604, we discuss breastfeeding and bottlefeeding. Read each section, make a list of questions about both types of feeding and talk them over with your healthcare provider at a prenatal visit.

Your Nutrition

If you're going to breastfeed, you need to begin thinking about your nutrition for the time you will nurse. It's important because it can affect the quality of your milk. You may have to avoid some foods because they can pass into breast milk and cause your baby stomach distress. And you'll need to continue to drink lots of fluids.

Keep up your calcium intake. Ask your healthcare provider about any vitamins you should take. For a discussion of nutrition during breastfeeding, see Appendix B.

If you choose to bottlefeed, you have a few more options. However, it's still important to follow a nutritious eating plan. You may need fewer calories, but don't drastically cut your calories in the hopes of losing weight quickly. You need good energy levels. Keep up your fluid intake. For a discussion of your nutrition if you bottlefeed, see Appendix C.

You Should Also Know

Pain Relief during Labor

Your uterus has to contract a lot so your baby can be born. Labor can be painful. Unfortunately, you won't have any idea what your labor is going to be like until it begins. When you're afraid of the pain you expect during labor and delivery, you tense up, which can make it worse. Listen to your body, and do what's necessary to get through labor and delivery. If you choose anesthesia, studies show it can speed up labor because you're more relaxed. Another study suggests anesthesia in early labor does *not* increase the Cesarean-delivery rate.

Labor-pain relief is approached in many ways. When you use medication, there are two patients to consider—you and your unborn baby. Find out in advance what options are available for pain control, then see how your labor goes before making a final decision.

Dad Tip

Who do you and your partner want in the delivery room? Having a baby is a personal experience. Some couples choose the intimacy and privacy of being alone during the birth. Other couples want family members and friends to share the experience with them. If you talk about it ahead of time, you can decide together what you both want. After all, it's your baby's birth.

Anesthesia is a complete block of all pain sensations and muscle movement. An *analgesic* is full or partial relief of pain. Narcotic analgesics pass to your baby through the placenta and may decrease respiratory function in a newborn. They can also affect baby's Apgar scores. These medications should not be given close to the time of delivery.

Anesthesia for delivery may be given as an injection of a particular medication to affect a particular area of the body. This is called a *block,* such as a *pudendal block*, an *epidural block* or a *cervical block*. Medication is similar to the type used to block pain when you have a tooth filled. The agents are xylocaine or xylocainelike medications.

Occasionally, it's necessary to use general anesthesia for delivery, usually for an emergency Cesarean delivery. A pediatrician attends the birth because the baby may be asleep following delivery.

What Is an Epidural Block?

An epidural block provides excellent relief by blocking painful sensations between the uterus and cervix, and your brain. Medication in the epidural prevents pain messages from traveling up your spinal cord to your brain.

Focusing on your breathing can help you stay relaxed during labor.

An epidural is one of the most popular anesthetics today and provides relief from the pain of uterine contractions and delivery. It should be administered only by someone trained and experienced in this type of anesthesia. Some obstetricians have this experience, but in most areas an anesthesiologist or nurse anesthetist administers it.

In 1986, only 10% of women in labor in the United States received an epidural. Today, over 70% of women in labor have an epidural.

While you are sitting up or lying on your side, an area of skin over your lower back in the middle of your spinal cord is numbed. A needle is placed through the numbed skin; anesthetic flows through the needle and around the spinal cord but not into the spinal canal. A catheter is left in place to deliver anesthesia. It can take up to 25 minutes before you experience pain relief.

Epidural pain medication may be delivered by a pump. The pump injects a small amount of medicine at regular intervals or as needed. Many hospitals use patient-controlled epidurals (PCEA)—you press a button for more medication when you need it.

On the average, epidurals slow labor by 45 minutes.

You may have heard various things about when an epidural can be given. Most healthcare providers believe an epidural block should be given based on your level of pain. Most agree a woman can have an epidural anytime after she begins active labor. You may not be required to be dilated to a specific point before getting an epidural.

Some medical conditions may keep you from having an epidural, such as a serious infection when you begin labor, scoliosis, previous back surgery or some blood-clotting problems. If you have one of these problems, discuss it at a prenatal visit.

You may have problems pushing if you have an epidural. But you should be able to feel enough pressure to push. An epidural may increase the chances forceps or a vacuum extractor may be needed during delivery.

An epidural block can make your blood pressure drop. Low blood pressure may affect blood flow to the baby. Fortunately, I.V. fluids given with the epidural help reduce the risk.

Studies have not shown epidural anesthesia increases the risk of Cesarean delivery. And no link between use of epidurals during labor and back pain after delivery has been established.

An epidural can cause shaking, as well as itching and headache. There are remedies for these problems. If you have trembling (nearly 50% of all laboring women do), ask for blankets, a heating pad or a hot-water bottle.

If you itch, wait a bit. Itching is usually mild and goes away on its own. Put pressure on the area with a towel, or apply lots of lotion. If itching doesn't go away, your healthcare provider may recommend medication, such as naloxone (Narcan).

Very occasionally, you'll get a headache. Drink a caffeinated beverage, such as coffee, tea or a caffeinated soda. Try resting on your back. If the headache persists for more than 24 hours, talk to your healthcare provider. If you become nauseous, breathing deeply can help. Inhale through your nose, and exhale through your mouth.

Combined Spinal-Epidural Analgesia (CSE). A *combined spinal-epidural analgesia (CSE)* uses epidural and spinal techniques to relieve pain. It is one of the most popular epidural options. The combination provides the quick relief of a spinal block, with the option of an epidural if your labor is longer. It is sometimes called a *walking epidural.*

A walking epidural doesn't have much to do with walking. It refers to regional labor-pain relief in which a woman maintains some strength in her legs. Few women actually walk after receiving pain relief, although some may walk to the toilet, while others use their legs to position themselves for delivery.

With CSE, there is a lower incidence of spinal headache. There may be less numbness with a CSE. CSE can also be delivered as PCEA.

Other Pain Blocks

When contractions are regular and the cervix begins to dilate, uterine contractions can be uncomfortable. For the early stage of labor, medication may be given through an I.V. or by injection into a muscle. A mixture of a narcotic analgesic drug, such as meperidine (Demerol), and a tranquilizer, such as promethazine (Phenergen), may be used. It reduces pain and may cause sleepiness or sedation. These medications also enter baby's bloodstream and can make baby groggy.

Spinal anesthesia is often used for a Cesarean delivery. It works within seconds and is effective for up to 45 minutes. Pain relief lasts long enough for the Cesarean delivery to be done.

Other types of blocks include a pudendal block, a paracervical block and intrathecal anesthesia. A pudendal block is given through the vaginal canal and decreases pain in the birth canal itself. You still feel contractions and pain in the uterus. A paracervical block provides pain relief for the dilating cervix but doesn't relieve contraction pain. Intrathecal anesthesia is delivered into the area surrounding the spinal cord. It isn't a total block; the woman feels contractions so she can push.

Tip for Week 39

Don't take tags off shower gifts and other gifts until after baby is born. You may need to exchange the gift if its size, color or "sex" isn't correct.

There is no perfect method for pain relief during labor and delivery. Discuss all the possibilities with your healthcare provider, and mention any concerns. Find out what types of anesthesia are available and the risks and benefits of each.

Anesthesia Problems and Complications

Complications are possible with anesthesia. Most affect the baby, including increased drugging of the baby with use of narcotics, such as Demerol, lower Apgar scores and depressed breathing. The baby may require resuscitation, or it may need to receive another drug, such as naloxone, to reverse effects of the first drug.

If a mother is given general anesthesia, increased sedation, slower respiration and a slower heartbeat may be observed in the baby. The mother is usually "out" for more than an hour and is unable to see her newborn infant until later.

Before labor, it may be impossible to determine which anesthesia will be best for you. But it's helpful to know what's available. If you're interested in nonmedical pain-relief methods, see the discussion in Week 40.

Cord-Blood Banking

You may have heard about storing blood from your baby's umbilical cord after birth. *Cord blood* is blood in the umbilical cord and placenta, which in the past were usually thrown away after delivery. Stem cells have proved useful in treating some diseases. Treatment corrects and/or replaces diseased or damaged cells.

Stem cells are present in cord blood. They are the forerunner of cells that make all blood cells. In cord blood, these special cells are undeveloped and can become many different kinds of blood cells. Cord blood doesn't need to be matched as closely for a transplant. This feature can be important for members of ethnic groups or people with rare blood types, who often have more difficulty finding acceptable donor matches.

How Cord Blood Is Used. Cord-blood transfers have been in use since about 1990. To date, over 10,000 cord-blood transfers have been done. Umbilical-cord blood (UCB) is good for treating diseases that affect the blood and immune systems.

UCB-derived stem cells are being studied as therapy for many disorders. Umbilical-cord blood has been used to treat over 75 life-threatening diseases, and more uses are likely to found in the future.

If you or your partner have a family history of some specific diseases, you may want to consider saving and banking your child's umbilical-cord blood, in case it's needed for treatment in the future. Blood can be used by siblings or parents. In fact, the most common use for stem cells from cord blood is between siblings. However, stored blood can't be used to treat a genetic disease in the child from whom the blood was collected. Those stem cells have the same genetic problems.

If you're interested, discuss this situation with your physician at a prenatal appointment. Today, over 600,000 family cord-blood units have been stored. You only have one chance to collect and save your baby's umbilical-cord blood.

Before making a decision, ask about how and where blood is stored and the cost of storing it. This is a decision you need to make together as a couple. But first you need good information, such as cost, because blood storage may not be covered by insurance.

In many hospitals, expecting mothers learn about cord-blood donation when they are admitted to the hospital. Donating cord blood is free.

If your baby is born this week, you may not finish reading this book. However, you may be interested in reading an excerpt from our baby book, *Your Baby's First Year, Week by Week*, which begins on page 637.

The book covers your baby's first year of life in a weekly format, similar to *Your Pregnancy Week by Week*. Information in the excerpt relates to the first week of your baby's life–we hope you find it helpful.

Collecting and Storing Blood. The cord-blood storage bank you choose sends you a collection kit; this is used to collect blood after delivery. It's collected within 9 minutes after birth, before you deliver the placenta. It's taken directly from the umbilical cord; there's no risk or pain to mom or baby. You can also bank the blood if you have a Cesarean delivery.

After cord blood is collected, it's usually picked up by a courier and taken to a banking facility where it is frozen and stored. At this time, we don't know how long frozen cells will last. Cord blood has been banked only since 1990; however, storage at this time is better than it was when freezing and storing blood first began.

It's expensive to collect and to store umbilical-cord blood. Collection and storage can run between $1000 and $2000. A single year's storage can cost around $100.

There are two types of banks—*private blood banking* and *public blood banking*. You may be advised to use private blood banking if you have a history of some illnesses. With private banking, access is guaranteed to your own or a relative's stored blood. Cord blood is available for you or a family member if you need it in the future.

Public UCB banks provide those who need stem cells from cord blood with donor cells. However, donors can't be guaranteed their own or a relative's cord blood. Anyone needing the cord-blood products may get the blood. In some areas, needs-based help is available.

If you donate your child's cord blood to a public bank, his or her name is added to the national registry. If the child ever needs cord blood, he or she is guaranteed it.

Most banks require the mother to be tested for various infections before blood is accepted. This can add to the cost of saving the blood. Your insurance company may pay for this testing, if you have a family history of a disease that might be treated with umbilical-cord blood. Call and ask them, if you're interested.

Some health-insurance companies pay the collection and storage fees for families at high risk of cancer or genetically based diseases. Cord-blood banking services may waive fees for at-risk families who are unable to afford them.

The blood bank you choose should be accredited by the American Association of Blood Banks. They have established procedures for collecting and storing umbilical-cord blood.

Donating Cord Blood. If you don't think you'll need the blood, you may want to donate it. If cord blood isn't used for patients, it may be used by researchers.

There are 18 public cord-blood banks in the United States at this time. They work with hospitals that ask women if they are willing to donate their baby's cord blood.

This is an expensive procedure, so not all hospitals participate in the program. In addition to increasing the amount of blood a public bank receives, many are attempting to increase their range of ethnic backgrounds and diversity by asking women of color to donate their baby's blood. If you're interested, ask your healthcare provider for information about cord-blood banking services and cord-blood donation in your area. In some states, the law requires information on UCB banking to be provided to you.

For a discussion of depression after pregnancy—Postpartum Distress Syndrome—see Appendix F, page 616.

Exercise for Week 39

Stand with your feet slightly apart and your knees soft. Hold onto a counter or a chair with your left hand for stability, if you need it. Holding in your tummy muscles, lift your right leg up behind you until you can touch your bottom with your foot. Return your foot to the floor, then turn around. Hold onto the support with your right hand, and lift your left foot. Repeat 8 times for each leg. *Tones quadriceps.*

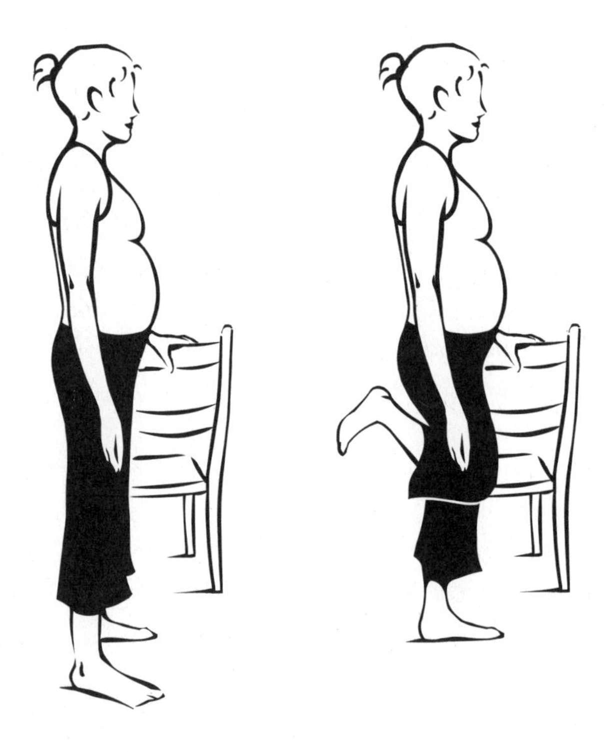

Week 40

Age of Fetus—38 Weeks

How Big Is Your Baby?

Your baby weighs about 7⅔ pounds (3.5kg). Its crown-to-rump length is about 14¾ to 15¼ inches (37 to 38cm). Total length is 20⅔ inches (51cm). Baby fills your uterus and has little room to move. See the illustration on page 559.

How Big Are You?

You probably don't care an awful lot about how much you measure. You feel you're as big as you could ever be, and you're ready to have your baby. From the pubic symphysis to the top of the uterus, you probably measure between 14½ and 16 inches (36 to 40cm). From your belly-button to the top of your uterus is 6½ to 8 inches (16 to 20cm).

How Your Baby Is Growing and Developing

Your baby is fully grown at this point. If you were correct about the date of your last period and your due date is this week, baby may be born very soon. However, it's helpful to realize only 5% of all babies are born on their due date. Don't get frustrated if you see your due date come and go. Baby will be here soon!

Changes in You

While You Wait to Go to the Hospital

If you're waiting to go to the hospital and are having pain, there are a few things you can do at home. The following actions may help you manage your pain. At the beginning of each contraction, take a deep breath. Exhale slowly. At the end of the contraction, again breathe deeply. When a contraction begins, try to distract yourself with mental pictures of pleasant or soothing images.

Your chances of having your baby on the way to the hospital are pretty small. Labor with a first baby often lasts between 12 and 14 hours.

Get up and move! It helps distract you and may relieve back pain. Ask your partner to massage your shoulders, neck, back and feet to help ease tension. It feels good! Hot and/or cold compresses can help reduce cramping and various aches and pains. A warm shower or bath can feel very good.

How Your Actions Affect Your Baby's Development

Going to the Hospital

If you preregistered at the hospital before your due date, it'll save time checking in and may help reduce your stress. If you didn't preregister, fill out forms early. If you wait until you're in labor, you may be concerned with other things.

Have your insurance card or insurance information readily at hand. It's helpful to know your blood type and Rh-factor, your healthcare provider's name, the pediatrician's name and your due date.

Ask your healthcare provider how you should prepare to go to the hospital; he or she may have specific instructions for you. You might want to ask the following questions.

- When should we go to the hospital once I'm in labor?
- Should we call you before we leave for the hospital?
- How can we reach you after regular office hours?

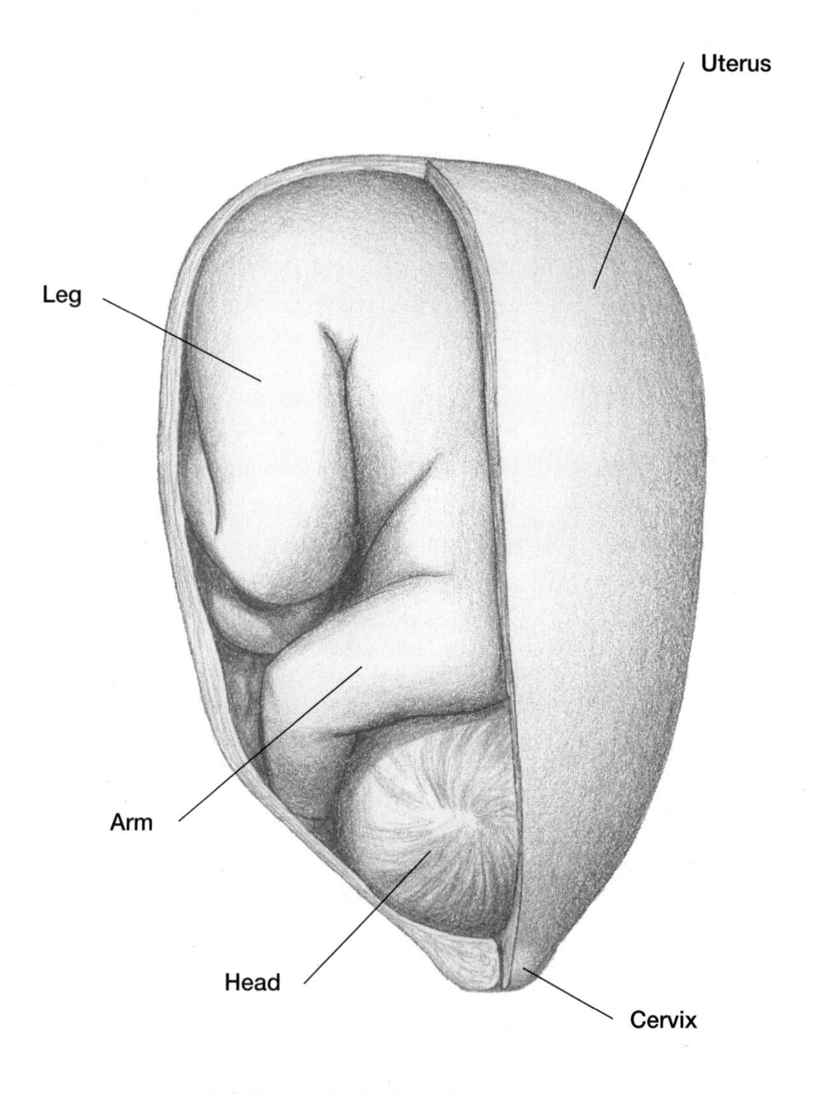

A full-term baby has little room to move.
This is one reason fetal movements may slow down in the last few weeks of pregnancy.

- Are there any particular instructions for me to follow during early labor?
- Where do we go—to the emergency room or the labor-and-delivery department?

Many couples are advised to go to the hospital after an hour of contractions that are 5 to 10 minutes apart. However, leave sooner if the hospital is far away or hard to get to, or if the weather is bad. When you get to the hospital, you'll be checked for signs of labor. See the discussion of the labor check in Week 38.

In the Hospital. A copy of your office chart is usually kept on record in labor and delivery. It contains basic information about your health and pregnancy. When you're admitted to labor and delivery (or a birthing center), you may also be asked many questions. They may include the following.

- Have your membranes ruptured? At what time?
- Are you bleeding?
- Are you having contractions? How often do they occur? How long do they last?
- When did you last eat, and what did you eat?

A brief pregnancy history is taken. Vital signs, including blood pressure, pulse, temperature and baby's heart rate, are noted. Tell them about any medical problems you have and any medications you take or have taken during pregnancy. If you've had complications, tell them when you first get to labor and delivery. This is also the time to tell them any information your healthcare provider gave you about your last pelvic exam.

A pelvic exam is done to see what stage of labor you're in and to use as a reference point for future exams during labor. This exam and vital signs are done by a labor-and-delivery nurse (the nurse can be male or female). Only in unusual situations, such as an emergency, will your healthcare provider do this initial exam. In fact, it may be quite a while before you see him or her. In many labors, the healthcare provider does not arrive until close to delivery.

Once You're Admitted. If you're in labor and remain at the hospital, your partner may have to admit you to the hospital if you haven't filled out preadmittance papers. After you are informed about the procedures that may be done for you and any risks involved, you may be asked to sign a form from the hospital, your healthcare provider and/or the anesthesiologist acknowledging you received this information.

After you're admitted, you may receive an enema. Blood may be drawn. Your healthcare provider may want to discuss pain relief, or you may have an epidural put in place, if you requested one. If you have decided to have an epidural or if it looks as if labor will last quite awhile, an I.V. will be started. You may still be able to walk around.

During this time, you and your partner may be alone, with nurses coming into the room to perform various tasks, then leaving. A monitoring belt may be placed on your tummy to record your contractions and the baby's heartbeat. The monitoring record can be seen in the room and at the nursing station.

Blood pressure is regularly checked, and pelvic exams are done to follow labor's progress. In most places, the healthcare provider is notified upon your admission to labor and delivery; he or she is then called at regular intervals as labor progresses. Your healthcare provider will also be called if any problem arises.

You may not realize it, but having a baby is hard work! You can do it.

In some cases, when you get to the hospital you may learn someone else will deliver your baby. If your healthcare provider believes he or she might be out of town when your baby is born, ask to meet those who "cover" when he or she is unavailable. It's not always possible for your healthcare provider to be there for the birth of your baby.

Keep Your Options Open

An important consideration in planning for your labor and delivery is the method(s) you may use to get through the process. Will you have epidural anesthesia? Are you going to attempt a drug-free delivery? Will you need an episiotomy or an enema?

Every woman is different, and every labor is different. You don't know what will happen and what you will need during labor and delivery for pain relief. It's impossible to know how long labor will last—3 hours or 20 hours. It's best to be flexible. Understand what's available and what options you can choose during labor.

During the last 2 months of pregnancy, discuss any concerns with your healthcare provider. Know what can be provided for you at the hospital you've chosen. Some medications may not be available in some areas.

Pain Relief without Medication

Some women do not want medication during labor to relieve pain. They prefer to use different techniques to relieve pain.

Nondrug techniques to manage labor pain include many things, such as continuous labor support, water therapy, hypnosis and acupuncture. *Continuous labor support* is often provided by a nurse, midwife or doula, and includes touch, massage, application of cold or heat, and other ways to provide physical comfort. It also includes emotional support, which gives you information and helps you communicate with those caring for you.

For some women, *water therapy (hydrotherapy)* during labor has been shown to reduce the amount of stress hormones released in the body. It may also decrease the frequency of contractions. Some women experience less pain and more relaxation in the water. The water also softens the perineal area, so it may stretch more easily. A warm (not hot) shower can relax and massage you. Water immersion involves a warm bath during early labor and is most often used then. Birth pools may be available in some hospitals. You may have to get out of the pool to give birth.

> If your labor slows down, your healthcare provider may give you oxytocin.

Hypnosis to relieve labor pain is sometimes called *hypnobirthing*; it may not be available everywhere. It can be effective for some women but may not be right for everyone. Visualization, relaxation and deep breathing help you enter a deep state of relaxation to help you deal with your fear of pain. However, understand that if you choose hypnotherapy to help you deal with pain, you must prepare and practice for months before baby's birth.

Acupuncture requires an acupuncturist willing to be on call to come to the labor and delivery room. It uses needles at specific points to relieve pain. It must usually be started at the beginning of labor. Acupressure uses pressure on specific parts of the body to help relieve pain and to relax you.

Swaying from side to side, changing positions and rolling on a birthing ball (like a big exercise ball) can help ease discomfort. Because you're upright, the force of gravity may help your labor progress. Walking also keeps you upright, which helps dilate the cervix naturally.

Aromatherapy, which consists of massage with certain aromatic oils, can be helpful for relaxation. Listening to instrumental music for at least 3 hours during early active labor may also help you deal with pain by helping you relax.

Massage for Relief

Massage is a wonderful, gentle way to help you feel better during labor. The touching and caressing of massage helps you relax and helps reduce pain. One study showed women who were massaged for 20 minutes every hour during active labor felt less anxiety and less pain.

Many parts of the body of a laboring woman can be massaged. Massaging the head, neck, back and feet can offer comfort and relaxation. The person doing the massage should pay close attention to the woman's responses to determine correct pressure.

Different types of massage affect a woman in various ways. You and your partner may want to practice the two types of massage described below *before* labor.

Effleurage is light, gentle fingertip massage over the abdomen and upper thighs; it is used during early labor. Stroking is light, but doesn't tickle, and fingertips never leave the skin. Place hands on either side of the navel. Move the hands upward and outward, and come back down to the pubic area. Then move the hands back up to the navel. Massage may extend down the thighs. It can also be done as a crosswise motion, around fetal-monitor belts. Move fingers across the abdomen from one side to the other, between the belts.

Counterpressure massage can relieve back-labor pain. Ask your labor coach to place the heel of his or her hand or the flat part of the fist (you can also use a tennis ball) against your tailbone. Firm pressure is applied in a small, circular motion.

Laboring Positions

Different laboring positions may allow you and your partner (or labor coach) to work together during labor to find relief. This interaction can help you feel closer, and it lets you share the experience. Some women say that using these methods brought them closer to their partner and made the birth experience a more joyful one.

Most women in North America and Europe give birth in bed, on their backs. However, some women are trying different positions to find relief from pain and to make the birth of their baby easier.

In the past, women often labored and gave birth in an upright position that kept the pelvis vertical. Kneeling, squatting, sitting or standing up lets the abdominal wall relax and the baby descend more rapidly. Because contractions are stronger and more regular, labor is often shorter.

Today, many women are asking to choose the birth position that is most comfortable for them. Freedom to do so can make a woman feel more confident about managing birth and labor. Women who choose their own methods may feel more satisfied with the entire experience.

If it's important to you, discuss it with your healthcare provider. Ask about the facilities at the hospital you will use; some have special equipment, such as birthing chairs, squatting bars or birthing beds. Positions you might consider for your labor are described below.

Walking and *standing* are good positions to use during early labor. Walking may help you breathe more easily and relax more. Standing in a warm shower may provide relief. When walking, be sure someone is with you to offer support.

There has been some debate about walking during labor. Some believe walking helps move the baby into position more quickly, dilates the cervix faster and makes labor more pain free. Others believe walking puts the woman at risk of falling and doesn't allow for fetal monitoring. One study of more than 1000 pregnant women showed walking had no effects. We believe the bottom line is that it's a personal decision on your part, and you should be allowed to decide what feels best for you.

Sitting can slow labor. Sitting to rest after walking or standing is OK, but sitting can be uncomfortable during a contraction.

Kneeling on hands and knees is a good way to relieve the pain of back labor. *Kneeling against a support,* such as a chair or your partner, stretches your back muscles. The effects of kneeling are similar to those of walking and standing.

Tip for Week 40

If you want to use a different labor position, massage, relaxation techniques and/or hypnotherapy to relieve labor pain, don't wait until you're in labor to ask about it. Discuss it with your healthcare provider at one of your prenatal visits.

When you can't stand, walk or kneel, *lie on your side.* If you receive pain medication, you'll need to lie down. Lie on your left side, then turn onto your right side.

Although *lying on your back* is the most common position used for labor, it can slow labor. It can also make your blood pressure drop and cause your baby's heart rate to drop. If you lie on your back, elevate the head of the bed and put a pillow under one hip so you are not flat on your back.

Your Nutrition

In the past, women in labor have only been allowed sips of water or a few ice chips to relieve thirst. This was because of concerns about vomiting and inhaling vomit into the lungs (aspiration) during labor and the risk of problems if anesthesia was needed for a Cesarean delivery.

ACOG has recently issued new guidelines. The new recommendations state if you have a normal, uncomplicated labor, you may drink modest amounts of *clear liquids*, such as water, fruit juice without pulp, carbonated beverages, clear tea, black coffee and sports drinks. If you have any risk factors, such as morbid obesity or diabetes, or if you may be at risk for a delivery involving forceps or a vacuum extractor, your fluid intake may be limited or curtailed.

If you're scheduled for a Cesarean delivery, you may drink clear liquids up to 2 hours before anesthesia is given. Don't eat solid food for 6 to 8 hours before surgery.

If your labor is long, your body may be hydrated with fluids through an I.V. After your baby's birth, if everything is OK, you maybe able to eat and drink without much restriction.

You Should Also Know

Your Labor Coach

Your labor coach may be one of your most valuable assets during labor and delivery. He (or she) can help you prepare. He can be there to support you as you go through the experience of labor together. He can share with you the joy of the birth of your baby.

In most instances, your partner is your labor coach. However, this isn't an absolute requirement. A close friend or relative, such as your mother or sister, may act as your labor coach. Or you may choose the services of a doula. Ask someone ahead of time; don't wait until the last minute. Give the person time to prepare for the experience and to make sure he or she will be able to be there with you.

Not everyone feels comfortable watching the entire labor and delivery. This may include your partner. Don't force your partner or labor coach to watch the delivery if he or she

> **Dad Tip**
>
> **Baby can come at any time. When your little one decides to make his or her appearance, be sure you take care of some things your partner might forget about. If she works outside the home, be sure to call her workplace and let them know she's at the hospital. Find out if she has any appointments or plans you may need to change for her. Ask her what might need to be done at home to finish preparing for baby's arrival.**

An important role of the labor coach is to make sure you get to the hospital! Work out a plan during the last 4 to 6 weeks of pregnancy so you know how to reach your coach. It's helpful to have an alternate driver, such as a family member, neighbor or friend, who's available in case you can't reach your labor coach immediately and need to be taken to the hospital.

doesn't want to. It's not unusual for a labor coach to get lightheaded, dizzy or pass out during labor and delivery. On more than one occasion, coaches or partners have fainted or become extremely lightheaded just from talking about plans for labor and delivery or a Cesarean delivery!

Before going to the hospital, your labor coach can time your contractions so you're aware of the progress of your labor. Once you arrive at the hospital, you both may be nervous. Your coach can do the following to help you both relax:

- talk to you while you're in labor to distract you and to help you relax
- encourage and reassure you during labor and when it comes time for you to push
- keep a watch on the door and protect your privacy
- help relieve tension during labor
- touch, hug and kiss (If you don't want to be touched during labor, tell your coach.)
- reassure you it's OK for you to deal vocally with your pain
- wipe your face or your mouth with a washcloth
- rub your abdomen or back
- support your back while you're pushing
- help create a mood in the labor room, including music and lighting (Discuss it ahead of time; bring things with you that you would like to have available during labor.)
- take pictures (Many couples find photographs taken of the baby after the delivery help them best remember these wonderful moments of joy.)

It's all right for your labor coach to rest or to take a break during labor, especially if labor lasts a long time. It's better if your coach eats in the lounge or hospital cafeteria. A labor coach should not bring work into the labor room—it shows little support for the laboring woman.

Many couples do different things to distract themselves and to help pass time during labor. These include picking names for the baby, playing games, watching TV or listening to music.

Talk to your healthcare provider about your coach's participation in the delivery, such as cutting the umbilical cord or bathing baby after birth. These things vary from one place to another. The responsibility of your healthcare provider is the well-being of you and your baby—don't make requests or demands that could cause complications.

Decide ahead of time about who needs to be called after baby's birth. Bring a list of names and phone numbers with you. There are some people you may want to call yourself. In most places, a telephone is available in the labor and delivery area, or you may be able to use your cell phones.

> Some couples choose to bring young children to see the birth of a new brother or sister. Ask your healthcare provider's opinion ahead of time. The delivery of the baby might be exciting and special to you and your partner, but it may be frightening to a young child. Many places offer special classes for older siblings to help prepare them for the new baby. This may be a better way to help your older children feel they're part of the birth experience.

If you want to be with your partner when friends or relatives first see the baby, make it clear. In most instances, you need some cleaning up. Take some time for yourselves with your new baby. After that you can show baby to friends and relatives, and share the joy with them.

Vaginal Delivery of Your Baby

We have already covered Cesarean delivery in Week 37. Most women don't have to have a Cesarean delivery—they have a vaginal birth.

There are three distinct stages of labor, as we've previously discussed. In the first stage of labor, your uterus contracts with enough intensity, duration and frequency to cause effacement and dilatation of the cervix.

The first stage of labor ends when the cervix is fully dilated and sufficiently open to allow the baby's head to come through it.

The second stage of labor begins when the cervix is completely dilated at 10cm. Once full dilatation is reached, pushing begins. Pushing can take 1 to 2 hours (first or second baby) to a few minutes (an experienced mom). This stage of labor ends with delivery of the baby. One study showed women who were able to bite down on a mouth guard had a significantly shorter second stage of labor than women who didn't use a mouth guard. Some experts believe a woman using a mouth guard can push harder and, therefore, shorten the second stage of labor.

Studies show if you wait about 3 or 4 minutes before cutting the umbilical cord, the extra blood flowing to your baby increases his or her iron levels for the first *6 months* of life.

The third stage of labor begins after delivery of the baby. It ends with delivery of the placenta and the membranes that have surrounded the fetus. Delivery of the baby and placenta, and repair of the episiotomy (if you have one) usually takes 20 to 30 minutes.

Following delivery, you and the baby are evaluated. During this time, you get to see and to hold your baby; you may even be able to feed him or her.

Depending on whether you deliver in a hospital or birthing center, you may deliver in the same room you've labored in. Or you may be moved to a delivery room nearby. After birth, you will go to recovery for a short time, then move to a hospital room until you're ready to go home.

You will probably stay in the hospital 24 to 48 hours after delivery, if you have no complications. If you do have any complications, you and your healthcare provider will decide what is best for you.

Exercise for Week 40

Stand with your feet slightly apart and your knees soft. Cross your chest with your right arm. With your left hand, gently push your right elbow toward you. Pat yourself on the back for a pregnancy job well done! Hold stretch for 10 seconds; repeat 4 times for each arm. *Provides a good stretch for the upper back.*

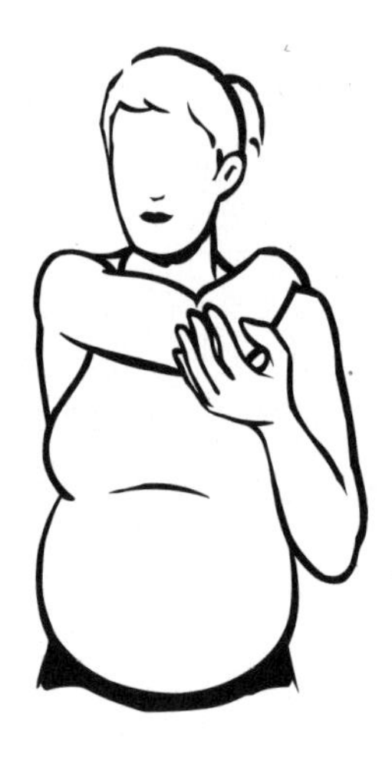

Week 41

When You're Overdue

Your due date has come and gone. You haven't delivered, and you're getting tired of being pregnant. You keep seeing your healthcare provider and hearing, "I'm sure it'll be soon. Just sit tight." You feel ready to scream. But hang in there. It *will* be over soon—the wait just seems never-ending right now.

What Happens When You Pass Your Due Date?

Your due date has come and gone, and still no baby! You're not alone—nearly 10% of all babies are born more than 2 weeks late.

A pregnancy is considered overdue (postterm) *only* when it exceeds 42 weeks or 294 days from the first day of the last menstrual period. (A baby born at 41 weeks, 6 days is *not* considered overdue, even if it feels like it to you!)

Being overdue has its own risks. The placenta may start to deteriorate, and baby may grow larger.

Your doctor can determine if baby is moving around in the uterus and if the amount of amniotic fluid is healthy and normal. If the baby is healthy and active, you're usually monitored until labor begins on its own.

Tests may be done as reassurance that an overdue baby is fine and can remain in the womb. If signs of fetal stress are found, labor may be induced.

Take Good Care of Yourself

It may be hard to keep a positive attitude when you're overdue. But don't give up yet! Eat healthfully, and keep up your fluid intake. If you can do so without problems, get some mild exercise, like walking or swimming. You may feel better.

The following exercise is easy to do, no matter how big you are! Lie on your left side on the floor or bed. Elevate your head with a pillow. Bend your knees, and pull your arms close to your body. While inhaling, reach your right arm over your head as you fully extend your right leg in front of you, leading with your heel. Hold for 3 seconds. Exhale as you return to the starting position. Do 4 times on each side; it helps stretch back muscles.

> ACOG does not recommend inducing labor for nonmedical reasons before 39 weeks.

One of the best exercises you can do at this point is water exercises. You can swim or exercise in the water without fear of falling or losing your balance. Even just walking back and forth in the pool can feel good!

Rest and relax now because your baby will be here soon, and you'll be very busy. Use the time to get things ready for baby so you'll be all set when you both come home from the hospital.

Postterm Pregnancies

Most babies born 2 weeks or more past their due date are delivered safely. However, carrying a baby longer than 42 weeks can cause some problems, so tests may be done on baby and labor may be induced, if necessary.

While baby is growing and developing, it depends on two important functions performed by the placenta—respiration and nutrition. When a pregnancy is overdue, the placenta may fail to provide the respiratory function and essential nutrients baby needs. A baby may begin to suffer nutritional loss. The baby is called *postmature.*

At birth, a postmature baby may have dry, cracked, peeling, wrinkled skin, long fingernails and abundant hair. It also has less vernix covering its body. The baby may have less fat and appear almost malnourished.

Because a postmature infant is in danger of losing nutritional support from the placenta, it's important to know the true dating of your pregnancy. This is another reason why it's important to go to all of your prenatal visits.

Tests You May Have

Various tests may be done to reassure you and your doctor your overdue baby is doing OK and can remain in the womb. In evaluating baby, the doctor looks at various pieces of data. For example, if you're having contractions, it's important to know how your baby is affected.

Tests are done on you to determine the health of your baby. One of the first tests is a vaginal exam. Your doctor will probably do this test every week to see if your cervix has begun to dilate. You may also be asked to record kick counts. A weekly ultrasound may be done to determine how big baby is and how much amniotic fluid is present. It also helps identify problems with the placenta, which could cause difficulties for baby.

Three other tests are often done when a baby is overdue. They check baby's well-being inside the womb. They are the *nonstress test,* the *contraction stress test* and the *biophysical profile.* Each is discussed below.

The Nonstress Test (NST)

A nonstress test (NST) is performed in your doctor's office or in the labor-and-delivery department of a hospital. While you're lying down, a fetal monitor is attached to your tummy. Every time you feel your baby move, you push a button that makes a mark on a strip of monitor paper. At the same time, the monitor records baby's heartbeat.

When baby moves, its heart rate usually goes up. The findings from the NST help your healthcare provider measure how well baby is tolerating life inside the uterus. Your doctor can decide if further action is necessary.

The Contraction Stress Test (CST)

A contraction stress test (CST), also called a *stress test,* gives an indication of how the baby is doing and how well the baby will tolerate contractions and labor. If the baby doesn't respond well to contractions, it can be a sign of fetal stress. Some believe this test is more accurate than the nonstress test in assessing baby's well-being.

To perform a CST, a monitor is placed on your abdomen. You are attached to an I.V. that dispenses small amounts of oxytocin to make your uterus contract. Sometimes nipple stimulation is used, which can cause the uterus to contract so an I.V. isn't necessary. The baby's heartbeat is monitored for its response to the contractions. If baby doesn't respond well to contractions, it can be a sign of fetal stress.

The Biophysical Profile (BPP)

A biophysical profile is done on baby to help determine fetal health; it's done when there is concern about baby's well-being. It uses a scoring system. The first four of the five tests listed below are done with ultrasound; the fifth is done with external fetal monitors. A score is given to each area. The five areas evaluated are:

- fetal breathing movements
- fetal body movements
- fetal tone
- amount of amniotic fluid
- reactive fetal heart rate (nonstress test [NST])

During the test, doctors evaluate fetal "breathing"—the movement or expansion of the baby's chest inside the uterus. This score is based on the amount of fetal breathing that occurs.

Movement of the baby's body is noted. A normal score indicates normal body movements. An abnormal score is applied when there are few or no body movements during the allotted time period.

Fetal tone and posture are evaluated. It is a good sign if baby has good tone.

Evaluation of the volume of amniotic fluid requires experience in ultrasound. A normal test shows adequate fluid around the baby. An abnormal test indicates little or no amniotic fluid around the baby.

Fetal heart-rate monitoring (nonstress test) is done with external monitors. It evaluates changes in the fetal heart rate associated with baby's movements. The amount of change and number of changes in the fetal heart rate can differ, depending on who's doing the test and their definition of normal.

An abnormal score is 0 for any of these tests; a normal score is 2. A score of 1 is a middle score. A total score is obtained by adding all the values together. Evaluation may vary depending on the sophistication of the equipment used and the expertise of the person doing the test. The higher the score, the better the baby's condition. A lower score may cause concern about the well-being of the fetus.

If the score is low, a recommendation may be made to deliver the baby. If the score is reassuring, the test may be repeated at a later date. If results fall between these two values, the test may be repeated the following day. Your doctor will evaluate all the information before making any decision.

Inducing Labor

There may come a point in your pregnancy that your doctor decides to induce labor, which means labor is started to deliver your baby. It's a fairly common practice; each year, doctors induce labor for about 450,000 births. In addition to inducing labor for overdue babies, it is also used when a woman has other problems or when baby is at risk.

When your doctor does a pelvic exam at this point in your pregnancy, it probably also includes an evaluation of how ready you are for induction. Indications for induction of labor include the following:

- pregnancy 2 weeks past the due date
- baby isn't thriving in the uterus (determined from tests)
- pre-eclampsia

- signs the placenta is no longer functioning as well as it should
- illness that threatens the well-being of mother-to-be or baby
- pregnancy-induced high blood pressure
- premature rupture of membranes
- bag of waters breaks but contractions don't begin in a reasonable amount of time
- infection of the uterine membranes

The *Bishop score* may also be used. It's a method of scoring used to predict the success of inducing labor. Scoring includes dilatation, effacement, station, consistency and position of the cervix. A score is given for each point, then they are added together to give a total score to help the doctor decide whether to induce labor.

Sometimes labor should *not* be induced. Your healthcare provider will take into account any contraindications to inducing labor.

Ripening the Cervix for Induction

Doctors often ripen the cervix before labor is induced. *Ripening the cervix* means medicine is used to help the cervix soften, thin and dilate.

Various preparations are used for this purpose. The two most common are Prepidil Gel and Cervidil. In most cases, doctors use Prepidil Gel and Cervidil to prepare the cervix the day before induction. Both preparations are placed in the top of the vagina, behind the cervix. Medication is released directly onto the cervix, which helps ripen it. This is done in the labor-and-delivery area of the hospital, so baby can be monitored.

> Research from the Centers for Disease Control and Prevention (CDC) indicates about 25% of all inductions are elective or medically unnecessary. If you're considering inducing your labor at 37 or 38 weeks for nonmedical reasons, you greatly increase baby's chances of having complications. Or you may end up having a Cesarean delivery.

Labor Induction

If your doctor induces labor, you may first have your cervix ripened, as described above, then you will receive oxytocin (Pitocin) through an I.V. The oxytocin starts contractions to help you go into labor. The length of the entire process—ripening your cervix until the birth of your baby—varies from woman to woman.

Oxytocin is gradually increased until contractions begin. The amount you receive is controlled by a pump, so you can't receive too much. While you receive oxytocin, you're also monitored for the baby's reaction to labor.

It's important to realize that being induced does not guarantee a vaginal delivery. In many instances, induction doesn't work. Inducing labor may increase your chances of having an emergency Cesarean delivery.

You may want to try some "natural" labor inducers that have been known to work for some women. They include:

- walking
- eating fresh pineapple (it contains bromelain, which may help soften cervical tissues)
- nipple stimulation
- sexual intercourse (semen contains prostaglandins, which help soften cervical tissues)

What Happens after Your Pregnancy?

After your baby is born, there will be a lot of changes in your life. Take a look at this overview so you'll have an idea of what to anticipate as you begin your life as a new mother. Our book, *Your Pregnancy Quick Guide: Postpartum Wellness,* is an in-depth look at you during the period after baby's birth. Reading it may answer many of your questions. You can also read our book, *Your Baby's First Year Week by Week,* which can answer many questions you and your partner may have about caring for your new baby. See the excerpt of this book that begins on page 637.

In the Hospital

- Muscles are sore from the effort of childbirth and labor.
- Your bottom is sore and swollen. If you had an episiotomy, it also hurts.
- Your incision may be uncomfortable, if you had a C-section or tubal ligation.
- Use the nurse-call button whenever necessary!
- Try different ways for you and your partner to bond with baby.
- Feeding (breast or bottle) the new miracle in your arms may be a little scary, but you'll soon be doing it like a pro!
- Heavy bleeding or passing blood clots larger than an egg can indicate a problem.

- High or low blood pressure may be a cause for further testing.
- Pain should be relieved by medication. If it isn't, tell the nurse.
- Fever over 101.5F (25.25C) may be a cause for concern.
- It's normal to cry or feel emotional.
- Ask for the paperwork so you can get baby a social security number. Fill it out, and be sure to send it in.
- Try to rest. Ask to turn off your phone and to restrict visitors.
- Even though you just lost 10 to 15 pounds with baby's birth, it'll take awhile for the rest of your weight to come off.
- Eat nutritiously to keep up energy and to produce milk, if you breastfeed.
- Write down thoughts and feelings about labor, delivery and the first hours with your new baby. Encourage your partner to do the same.
- Watch hospital videos about baby care. Ask staff for clarification or help.
- Get the name, address and telephone number of your pediatrician.
- Ask questions, and get help from the nurses and staff in the hospital.
- Ask your partner to take you for a walk outside your hospital room.
- Take time for you, your partner and your baby to bond as a family.

1st Week Home

- You'll still have painful uterine contractions, especially during nursing.
- It's normal for your breasts to be full of milk, engorged and leaking.
- The area of your episiotomy or tear is probably still sore.
- Muscles may also be sore.
- Maternity clothes may be the most comfortable clothes to wear.
- Your legs may be still swollen.
- You may leak urine or stool and can't control it.
- If bleeding gets heavier, or you pass blood clots, call your doctor.

- It may indicate a problem if you get red streaks or hard spots in your breasts.
- Call your doctor if you develop a fever.
- Take it easy; don't worry about the housework.
- It's normal to cry, sigh or laugh for no reason.
- Be sure to ask for help from friends and family.
- You may still look a little pregnant from the side.
- You still carry some of the extra weight you gained during pregnancy.
- Make baby's first appointment with the pediatrician.
- Have baby added to your insurance policy. There may be a time limit, so don't delay.
- Keep important "baby" documents together, such as the birth certificate, immunization record (when you get it at baby's first pediatrician's visit) and baby's social security card.
- Make your 6-week postpartum checkup appointment.
- Begin making plans for day-care arrangements, if you haven't started already.
- Give your partner a job or assignment to help you and to make him feel useful.
- Contact La Leche League, if you have any problems breastfeeding.

2nd Week Home

- Your breasts (whether or not you breastfeed) are full and uncomfortable.
- Hemorrhoids still hurt, but they should be getting better.
- With swelling and water retention diminishing, you can wear some of your clothes and shoes again.
- Feeding baby is starting to work better.
- When you cough, laugh, sneeze or lift something heavy, you may lose stool or urine and not be able to control it.
- You are probably fatigued. Taking care of baby requires a lot of time and energy.

- A foul odor or yellow-green vaginal discharge may indicate a problem; it should be decreasing at this point. If it isn't, contact your doctor.
- It's OK to let baby cry a little before checking on him or her.
- You can almost see your feet when you look down (your tummy is getting smaller).
- Write down any questions for your visit with your pediatrician.
- Keep your appointment with your doctor if you had a C-section or tubal ligation; you need to have your incision checked.
- Write down some of your thoughts and feelings in your journal.

3rd Week Home

- Swelling and soreness around your bottom are decreasing, but sitting for a long time still may not feel very comfortable.
- Swelling in hands decreases. If you took off your rings during pregnancy, try them on again.
- Baby doesn't know the difference between night and day, so your sleep patterns are also disturbed.
- Getting ready to go anywhere is like planning a major trip. It takes three times longer to get ready with baby.
- Call your doctor if you develop red streaks or tender, hard spots on your legs, particularly the back of the calves. It could be a blood clot.
- You may feel sad or depressed some of the time. You may even cry.
- You may have varicose veins, just like your mother! They'll get better as you recover from pregnancy and begin exercising again.
- Skin on your abdomen still looks stretched out when you stand up.
- You may be seeing the pediatrician again this week. You'll probably receive his or her immunization record at this visit. Put it in a safe place with baby's other important papers.
- Take lots of pictures and videos! You'll be amazed how quickly baby will change and grow.

- Keep your partner involved. Let him try his hand at caring for baby. Ask for his help with household chores.
- By this point, you've changed over 200 diapers—you're a pro!

4th Week Home

- Muscles feel better, and you can do more now. Be aware—it's easy to pull or to strain muscles you haven't used for a while.
- Control of urine and stool are improving. Doing your Kegel exercise is paying off.
- Baby is showing signs of adjusting to a regular schedule.
- Bending over or lifting may still be difficult. Take things slowly, and allow yourself plenty of time for even the easiest chores.
- Your first menstrual period after delivery could happen at any time. If you don't breastfeed, your first period is usually 4 to 9 weeks after delivery, but it can happen earlier.
- Blood in your urine, dark or cloudy urine, or severe cramping or pain with urination may be symptoms of a urinary-tract infection (UTI). Call your doctor.
- You've been walking and doing light exercise, and it feels OK. Keep it up!
- Prepare for your 6-week postpartum appointment. Write down any questions you have as they come to you.
- A night out with your partner is a good plan. Ask grandparents, other family members and friends to babysit.
- Time with your new baby is precious. Soon you may be going back to work or returning to other activities.

5th Week Home

- As you get back to regular activities, sore muscles and a sore back may be expected.

- Bowel movements may occasionally be uncomfortable in the area of your episiotomy or rectum.
- Bladder and bowel control have returned.
- You may be getting a little anxious to go back to work. You may have missed your friends and the work you do.
- It may be hard to go back to work and not be there for every moment with your baby.
- Plan for after-birth contraception. Decide on some type of birth control, and be ready to start it.
- Baby blues should be getting much better, if they haven't disappeared already.
- You may be a little nervous about going back to work.
- Clothes may still be snug, even if they were loose before pregnancy.
- Remind yourself that it took you 9 months of pregnancy to gain the weight you did. It will take awhile to return to your prepregnancy figure.
- Returning to work requires planning. Start now to put your "back-to-work" schedule into effect.
- Plans for day-care, tending, nursing and other things need to be in place soon. Family and friends can be an important ingredient.

6th Week Home

- Having a pelvic exam at your 6-week checkup isn't usually as bad as you might expect.
- In the 6 weeks since baby's birth, your uterus has gone from the size of a watermelon to the size of your fist; it now weighs about 2 ounces.
- At your 6-week postpartum appointment, plan to discuss several important subjects, such as contraception, your current activity level, limitations and future pregnancies.
- People in your OB's office have probably been helpful to you. Thank them, and ask if you can call with future questions.

- If you still have baby blues or feel depressed every day, tell your doctor.
- If you bleed vaginally or have a foul-smelling discharge, inform you doctor.
- If you have pain or swelling in your legs or your breasts are red or tender, bring it up at your visit.
- Ask questions; make a list. Good questions include the following.
    - What are my choices for contraception?
    - Do I have any limitations as far as exercise or sex?
    - Is there anything I should know from this pregnancy and delivery if I decide to get pregnant again?
- If you take baby with you to your postpartum checkup, take plenty of supplies. You may have to wait.
- If you're going back to work soon, check on child-care arrangements.
- Continue to involve your partner as much as possible.
- Keep writing your thoughts and feelings in your journal. Encourage your partner to do the same.

3 Months

- Muscles may be sore from exercising—a little more than a month ago, you were given the OK to do any exercises you wanted.
- You may have your first period around this time. It could be heavier, longer and different from those before pregnancy.
- If you haven't done anything about contraception, do it now! (Unless you want to celebrate two birthdays in the same year.)
- It's OK to let baby cry when she's a little fussy and needs to soothe herself.
- Your pounds and inches may not be disappearing as quickly as you would like. Keep exercising and eating nutritiously. You'll get there!
- Write down baby's milestones as they happen; write them in baby's book or keep a journal.

- Look for things your partner can do to be involved in baby's care. Let him help out when he can.
- If you've stopped breastfeeding, let baby's dad give him a bottle.

6 Months

- Getting on the scale may still be a daunting task. But hang in there, and keep working hard on eating well and exercising!
- Your first period may occur around this time, if you are breast-feeding. It could be heavier, longer and different from those before pregnancy.
- Don't try to do it all yourself. Let your partner and others help.
- Baby's feeding schedule should be well established by now.
- Take time for yourself.
- Arrange time for regular activities, such as exercising, baby play groups and meeting with other new moms.
- You're starting to fit into some of your clothing from before pregnancy.
- Share special baby moments with your partner.
- Record baby's noises, or take pictures. A recorder and video camera are great for this!
- Find a friend with a baby, and trade child-care duties. It's a good way for each of you to have some time for yourself.

1 Year

- All systems are go! It's taken time, energy and hard work, but your life is going smoothly now.
- Baby sleeps through the night most of the time.
- Don't miss your yearly exam or your Pap smear.
- Your body is returning to its prepregnancy shape. Your tummy is flat, you've lost most of the pregnancy weight and you feel great.

- Continue taking care of yourself. Eat nutritiously, get enough rest and exercise.
- Write down feelings about this time in your life. Encourage your partner to do the same.
- Sharing child care can be a good way to develop baby play groups. Interacting with other children is good for baby.
- Baby's first birthday is just around the corner. Celebrate!
- Enjoy baby's first words, first steps and every other first that will happen.
- Continue taking pictures of baby.
- You may be considering another pregnancy.

From the authors of the bestselling Your Pregnancy™ series, the revised and expanded edition of the book new parents trust.

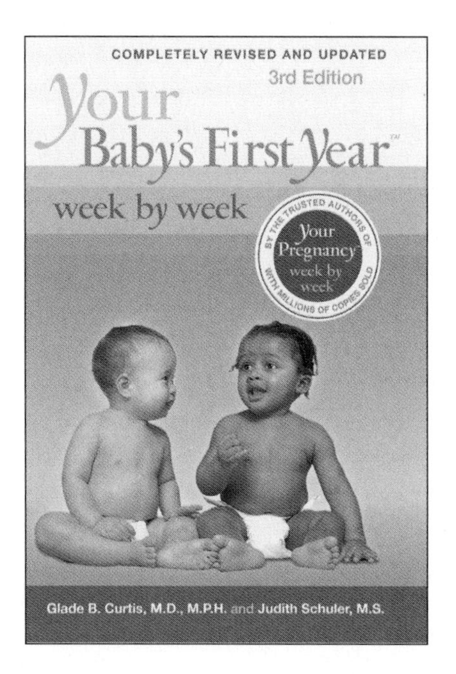

Bringing your baby home is exciting—it can also be intimidating and mind boggling!

- How do you know what baby's cries mean?
- How do you know if she's sick?
- How do you diaper him?
- Is she getting enough milk?
- How do you give him a bath?

Most new parents have questions and concerns about the wonderful, sometimes scary, experience of caring for their new baby. To that end, we have written a companion book, *Your Baby's First Year Week by Week*, in which we answer many of the questions you may have about the incredible first year you will spend with your baby. We have included an excerpt from it dealing with some of the issues you and your partner may have as you begin your parenting journey. See page 637.

Appendix A: Getting Pregnant

Some couples have issues with infertility. *Infertility* is defined as the inability or decreased ability to achieve pregnancy. Problems that affect fertility can be present in either partner. When evaluating fertility, both parents-to-be should be examined. This discussion explores some of the reasons a couple may have trouble conceiving.

Before you start to worry about not getting pregnant, look at your age. If you're healthy and in your 20s, don't get concerned unless a year has passed and you aren't pregnant. If you're over 30, talk to your doctor if you aren't pregnant in 6 months. Studies show fertility decreases as a couple gets older. Your best chance of becoming pregnant is between the ages of 18 and 25.

A woman's eggs decrease in quality and quantity as she ages. However, new research suggests a woman may produce new eggs throughout her lifetime, indicating she is *not* born with all the eggs she will ever produce. More research needs to be done, but these findings may have an impact on a woman's fertility in the future.

If you have health issues, you may want to talk to your doctor after unsuccessfully trying to get pregnant for 6 months. If you have any of the following, consult your physician:

- endometriosis
- PID—pelvic inflammatory disease
- painful or irregular periods
- recurrent miscarriages
- sexually transmitted disease

Endometriosis is most common in women in their 30s and 40s, especially in women who have not had children. It also runs in families, so if a sister or your mother had the problem, you may also experience it.

Check your diet; what you eat and drink is important. Eating at least two servings a day of full-fat dairy products has been shown to help increase fertility by as much as 25%! If you eat low-fat dairy foods every day, you may actually be *reducing* your chances of conceiving.

Fertility may be impaired if 25% or more of your food comes from protein sources. High protein intake could interfere with embryonic development. Recent studies show taking in more than 300mg/day of caffeine can also impact fertility. In addition, eating disorders can cause infertility.

Taking specific vitamins and minerals may help increase your chances of pregnancy. Decreased levels of iron, protein, vitamin C and zinc have been tied to less-frequent ovulation and an increased risk of early miscarriage. A daily multivitamin can help you increase your levels of these important vitamins and nutrients.

Studies show depression and stress may affect your fertility. In addition, alcohol decreases fertility. An occasional glass of wine is OK, but don't drink every day.

Ovulation Monitors and Other Tests

You may be advised to use a test to predict when ovulation occurs. Many are available. Ovulation test sticks and test strips detect a surge in luteinizing hormone (LH). So do other tests that test urine from the beginning of your cycle.

Most tests can be done at home and are easy to use. All the tests work well if you have a fairly regular menstrual cycle. But you need to be consistent in your testing.

If your menstrual cycle is *not* regular, consider using a daily ovulation test. It provides testing for 20 days every month to help ensure you don't miss a surge in luteinizing hormone.

Your best chance of getting pregnant is actually the day *before* a surge in LH. The second best day is the day of the surge, and the third best day is the day after the surge.

Types of Tests

Today we're lucky to have many tests available to predict when ovulation occurs to help a woman conceive. Below is a discussion of some ovulation-predictor tests available.

- The *First Response Easy-Read Ovulation Test* may help you learn the most fertile time during your cycle. You use it for 7 days, during the time you believe you're ovulating, and it shows the day you are most fertile.
- The *Clear-Plan Easy Fertility Monitor* helps you track where you are in your menstrual cycle. All you have to do is press a button at the start of a new menstrual period to begin tracking your cycle. For 10 days during the cycle, you use a urine sample to test hormone levels. The monitor judges where you are in your fertility cycle.
- The *Donna Saliva Ovulation Tester* uses your saliva to predict ovulation. In the 1940s, researchers found the salt content of a woman's saliva is the same as the woman's cervical fluid when she ovulates. Using this information, a test was developed to help predict ovulation. Saliva is placed on the microscope lens, and the crystallized pattern is examined after it dries. When a woman is *not* ovulating, random dots appear; however, 1 to 3 days before ovulation, short hairlike structures can be seen. On the day of

ovulation, a fernlike pattern appears which makes it easy to distinguish from the other patterns.

- *OV-Watch* is a device you wear on your wrist, like a wrist watch, to help you find out when you're most fertile. The device measures the concentration of chloride on your skin—chloride can be an indicator of increased fertility. When you read the OV-Watch, it tells you whether you are fertile (preovulation), ovulating, less fertile (after ovulation) or not fertile. It is lightweight and worn at night. When you wake up in the morning, you read the results. If you're interested, ask your healthcare provider about it.
- The *TCI Ovulation Tester* measures the level of estrogen throughout your cycle by using a sample of your saliva. Some saliva is placed on a slide, and when it's dry, you examine it with a small lens or eye piece. When your saliva has a fernlike appearance, you're fertile.
- The *Ovulite* microscope is similar to the TCI test; however, it allows for unlimited testing of your saliva. You sample your saliva daily, and when you see a change, you know you're ovulating.

Other Fertility Tests. Home tests for men measure whether sperm is moving and provide an approximate sperm count (sperm concentration). Sperm concentration is one of the factors used by doctors to help determine male fertility.

One test for men is a home screening test called *Baby Start*. It's a quick test that looks at sperm concentration in semen. It measures sperm as above or below the cutoff of 20 million sperm cells per milliliter (ml). Two test results of less than 20 million cells/ml may indicate male infertility.

Sperm concentration is one element used to help determine fertility. However, because many additional factors play a role in male fertility, a positive test result is *not* a guarantee of fertility. It's a screening test. If your partner uses this test and results indicate a low sperm count, suggest he see a urologist for further testing.

There's a fertility test for couples to use at home; it is called *Fertell* and contains tests for each partner. The tests measure the number of sperm that can swim through mucus in the man and the level of follicle-stimulating hormone (FSH) in a woman at a particular point in her cycle. FSH is important in a woman's ovulation and fertility. The test is available without a prescription and costs about $100.

Your Partner's Health and Fertility

Your partner can affect your ability to get pregnant and may also have an impact on your pregnancy. We know about 40% of all infertility problems can be placed directly on the shoulders of the male partner.

Men have a biological clock. After age 30, a man's level of testosterone decreases about 1% each year. Men over 40 are at increased risk for infertility. In addition, if a man fathers a child after he reaches 40, the child has a greater chance of problems. Risks are even higher for men 55 and older.

Women who have a partner over age 40 have an increased risk of miscarriage, no matter what the woman's age. The miscarriage rate for partners of men under 30 is about 14%. For men over 45, that rate is over 30%!

If your partner's parents underwent fertility treatments to conceive him, he may have fertility issues. Some problems in men born after fertility treatments include lower sperm count, smaller testicles and fewer motile sperm.

Other things can impact on a man's fertility. Below is a discussion of some of the elements that can affect a man.

Foods and Supplements

Your partner's eating habits can affect your chances of getting pregnant. Studies show men who eat and/or avoid certain foods for at least 3 months may increase fertility. Beneficial foods to eat and foods to avoid include those listed in the box on page 593.

Supplements can also affect fertility. Your partner should take a multivitamin every day, especially one with zinc. Avoid zinc supplements that contain cadmium, which can damage the testes. Your partner needs an adequate intake of selenium, either in the foods he eats or as a 60mcg supplement every day. Selenium-rich foods include garlic, fish and eggs.

It's important for a man to consume folate (the folic acid found in food) before conception. One study showed men who took in more than 700mcg each day from food sources passed on 20% fewer chromosomal abnormalities. Good sources of folate include asparagus, bananas, tuna and spinach.

Be careful with manganese—higher blood levels have been found to lower sperm quality. Calcium supplements made from seashells may be contaminated with metals.

Lifestyle Issues

Your partner's lifestyle choices and changes may increase your chances of pregnancy. They may provide your growing baby a healthy start in life when you do get pregnant.

Fertility Food Facts

Foods Beneficial to Fertility

- Grains and seeds
- Nuts, such as cashews and almonds
- Chocolate
- Vitamin-C-rich organic fruits and vegetables, grown without pesticides
- Dark, green, leafy vegetables
- Total of 6 to 8 ounces a day of chicken, meat or fish, including red meat and cooked oysters (but keep total weekly fish intake to 12 ounces or less)
- Calcium-rich foods, such as yogurt, cheese and milk
- Fortified breakfast cereals

Foods that May Contribute to Infertility

- Chips, cookies and crackers made with partially hydrogenated oils
- Fruits and vegetables commercially grown with pesticides
- Fried foods
- High-meat diet

Use of tobacco products can affect sperm production. Smoking one or two packs of cigarettes a day may cause sperm to move slowly and be misshapen. Second-hand and third-hand smoke can also affect a man's fertility.

Smoking marijuana can damage sperm and lower the number of sperm produced. It takes up to several months to rid the body of THC (tetrahydrocannabinol), even after a person quits smoking marijuana.

Alcohol use can lower testosterone levels and contribute to erectile dysfunction. One study showed men who reported drinking heavily around the time of conception increased their partner's risk of miscarriage. Alcohol can cause chromosomal abnormalities in sperm cells.

A man who is too thin or too heavy may have a lower sperm count. Men who are too thin may be malnourished. Men who are too heavy may have lower testosterone levels.

Long-term exposure to solvents in water-based paint has been shown to affect a man's sperm. The culprit is glycol ether. Use of anabolic steroids and nonsteroidal anti-inflammatory medications may slow or reduce sperm production. Even antibiotics can affect sperm production.

Limit time in the hot tub. The scrotum is a few degrees cooler than the rest of the body, so soaking a long time in hot spa water may affect sperm.

Medical Problems

About 10% of American men who are trying to achieve a pregnancy with their partner experience some sort of fertility problem. However, many men don't know they have a problem.

A low sperm count may be caused by infection, hormone problems, certain medications or undescended testicles. Your partner's doctor can explore these conditions with him.

One of the most common situations is a *varicocele*, a collection of enlarged veins in the scrotum that leads to lower sperm production. Another problem is an obstruction in the ducts that carry sperm from the testes. Often, both of these can be taken care of with microsurgical techniques. Taking care of these problems can improve a man's sperm count and increase your chances of achieving pregnancy as a couple.

Treatments for Infertility

If your doctor suggests a *fertility workup* for you and your partner, it helps to understand what's involved. For your partner, a physical and semen analysis may be done and a detailed medical history may be taken.

More is involved in testing you. You are asked for a detailed medical history, and you will probably have a pelvic exam. Blood work may be done to check hormone levels. A vaginal ultrasound to examine your ovaries and uterus may also be done. If your doctor wants to check your Fallopian tubes, a hysterosalpingogram (HSG) may be performed.

Preimplantation Genetic Diagnosis (PGD)

A test that may be done before pregnancy is called *preimplantation genetic diagnosis* (PGD). It's a type of genetic test and is often done if a woman has in-vitro fertilization (IVF). With IVF, an embryo is created outside the womb (*in vitro*) by mixing together an egg and a sperm, then the resulting embryo is implanted in the woman's uterus.

With PGD, a few cells from the embryo are removed and tested *before* the embryo is implanted. The test is done to identify genes responsible for some severe hereditary diseases. The technique has been used to diagnose various disorders, such as cystic fibrosis, Down syndrome, Duchenne muscular dystrophy, hemophilia, Tay-Sachs disease, sickle-cell disease and Turner syndrome.

The goal with PGD is to select healthy embryos for implantation to avoid serious genetic disease. Using this test, a normal embryo can be implanted in the uterus.

After test results are back for you both, you meet with your doctor to discuss results. Then together with your doctor, you examine options for care and/or treatment, if it is necessary for either of you.

Assisted Reproductive Technologies (ART)

Assisted reproductive technologies (ART) can often help a couple achieve pregnancy. ART account for more births today and include the following techniques:

- ovarian stimulation
- superovulation
- in-vitro fertilization

Ovarian stimulation is used to stimulate ovaries to produce an egg. Several different medications are used for this purpose. One of the more common ones is clomiphene (Clomid); it is used most often in women who aren't ovulating and may result in controlled ovarian hyperstimulation. The chance of twin fetuses is somewhat less with clomiphene than with other fertility medicine, but an increased chance still exists.

A complication that may occur is ovarian hyperstimulation syndrome. It is usually mild but can be severe. Ovaries become enlarged and the abdomen becomes distended. Severity can range from moderate discomfort to life-threatening ovarian enlargement and fluid shifts.

The use of fertility drugs can result in *superovulation,* which results in multiple eggs and increases the chance of multiple pregnancies. A large percentage of births resulting from assisted-reproductive techniques are multiples.

In-vitro fertilization (IVF) is the process in which eggs are placed in a medium and sperm are added for fertilization. The zygote produced is then placed inside the uterus in an attempt to result in pregnancy.

Assisted-reproductive techniques account for nearly 65% of all multiple births today. Twins are more common if more than one embryo is inserted. This results when several fertilized eggs are inserted into a woman's uterus in hopes at least one will implant. Today, many experts recommend transferring only one embryo because it improves the live-birth rate and decreases costs.

Fertility treatments are expensive and can cost up to $15,000 for each attempt at conception. Often, fertility treatments are not covered by health insurance.

Appendix B: Breastfeeding Your Baby

Until the 1940s, babies were breastfed almost exclusively. Today, about 70% of all new moms start out breastfeeding their babies. Breastfeeding is the healthiest way to feed baby. For many women, it's a wonderful, loving time and often completes the birth experience.

Breast milk provides many benefits for baby that can't be duplicated by formula feeding. Breast milk provides the best nutrition for your baby.

You can usually begin breastfeeding within an hour (or sooner) after birth. When you do, you begin to establish your milk supply. You can also take advantage of baby's natural sucking instinct. Starting as soon as possible provides your baby with *colostrum,* the first milk your breasts produce. Colostrum helps boost baby's immune system. Breast milk comes in 12 to 48 hours after birth.

For a more complete discussion of breastfeeding baby, read our books *Your Baby's First Year Week by Week* and *Your Pregnancy Quick Guide to Feeding Your Baby.*

Breastfeeding Counselors and Lactation Consultants

If you have problems breastfeeding after baby's birth, people are available to help you. Contact your local La Leche League to be put in contact with a *breastfeeding counselor* who can offer support and share experiences, usually for no fee. She may be available by telephone to answer questions, or she may visit you at home.

When a breastfeeding counselor comes across a problem beyond her scope, she can refer you to a *lactation consultant.* Breastfeeding counselors and lactation consultants often work closely together. A lactation consultant is a qualified professional who may work in hospitals, home-care services, health agencies and pri-

If you smoke, it's best to breastfeed. The benefits of breastfeeding outweigh the hazards from smoke that a baby is exposed to. Nicotine passes through breast milk, but the cancer-causing agents in cigarettes do *not* pass to baby. If you must smoke, wait 90 minutes after smoking to breastfeed. And be sure *not* to smoke around baby!

vate practice. A consultant can help with basic breastfeeding issues, assess and observe you and your baby, develop a care plan, inform healthcare providers of the situation and follow up with you as needed. You can even contact a lactation consultant before baby's birth.

Contact the International Lactation Consultant Association for further information. They can be reached at 919-861-5577 or through their website at www.ilca.org.

Benefits of Breastfeeding

All babies receive some protection from mom against disease before birth. During pregnancy, antibodies pass from mother to baby through the placenta. They circulate through baby's blood for a few months after birth. Breastfed babies receive continued protection in breast milk.

Nursing the first 4 weeks of baby's life provides the most protection for baby and the best hormone release for you. Breastfeeding for as short as 3 months may reduce baby's risk of developing allergies and infections. Breastfeeding for the first 6 months may help reduce the risks of asthma, juvenile diabetes, childhood leukemia, stomach viruses and ear infections in baby. And you may lower your child's risk of SIDS by 50%!

The American Academy of Pediatrics (AAP) recommends breastfeeding exclusively for the first 6 months. However, by the time a baby reaches 3 months, only one in three will still be breastfed. By this age, about 35% of all breastfed babies also receive formula. By the age of 6 months, only 12% of all babies receive breast milk exclusively.

Breast milk contains many substances to help prevent infection. Breastfeeding may reduce the intensity and length of time a problem lasts. For a while, breast milk gives baby immunity against illnesses *you've* had. However, microwaving breast milk can kill antibodies that help protect baby from illness and disease, so *never* microwave breast milk.

DHA (docosahexaenoic acid) and ARA (arachidonic acid) in breast milk are important for baby. Studies show a baby who has them in his diet may have a higher IQ and greater visual development.

Breastfeeding and You

Breastfeeding your baby will definitely have some effects on you. It may help you lose weight, but studies show you need to breastfeed baby for at least 3 months to get any benefit. After your milk supply is well established (about 6 weeks), strenuous exercise shouldn't impact your milk supply. However, sleep loss can affect your milk supply.

Breastfeeding may reduce your risks of diabetes, high blood pressure and heart disease in later life. In addition, new research shows it may cut your breast-cancer risk by nearly 60%! If there's a history of breast cancer in your family, especially your mother or sisters, breastfeeding may help protect you against developing breast cancer. One study recommends women with a family history of breast cancer should be strongly encouraged to breastfeed.

Breastfeeding does *not* make your breasts sag. Your age, weight before pregnancy, your breast size and whether you smoke are greater factors in determining whether your breasts will sag after baby's arrival.

Still being careful with caffeine consumption? Drinking one to two cups of coffee a day shouldn't affect baby. However, if you notice baby becoming agitated, cut down your intake.

Be careful with alcohol consumption. Don't believe the old wives' tale that drinking beer will help increase your milk supply. When you do have an alcoholic drink, drink it immediately after breastfeeding and don't have more than one. Choose wine or beer because the percentage of alcohol in beer and wine is lower than that for hard liquor. Beer and wine pass from your body in about 3 hours. Studies show it takes up to 13 hours for hard liquor to leave the body.

Disadvantages of Breastfeeding

Let's be honest—there are disadvantages to breastfeeding. Breastfeeding ties you completely to baby. Because you must be available when baby is hungry, other family members may feel left out.

Because breast milk empties rapidly from baby's stomach, most newborns need to feed every couple of hours. You may spend more time feeding baby than you anticipated. Pay careful attention to your diet. Most substances you eat or drink (or take orally, such as medicine) can pass to baby in your breast milk and might cause problems.

Problems You May Have during Breastfeeding

Problems during breastfeeding are not uncommon. On the opposite page is a discussion of the three most common medical situations you may encounter.

Engorgement

A common breastfeeding problem for some women is *breast engorgement.* Breasts become swollen, tender and filled with breast milk. What can you do to relieve this problem?

The best cure is to drain the breasts, if possible, as you do when breastfeeding. Some women take a hot shower and empty their breasts in the warm water. Ice packs may also help.

Feed your baby from both breasts *each time* you feed. Don't feed on only one side.

When you're away from your baby, try to express some breast milk to keep your milk flowing and breast ducts open. You'll also feel more comfortable.

Over-the-counter medicines, such as acetaminophen, are often useful in relieving the pain of engorgement. Acetaminophen is recommended by the American Academy of Pediatrics as safe to use while breastfeeding.

You might need to use stronger medications, such as acetaminophen with codeine, if pain is more severe. Call your healthcare provider; he or she will decide on treatment.

Breast Infections

It is possible to get an infection in your breast while breastfeeding. An infection may cause pain in the breast, and the breast may turn red and become swollen. You may have streaks of red discoloration on the breast; you may also feel as though you have the flu.

If you think you have an infection, call your healthcare provider. He or she can devise a treatment plan and/or prescribe medication for you, if necessary.

Sore Nipples

Most nursing mothers have sore nipples at some point, particularly when they begin breastfeeding. You can take steps to lessen or to relieve the soreness. Try the following.

- Keep your breasts dry and clean.
- Do *not* air dry—it encourages scab formation and can take quite a while for a sore breast to heal.
- Moist healing is best, such as applying lanolin.
- Cover the entire nipple area with lanolin every time baby finishes nursing.
- Express a little breast milk after breastfeeding, and rub it over your nipples. Research shows that breast milk contains antibiotic qualities that can help prevent and/or heal sore, cracked nipples.

Good news! Before too long—a few days to a few weeks—your breasts will become accustomed to breastfeeding, and problems will lessen.

Your Nutrition If You Breastfeed

You need to think about your nutrition when you breastfeed. It's important in making breast milk.

You will probably be advised to eat about 500 extra calories each day. Your breast milk provides 425 to 700 calories to your baby every day! The extra calories help you maintain good health, so they should be nutritious, like the ones you ate during pregnancy. Choose 9 servings from the bread/cereal/pasta/rice group and 3 servings from the dairy group. Fruit servings should number 4, and vegetable servings should number 5. The amount of protein in your diet should be 8 ounces a day during breastfeeding. Be careful with fats, oils and sugars; limit intake to 4 teaspoons.

Some foods can pass into breast milk and cause baby stomach distress. Avoid chocolate, foods that produce gas in you, highly spiced foods and any other foods you have problems with. Discuss the situation with your healthcare provider and your pediatrician if you have questions.

You also need to continue to drink lots of fluids. Keeping hydrated can help increase your milk production and energy levels. Drink at least *2 quarts* of fluid every day. You'll need more fluid in hot weather. Avoid caffeine-containing foods and drinks; they can act as diuretics.

Keep up your calcium intake. Ask about the kind of vitamin supplement you should take. Some mothers take a prenatal vitamin as long as they breastfeed. Some new moms take lactation supplements that contain higher doses of some vitamins and minerals than prenatal vitamins, and lower doses of iron.

Breastfeeding depletes your supply of choline. You need 550mg a day to replace it.

Breastfeed with Confidence—Tips to Get Started

You may have some problems when you begin breastfeeding. Don't be discouraged if you do. It takes some time to discover what works for you and baby. There are things to do to help make breastfeeding a success. Below are some things to keep in mind as you begin nursing.

> Breastfed babies need extra vitamin D because breast milk doesn't contain enough of this important vitamin. Talk to your pediatrician about giving baby 400IU of a liquid vitamin-D supplement every day, beginning at birth.

It takes practice! Although breastfeeding is a natural way to feed baby, it takes time and practice to get the hang of it.

Feed baby on demand—this could be as many as 8 to 10 times a day or more! A baby usually cuts back to eating 4 to 6 times a day by age 4 months. A breastfed baby will take in only as much breast milk as he needs, so your milk production will usually adjust to his needs.

Hold baby so he can easily reach your breast while nursing. Hold him across your chest, or lie in bed. His tummy should touch you; tuck his lower arm between your arm and your side.

Help him latch on to your breast. Brush your nipple across his lips. When he opens his mouth, place your nipple and as much of the areola as possible in his mouth. You should feel him pull the breast while sucking, but it shouldn't hurt.

If you're having problems with breastfeeding, keep a log of the time and length of each feeding and which side you nursed on. This may help you see more clearly how much time you're spending feeding baby every day.

Nurse baby 5 to 10 minutes on each breast; he gets most of his milk at the beginning of the feeding. Don't rush him—it can take as long as 30 minutes for him to finish. Baby may not need burping. As you begin, burp between feedings at each breast and when baby finishes. If he doesn't burp, don't force it. He may not need to.

Some experts believe you can start feeding baby a bottle almost as soon as you get home from the hospital. If you're going to give baby a bottle, give him expressed breast milk because he's familiar with the taste. In addition, feed a bottle an hour or two *after* breastfeeding. It's easier to get baby to try a bottle when he's not starving.

Breastfeeding More than One Baby

Feeding multiples can be a challenge. Even if you have more than one baby, you should be able to breastfeed them. Breastfeeding for one or two feedings a day gives them the protection from infection that breast milk provides. Research has shown that even the smallest dose of breast milk gives baby an advantage over babies only fed formula.

If babies are early, and you can't nurse them, begin pumping! Pump from day one, and store your breast milk for the time babies are able to receive it. In addition, pumping tells the body to produce breast milk—pump and the milk will come. It just takes some time.

You may find your babies do well with breast *and* bottlefeeding. Bottlefeeding doesn't always mean feeding formula. You can bottlefeed expressed breast milk.

Supplementing with formula allows your partner and others to help you feed the babies. You can breastfeed one while someone else bottlefeeds the other. Or you can nurse each one for a time, then finish the feeding with formula. In either case, someone else can help you.

Medications You May Take while Breastfeeding

Be very careful with any medicine you take if you breastfeed, even in the hospital. If you take codeine for pain after delivery, watch baby for signs of difficulty breathing, limpness and extreme drowsiness.

Take a medication *only* when you need it, and take it *only* as prescribed. Ask for the smallest dose possible. Ask about possible effects on the baby, so you can be alert for them. Wait to get treatment, if possible. Consider taking medication immediately after nursing; it may have less of an effect on baby.

Many new moms worry about taking antibiotics while breastfeeding. Most commonly used antibiotics are safe for breastfeeding moms. There is some concern about metronidazole (Flagyl). The AAP suggests a woman shouldn't breastfeed while taking it. She should also throw out milk for 24 hours after finishing the medicine, before breastfeeding again.

Safe antibiotics to take during nursing include acyclovir, amoxicillin, aztreonam, cefazolin, cefotaxime, cefoxitin, cefprozil, ceftazidime, ceftriaxone, chloroquine, ciprofloxacin, clindamycin, dapsone, erythromycin, ethambutol, fluconazole and gentamicin. Also safe to use are isoniazid, kanamycin, nitrofurantoin, ofloxacin, quinidine, quinine, rifampin, streptomycin, sulbactam, sulfadiazine, sulfisoxazole, tetracycline and trimethoprim-sulfamethoxazole.

If a medicine could have serious effects on your baby, you may decide to bottle-feed while you take the medication. You can maintain your milk supply by pumping (then throwing away) expressed milk.

Is Baby Getting Enough Milk?

You may be concerned about how much breast milk your baby gets at a feeding. There are clues to look for. Watch his jaws and ears while he eats—is he actively sucking? At the end of a feeding, does he fall asleep or settle down easily? Can he go 1½ hours between feedings? You'll know your baby is getting enough to eat if he:

- nurses frequently, such as every 2 to 3 hours or 8 to 12 times in 24 hours
- has 6 to 8 wet diapers and/or 2 to 5 bowel movements a day
- gains 4 to 7 ounces a week or at least 1 pound a month
- appears healthy, has good muscle tone and is alert and active

There are some warning signs to watch for. Be concerned if your breasts show little or no change during pregnancy, there's no engorgement after birth or no breast milk by the fifth day. If you can't hear baby gulping while he feeds or he loses more than 10% of his birth weight, it's cause for concern. If baby never seems satisfied, discuss it with your pediatrician.

If your baby is a boy, your breast milk contains 25% more calories than if baby is a girl.

Appendix C: Bottlefeeding Your Baby

Many women choose to bottlefeed baby—studies show more women bottlefeed than breastfeed. In fact, many new moms begin by breastfeeding, but by 3 months, over 65% of all babies are bottlefed exclusively. By the age of 6 months, only 12% of all babies receive only breast milk.

Don't feel guilty if you decide to bottlefeed—it's a personal decision you're entitled to make. You won't be considered a "terrible mother" because you choose not to, or cannot, breastfeed. Baby will be OK if you bottlefeed her.

Sometimes a woman can't breastfeed. You may be very underweight or have a medical condition so you can't breastfeed. Some babies have problems breastfeeding or can't breastfeed due to a physical problem. Lactose intolerance can also cause breastfeeding problems.

Some women try to breastfeed, but it doesn't work out. You may choose not to breastfeed because of other demands on your time, such as a job or other children to care for. Your baby can still get all the love, attention and nutrition she needs by bottlefeeding. Don't worry about it. It's OK!

Bottlefeeding doesn't always mean feeding baby formula. You can also bottlefeed expressed breast milk. There may be many reasons you may choose to introduce your baby to the bottle. One is so Dad can feed baby. Another is so Mom can get a bit of rest. This is especially important if the new mother is ill or suffers from postpartum distress syndrome.

For a more-complete discussion of bottlefeeding baby, read our books *Your Baby's First Year Week by Week* and *Your Pregnancy Quick Guide to Feeding Your Baby.*

Advantages to Bottlefeeding

Your baby can receive good nutrition if you bottlefeed her iron-fortified formula. Some women enjoy the freedom bottlefeeding provides. It can make it easier for someone else to help care for the baby. You can determine exactly how much formula your baby is taking in at each feeding. There are also other advantages to bottlefeeding.

- Bottlefeeding is easy to learn; it never hurts if it's done incorrectly.
- Dad can be more involved in caring for baby.

- Bottlefed babies may go longer between feedings because formula is usually digested more slowly than breast milk.
- A day's supply of formula can be mixed at one time, saving time and effort.
- You don't have to be concerned about feeding baby in front of other people.
- It may be easier to bottlefeed if you plan to return to work soon after baby's birth.
- If you feed iron-fortified formula, baby won't need iron supplements.
- If you use fluoridated tap water to mix formula, you may not have to give baby fluoride supplements.
- Premeasured formula containers are great when you're on the go.

It takes about 10 to 15 days for your milk production to decline and stop if you don't breastfeed. The greatest discomfort is usually experienced between the third and fifth day after delivery. To help ease soreness, wear a sports bra day *and* night, take acetaminophen or ibuprofen, and use cold packs.

Bottlefeeding is not cheap—you'll spend $1500 to $2000 to feed your baby formula for the first year.

Most parents want to establish a strong bond with baby. However, some fear bottlefeeding won't encourage closeness with their child. They fear bonding won't happen between parent and baby. It's not true that a woman must breastfeed her baby to bond with her.

Skin-to-skin contact while bottlefeeding helps bring mom (or anyone else feeding baby) and baby closer. When feeding baby, choose a quiet place—this helps her concentrate on eating and helps you bond.

Your Nutrition If You Bottlefeed

Even if you bottlefeed, it's important to follow a nutritious eating plan, such as the one you followed during pregnancy. Continue to eat foods high in complex carbohydrates, such as grain products, fruits and vegetables. Lean meats, chicken and fish are good sources of protein. For your dairy products, choose the low-fat or skim types.

You need fewer calories than you would if you were breastfeeding. But don't drastically cut your calories in the hopes of losing weight quickly. You still need to eat nutritiously to maintain good energy levels. Be sure the calories you eat are not from junk foods.

Here is a list of the types and quantities of foods you should try to eat each day. Choose 6 servings from the bread/cereal/pasta/rice group and 3 servings of fruit. Eat 3 servings of vegetables. From the dairy group, choose 2 servings. Eat about 6 ounces of protein each day. We still advise caution with fats, oils and sugars; limit intake to 3 teaspoons. And keep up your fluid intake. You can also use the pregnancy nutrition plan as a reference; see Week 6.

Formulas to Consider

Commercial formula first became available in the 1930s. Today, we have many types and brands of formula available to feed baby. Ask your pediatrician about the type of formula you should feed your baby.

When choosing formula, there isn't much difference among the brands of regular formula available. Most babies do well on milk-based formula. Basic infant formula comes from cow's milk and is modified to make it more similar to breast milk. It's also easier to digest than regular cow's milk. Most formulas are iron fortified. A baby needs iron for normal growth; a recent study showed that too little iron can lead to problems.

Formulas are packaged in powder form, concentrated liquid and ready-to-feed. Powdered formula is the least expensive. The end product is the same. When choosing formula, go for the powdered type in cans. Cans containing liquid formula often are lined with plastic containing BPA. To avoid BPA exposure, many companies sell products in glass or BPA-free containers.

All formulas sold in the United States must meet the same minimum standards set by the FDA, so they are all nutritionally complete. You don't need to worry about contaminated formula. Formula production is strictly controlled, so the risk of contamination is very low. It's illegal to import formula from other countries. If you know of a grocery store selling foreign formula, don't buy it!

Many formulas on the market include two nutrients found in breast milk—DHA and ARA. DHA (docosahexaenoic acid) contributes to baby's eye development. ARA (arachidonic acid) is important in baby's brain development. Studies show babies fed with formula supplemented with DHA and ARA do better on cognitive tests than babies fed formula without them. They also have better visual sharpness.

If you make formula from tap water, use cold water. Many pipes can contain lead; heated tap water releases lead from pipes. If you want to warm up the formula, use hot water on the *outside* of the bottle.

The American Academy of Pediatrics recommends a baby be fed iron-fortified formula for the first year of her life. Feeding for this length of time helps maintain adequate iron intake.

Feeding Equipment to Use

Don't buy plastic bottles or containers with the number 7 on the label or bottom. This helps avoid exposing baby to BPA. When you feed her a bottle, you may want to use a slanted one. Research shows this design keeps the nipple full of milk, which means baby takes in less air. A slanted bottle also helps ensure baby is sitting up to drink. When a baby drinks lying down, milk can pool in the eustachian tube, which may lead to ear infections.

You'll also have to choose a nipple for baby's bottle. A wide, round, soft flexible nipple helps baby latch on with her mouth opened wide, similar to nursing. Another type of nipple allows formula or pumped breast milk to be released at the same rate as breast milk flows during nursing. A twist adjusts the nipple to a flow that is slow, medium or fast. In this way, you can find the flow that works best for your baby. The nipple fits on most bottles. Check your local stores if you're interested.

Bottlefeeding Pointers

Bottlefed babies take from 2 to 5 ounces of formula at a feeding. They feed about every 3 to 4 hours for the first month (6 to 8 times a day). If baby fusses when her bottle is empty, it's OK to give her a little more. When baby is older, the number of feedings decreases, but the amount of formula you feed at each feeding increases.

If baby pulls away from the bottle, it's usually a sign she's finished feeding. However, you may want to try burping her before ending the feeding.

You know baby's getting enough formula if she has 6 to 8 wet diapers a day. She may also have 1 or 2 bowel movements. Stools of a bottlefed baby are more solid and greener in color than a breastfed baby's.

If your baby poops after a feeding, it's caused by the *gastrocolic reflex*. This reflex causes squeezing of the intestines when the stomach is stretched, as with feeding. It's very pronounced in newborns and usually decreases after 2 or 3 months of age.

After baby drinks 2 ounces, burp her. Burp baby after every feeding to help her get rid of excess air. If baby doesn't want a feeding, don't force it. Try again in a couple of hours. But if she refuses two feedings in a row, contact your pediatrician. Baby may be sick.

Appendix D: If Your Baby Is Premature

Over 475,000 babies are born prematurely in the United States every year. *Premature birth* is defined as birth before 37 weeks of pregnancy. About 12% of all births are considered premature or preterm; in the past 30 years, the number of preterm births has increased by 30%. Research shows about 25% of preterm births are a result of a pregnancy problem. However, for nearly 50% of all premature births, the cause is unknown.

A baby born prematurely is often called a *preemie*; the type of care he receives depends on how early he was born. Some babies are not extremely early and won't require extensive care. Other babies need long-term care and won't go home for weeks or months. The rule of thumb is the earlier a baby is born, the longer he'll need care.

All premature babies are individuals. Your baby will be evaluated and tended to based on his unique needs. For a more complete discussion of your premature baby, read our book *Your Baby's First Year Week by Week.*

Immediate Care for Your Newborn

When a baby is born early, many things can happen very quickly. A preemie needs more care because his body can't take over and perform some normal body functions. If baby has difficulty breathing, the nursing staff will help him, which can be done in many ways. After baby is tended to in the delivery room, he will be moved to the infant-care nursery or to a special unit for treatment, evaluation and care.

If baby needs wide-ranging, in-depth care, he will be moved to the neonatal intensive-care unit, also called the NICU (pronounced *NICK-U*). The nurses and physicians who work in these units have received specialized education and training so they may care for preemies.

The first time you see baby for any length of time may be after he has been moved to the NICU. You may be amazed by his size. The earlier he was born, the smaller he will be.

As time passes and baby grows, you'll probably be able to hold him. You will also be encouraged to care for him, such as giving him a bath, changing him and feeding him. Kangaroo care—holding a naked baby against your naked chest—for 1 hour a day, several times a week, provides many health benefits for a preemie.

You'll see many pieces of equipment and machines in the unit. They are there to help provide the best care possible for your baby. Monitors record various information, ventilators help baby breathe, lights warm baby or help treat jaundice. Even baby's bed may be unique.

Feeding Your Preemie

Feeding is very important in a premature baby. In fact, a baby being able to feed on his own for all of his feedings may be one of the milestones the doctor looks for when considering when to release him. Breastfeeding or bottlefeeding for every feeding is a major accomplishment.

For the first few days or weeks after birth, a premature baby is often fed intravenously. When a baby is premature, he may not have the ability to suck and to swallow, so he can't breastfeed or bottlefeed. His gastrointestinal system is too immature to absorb nutrients. Feeding him by I.V. gives him the nutrition he needs in a form he can digest.

Premature babies often have digestive problems. They need to be fed small amounts at each feeding, so they must be fed often.

If you're going to breastfeed baby, you'll need to supply your breast milk. Pumping may be the answer. Studies have shown any amount of breast milk is good for a preemie, so seriously consider this important task.

DHA (docosahexaenoic acid) and ARA (arachidonic acid) are two nutrients present in breast milk that can really help a preemie. If you can't breastfeed, ask the NICU nurses if baby will be fed a special preemie formula that contains these nutrients.

The composition of your breast milk when baby is born prematurely is different from the breast milk when baby is full-term. Because of this difference, baby may also be supplemented with formula.

Choosing a Pediatrician for Your Preemie

The care your baby receives after he leaves the hospital is very important. Try to find a pediatrician who has had experience caring for premature babies. You'll probably be seeing this doctor quite frequently during the first year, so it's important to feel comfortable with him or her.

Problems Some Preemies May Have

When a baby is born prematurely, he hasn't had time to finish growing and developing inside the womb. Being born too early can impact on baby's health in many ways. Today, with all the medical and technological advances medicine has made in the care of premature babies, we are fortunate that many children have few long-term difficulties.

Some immediate problems your baby may have are listed below. Some are short term; others may need to be dealt with for the rest of the child's life.

- jaundice
- apnea
- respiratory distress syndrome (RDS)
- broncho-pulmonary dysplasia (BPD)
- undescended testicles
- patent ductus arteriosus
- intracranial hemorrhage (ICH)
- retinopathy of prematurity (ROP)
- respiratory syncytial virus (RSV)

Taking Baby Home

At some point, you'll be able to take baby home. Your baby will be ready to go home when he has no medical problems that require him to be in the hospital, can maintain a stable body temperature, takes all of his feedings on his own (no tube feeding) and is gaining weight.

People in the NICU will help you prepare for this important event. They can help you plan for any special-care needs before you take baby home. Once home, most preemies do well.

Your premature baby may be at an increased risk for SIDS. To help protect him, follow established guidelines for reducing SIDS for the entire *first year* of your baby's life. It's important to put baby *on his back* every time you put him in his crib or bassinet!

Mental and Physical Development of Your Baby

As baby grows and develops, you must always keep in mind that he was born early. For as long as the first 2 years of his life, development may be slower than the development of children who were born close to their due date. Your baby will have two ages—his *chronological age* (when he was born) and his *developmental age,* which is based on the date he was due. Developmental age is also called *adjusted age.*

Experts believe children born early may need help well beyond the early years. As parents, you'll want to be involved in measuring your child's learning and behavior activities. Discuss this with your physician so you can work together as a team to help your child.

When a baby is born early, it may take him longer to reach an event marking a new development or stage. These are called *milestones* and help you determine how baby is advancing. It really doesn't matter *when* your child reaches a milestone as long as he eventually reaches it!

When you evaluate how your child is developing, correct his age for the weeks of prematurity. Consider his developmental age from his due date, not his actual date of birth! For example, if baby was born on April 18th but his due date was actually June 6th, begin measuring his development from June 6th. Consider this his "developmental birthday."

Appendix E: Choosing Child Care for Baby

If you and your partner work, child care may be one of the most important decisions you must make for baby. You're not alone. Nearly 65% of all working mothers have children under age 6.

Finding the best situation for your baby can take time. Begin the process long before you need it. Often this means finding child care before baby is born. Some places have a waiting list.

There is a shortage of quality child care for children under age 2. If you find a care provider you're comfortable with, but it's not time to leave your baby, ask to put down a deposit and set a date for child care to begin. Keep in touch with the care provider, and plan to meet before you place your child in daily care.

Many decisions must be made when selecting someone to care for your baby. You want the best setting and the best caregiver for your child. The way to do that is to know what your options are before you begin. There are many choices when it comes to child care. Any of a variety of situations could be right for you. Examine your needs and the needs of your child before you decide which one to pursue.

Always check references before you make a final decision! This applies to centers as well as in-home caregivers (your home or theirs).

Checklist for Child-Care Situations

When you're choosing child care for your baby, keep the following in mind as you check out various places.

- Be sure the place is clean and childproofed, and the play area is fenced in. Look at equipment and toys to make sure they are safe, clean and well-maintained.
- Watch how child-care providers interact with the children. Are they actively involved with them? The ratio of infants to care givers should be 3 to 1, with no more than 6 babies in a group.
- Ask about the turnover rate of employees. See how the director interacts with his or her staff. Check to see that all caregivers have been checked out thoroughly by the center before they were employed.
- Are visits to your child permitted at any time, or are you asked to come only at certain times so you don't disrupt routines?

- Check snacks to see if they are nutritious and prepared in a clean kitchen or prep area.

In-Home Child Care

In-home child care involves either someone coming to your home to take care of baby or you taking baby to someone else's house. With in-home care, the caregiver can be a relative or nonrelative.

When you have someone come to your home, it makes things easier for you. You don't have to get baby ready in the morning. You never have to take your child out in bad weather. If she's sick, you don't have to take time off from work or try to find someone to stay with her. It takes less time in the morning and evening if you don't have to drop off baby or pick her up.

Care in your own home may be an excellent choice for a baby or small child because it provides one-on-one attention (if you only have one child at home). The environment is also familiar to the child.

Taking your child to someone else's home is another in-home care option. Often homes have small group sizes and offer more flexibility for parents, such as keeping the child longer on a day you have a late meeting. They may offer a homelike setting, and your child may receive lots of attention. In a group-home situation, there should be a maximum of two children under age 2.

Whether you choose to have someone come to your home or take your child to another person's home, there are some steps you can use to find a care provider. Following the suggestions below can help you find the best caregiver for your child.

Advertise in local newspapers and church bulletins to find someone to interview. State how many children are to be cared for and their ages. Include information on the days and hours care is needed, experience you're seeking and any other particulars. State that references are required and you will check them.

Talk to people on the telephone first to determine whether you want to interview them. Ask about their experience, qualifications, child-care philosophy and what they are seeking in a position. Then decide if you want to pursue the contact with an in-person interview. Make a list of all your concerns, including days and hours someone is needed, duties to be performed and need for a driver's license. Discuss these with the potential caregiver.

Check references for anyone you're considering! Have the potential caregiver give you the names and phone numbers of people he or she has worked for in the past. Call each family, let them know you're considering this person as a caregiver and discuss it with them.

Care for an Infant

Be sure the place you choose for your infant can meet her needs. A baby must be changed and fed, but she also needs to be held and interacted with. She needs to be comforted when she's afraid. She needs to rest at certain times each day.

When searching for a place, keep in mind what will be required for your child. Evaluate every situation as to how it can respond to the needs of your baby.

After you hire someone, drop by occasionally unannounced. See how everything is when you do. Pay attention to how your child reacts when you leave or arrive. This can give you a clue as to how your child feels about the caregiver. Do this for any type of child care you choose.

Child-Care Centers

At a child-care center, many children are cared for in a larger setting. Centers vary widely in the facilities and activities they provide, the amount of attention they give each child, group sizes and child-care philosophy. Day-care centers usually provide care to many children.

You may find some child-care centers don't accept infants. Often centers focus more on older children; babies take a lot of time and attention. If the center accepts infants, the ratio of caregivers to children should be about one adult to every three or four children (up to age 2).

Inquire about training required for each child-care provider or teacher. Some facilities expect more from a caregiver than others. In some cases, a facility hires only trained, qualified personnel, or they train them and provide additional training.

The Cost of Child Care

Paying for child care can be a big-budget item in household expenses. For some families, it can cost as much as 25% or more of their household budget. Public funding is available for some families. Title EE is a program paid for with federal funds. Call your local Department of Social Services to see if you're eligible.

Other programs that can help with child-care costs include a federal tax-credit program, the dependent-care-assistance program and earned-income tax credit.

These programs are regulated by the federal government. Contact the Internal Revenue Service at 800-829-1040 for further information.

Special-Care Needs

In some situations, your child may have special needs. If your baby is born with a problem and needs one-on-one care, you may have a harder time finding child care. In these special cases, you may have to spend extra time seeking a qualified care provider.

Contact the hospital where your child has been cared for, and ask for references. Or contact your pediatrician. The office staff may be in contact with someone who can help you. It may be better for a child with special needs for the care provider to come to your home.

Appendix F: Postpartum Distress Syndrome (PPDS)

You may experience many emotional changes after baby is born. Mood swings, mild distress or bouts of crying are not uncommon. Changes in moods are often a result of hormonal changes you experience after birth, just as they were when you were pregnant.

Many women are surprised by how tired they are emotionally *and* physically in the first few months after their baby's birth. Make sure you take time for yourself. Sleep and rest can help you deal with mood shifts, which seem to occur more often when a woman is exhausted.

After pregnancy, many women experience some degree of depression. This is called *postpartum distress syndrome (PPDS).* Some experts believe postpartum depression may begin *during* pregnancy, but symptoms may not appear until several months *after* delivery. They may occur when a woman starts getting her period again and experiences hormonal changes.

Postpartum distress syndrome can resolve on its own, but it can often take as long as a year. With more severe problems, treatment may relieve symptoms in a matter of weeks, and improvement should be significant within 6 to 8 months. Often medication is necessary for complete recovery.

If your baby blues don't get better in a few weeks, or if you feel extremely depressed, call your healthcare provider. You may need medication to help deal with the problem.

Different Degrees of Depression

There are different degrees of depression. The mildest form is *baby blues.* Up to 80% of all women have "baby blues." They usually appear between 2 days and 2 weeks after the baby is born. They are temporary and usually leave as quickly as they come. This situation lasts only a couple of weeks, and symptoms do not worsen.

A more serious version of postpartum distress is called *postpartum depression (PPD).* It affects about 10% of all new mothers. The difference between baby blues and postpartum depression lies in the frequency, intensity and duration of the symptoms.

PPD can occur from 2 weeks to 1 year after the birth. A mother may have feelings of anger, confusion, panic and hopelessness. She may experience changes in her eating and sleeping patterns. She may fear she will hurt her baby or feel as if she is going crazy. Anxiety is one of the major symptoms of PPD.

The most serious form of postpartum distress is *postpartum psychosis (PPP)*. The woman may have hallucinations, think about suicide or try to harm the baby. Many women who develop postpartum psychosis also exhibit signs of bipolar mood disorder, which is unrelated to childbirth. Discuss this situation with your physician if you are concerned.

After you give birth, if you believe you are suffering from some form of postpartum distress syndrome, contact your healthcare provider. Every postpartum reaction, whether mild or severe, is usually temporary and treatable.

It's normal to feel extremely tired, especially after the hard work of labor and delivery and adjusting to the demands of being a new mom. However, if after 2 weeks of motherhood you're just as exhausted as you were shortly after you delivered, you may be at risk of developing postpartum depression.

Causes of Postpartum Distress Syndrome

Researchers aren't sure what causes postpartum distress; not all women experience it. A woman's individual sensitivity to hormonal changes may be part of the cause; the drop in estrogen and progesterone after delivery may contribute to postpartum distress syndrome.

A new mother must make many adjustments, and many demands are placed on her. Either or both of these situations may cause distress. If you had a Cesarean delivery, you may also be at greater risk for postpartum depression.

Other possible factors include a family history of depression, lack of familial support after the birth, isolation and chronic fatigue. You may also be at higher risk of suffering from PPDS if:

- your mother or sister suffered from the problem—it seems to run in families
- you suffered from PPDS with a previous pregnancy—chances are you'll have the problem again
- you had fertility treatments to achieve this pregnancy—hormone fluctuations may be more severe, which may cause PPDS
- you suffered extreme PMS before the pregnancy—hormonal imbalances may be greater after the birth
- you have a personal history of depression, or you suffered from untreated depression before pregnancy
- a hormonal drop as a result
- you are anxious or have low self-esteem
- you have a struggling relationship with baby's father

- your access to finances and health care are limited
- you experience little social support
- you had more than one baby or you have a colicky or high-maintenance baby
- you experienced a lack of sleep during pregnancy, you sleep less than 6 hours in a 24-hour period or you wake 3 or more times a night

In addition, if you answer "most of the time" or "some of the time" to any of the following questions, you may be at increased risk.

- I blame myself when things go wrong (even if you have nothing to do with them).
- I often feel scared or panicked without good reason.
- I am anxious or worried without good reason.

Handling the Baby Blues

One of the most important ways you can help yourself handle baby blues is to have a good support system near at hand. Ask family members and friends to help. Ask your mother or mother-in-law to stay for a while. Ask your husband to take some work leave, or hire someone to come in and help each day.

Rest when your baby sleeps. Find other mothers who are in the same situation; it helps to share your feelings and experiences. Don't try to be perfect. Pamper yourself.

Do some form of moderate exercise every day, even if it's just going for a walk. Eat nutritiously, and drink plenty of fluids. Get out of the house every day. Eating more complex carbohydrates may help raise your mood. And giving baby a massage may help *you* because it helps you connect with your baby.

Talk to your healthcare provider about temporarily using antidepressants if the above steps don't work for you. About 85% of all women who suffer from postpartum depression require medication for up to 1 year.

Dealing with More Serious Forms of PPDS

Beyond the relatively minor symptoms of baby blues, postpartum distress syndrome can appear in two ways. Some women experience acute depression that can last for weeks or months; they cannot sleep or eat, they feel worthless and isolated, they are sad and they cry a great deal. For other women, they are extremely anxious, restless and agitated. Their heart rate increases. Some unfortunate women experience both sets of symptoms at the same time.

If you experience any symptoms, call your healthcare provider immediately. He or she will probably see you in the office, then prescribe a course of treatment. Do it for yourself and your family.

Your Distress Can Affect Your Partner

If you experience baby blues or PPD, it can also affect your partner. Prepare him for this situation before baby is born. Explain to him that if it happens to you, it's only temporary.

There are some things you might suggest to your partner that he can do for himself, if you get blue or depressed. Tell him not to take the situation personally. Suggest he talk to friends, family members, other fathers or a professional. He should eat well, get enough rest and exercise. Ask him to be patient with you, and ask him to provide his love and support to you during this difficult time.

Glossary

Abdominal measurement—Measurement at prenatal visits of baby's growth inside the uterus. Made from pubic symphysis to fundus; also called *fundal measurement.* Too much growth or too little growth may indicate problems.

Abnormal placentation—Complication of multiple Cesarean deliveries; of concern to medical experts with increasing rate of Cesarean delivery.

Abruptio placenta—See *placental abruption.*

Acquired immunodeficiency syndrome (AIDS)—Debilitating, frequently fatal illness that affects the body's ability to respond to infection. Caused by the human immune deficiency virus (HIV).

Active labor—Woman's cervix is dilated between 4 and 8cm. Contractions are usually 3 to 5 minutes apart.

Advance-practice nurse—Nurse who has received postgraduate education in a medical specialty; must be nationally certified, such as in women's health. Licensed through a state nursing board. Also called a *nurse practitioner (NP).*

Aerobic exercise—Exercise that increases heart rate and causes person to consume oxygen.

Afterbirth—Placenta and membranes expelled after baby is delivered. See *placenta.*

Alpha-fetoprotein (AFP)—Substance produced by unborn baby as it grows inside the uterus. Large amounts of AFP are found in amniotic fluid. Part of triple- or quad-screen test.

Alveolar gland—Grapelike cluster of cells in the breast where milk is produced.

Amino acids—Substances that act as building blocks in developing baby.

Amniocentesis—Procedure in which amniotic fluid is removed from amniotic sac for testing for some genetic defects and for fetal lung maturity.

Amniotic fluid—Fluid surrounding baby inside the amniotic sac.

Amnioinfusion—Injection of sterile saline solution into the amniotic sac.

Amniotic sac—Membrane that surrounds the baby inside the uterus; contains baby, placenta and amniotic fluid. Also called *amnion.*

Ampulla—Dilated opening of a tube or duct.

Anatomy scan—Ultrasound that measures baby's length and head size, and checks for organ development. Also called a *level-2 ultrasound.*

Anemia—Condition in which the number of red blood cells is less than normal.

Anencephaly—Defective development of baby's brain, combined with absence of bones normally surrounding the brain.

Aneuploidy—Abnormal number of chromosomes.

Angioma—Tumor or swelling; composed of lymph and blood vessels. Usually benign.

Anovulatory—Woman doesn't ovulate.
Anti-inflammatory medications—Drugs to relieve pain and/or inflammation.
Apgar scores—Measurement of baby's response to birth and life on its own. Taken 1 minute and 5 minutes after birth.
Areola—Colored ring surrounding the nipple of the breast.
Arrhythmia—Irregular or missed heartbeat.
Aspiration—Swallowing or sucking foreign body or fluid, such as vomit, into an airway.
Asthma—Disease marked by recurrent attacks of shortness of breath and difficulty breathing. Often caused by allergic reaction.
Atonic uterus—Uterus that lacks tone.
Atopic—Inherited tendency to develop allergies; caused by an oversensitive immune system.
Augmented labor—When labor is "stalled" or progress is not being made, medication (oxytocin) is given.
Autoantibodies—Antibodies that attack parts of the body or tissues.

Baby blues—Mild depression in a woman after delivery.
Back labor—Labor pain felt in the lower back.
Beta-adrenergics—Substances that interfere with transmission of stimuli; affects autonomic nervous system.
Bicornuate uterus—Uterus is divided into two halves; a woman may have one cervix or two cervices.
Bilirubin—Product formed in the liver from hemoglobin when red blood cells are destroyed.
Biophysical profile (BPP)—Method of evaluating baby before birth.
Biopsy—Removal of a small piece of tissue for microscopic study.
Birthing center—Facility specializing in delivering babies. Usually a woman labors, delivers and recovers in same room. May be part of hospital or a free-standing unit. Sometimes called *LDRP,* for labor, delivery, recovery and postpartum.
Bishop score—Method used to predict success of inducing labor. Includes dilatation, station, effacement, consistency and position of cervix. Score is given for each point, then all are added together to give a total score to help doctor decide whether to induce labor.
Blood pressure—Push of blood against artery walls; arteries which carry blood away from the heart. Changes in blood pressure may indicate problems.
Blood typing—Test to determine if a woman's blood type is A, B, AB or O.
Blood-pressure check—Checking a woman's blood pressure. Changes in blood pressure can be an alert for potential problems. High blood pressure can be significant during pregnancy, especially nearer the due date.
Blood-sugar tests—See *glucose-tolerance test.*
Bloody show—Small amount of vaginal bleeding late in pregnancy; often precedes labor.

Board certification (of physician)—Doctor has received additional training and testing in a particular specialty. In obstetrics, the American College of Obstetricians and Gynecologists offers certification. Certification requires expertise in care of women. *FACOG* following doctor's name means he or she is a Fellow of the American College of Obstetricians and Gynecologists.
Braxton-Hicks contractions—Irregular, painless tightening of the uterus during pregnancy.
Breech presentation—Abnormal birth position of fetus. Buttocks or legs come into the birth canal before the head.

Carrier—Person with recessive disease-causing gene. A carrier usually shows no symptoms but can pass mutant gene on to his or her children.
Cataract, congenital—Cloudiness of the eye lens; present at birth.
Cell antibodies—See *autoantibodies.*
Certified nurse-midwife (CNM)—Registered nurse who has received additional training delivering babies and providing prenatal and postpartum care to women.
Cephalo-pelvic disproportion—Baby is too big to fit through the birth canal.
Cervical cultures—To test for STDs; when Pap smear is done, a sample may be taken to check for chlamydia, gonorrhea and other STDs.
Cervix—Opening of the uterus.
Cesarean section or delivery—Delivery of a baby through an abdominal incision rather than through the vagina. Also called *C-section.*
Chadwick's sign—Dark-blue or purple discoloration of vagina and cervix during pregnancy.
Chemotherapy—Treatment of a disease with chemical substances or medication.
Chlamydia—Sexually transmitted venereal infection.
Chloasma—Colored patches of irregular shape and size on the face (may have the appearance of a butterfly) or other body parts. Can be extensive. Also called *mask of pregnancy.*
Chorion—Outermost fetal membrane around amniotic sac.
Chorionic villus sampling (CVS)—Diagnostic test done early in pregnancy to determine some pregnancy problems. Tissue is taken from area of the placenta inside the uterus through the abdomen or cervix.
Chromosomal abnormality—Abnormal number or abnormal makeup of chromosomes.
Chromosomes—Structures within cells that carry genetic information in the form of DNA. Humans have 22 pairs of chromosomes and 2 sex chromosomes. One chromosome of each pair is inherited from the mother; the other is inherited from the father.
Cleft lip—Birth defect of the lip.
Cleft palate—Birth defect in part of the roof of the mouth.
Clubfoot—Birth defect in which a foot is misshaped and twisted.

Colostrum—Thin yellow fluid; first milk to come from the breast. Most often seen toward the end of pregnancy. Different in content from milk produced later during nursing.

Complete blood count (CBC)—Blood test to check cellular elements of the blood, iron stores, and to check for infections.

Condyloma acuminatum—Sexually transmitted skin tags or warts; caused by human papilloma virus (HPV). Also called *venereal warts.*

Congenital deafness screening—Blood test to help identify problem in a baby if a couple has a family history of inherited deafness.

Congenital problem—Problem present at birth.

Conization of the cervix—Large biopsy of the cervix that is taken in the shape of a cone.

Conjoined twins—Twins connected at some point on their bodies; may share vital organs. Previously called *Siamese twins.*

Constipation—Infrequent or incomplete bowel movements.

Contraction stress test (CST)—Test of baby's response to uterine contractions to evaluate baby's well-being.

Contractions—Uterus squeezes or tightens to push baby out during birth.

Corpus luteum—Area in the ovary where an egg is released at ovulation. Cyst may form in area after ovulation, called *corpus luteum cyst.*

Crown-to-rump length—Measurement from top of baby's head (crown) to baby's buttocks (rump).

Cystic fibrosis—Inherited disorder that causes breathing and digestion problems.

Cystitis—Bladder inflammation.

Cytomegalovirus (CMV) infection—Most common virus passed from mom to baby during pregnancy; infects about 1% of all newborns.

Cytotoxic—Substance that can terminate a pregnancy.

D&C (dilatation and curettage)—Surgical procedure in which the cervix is dilated and the lining of the uterus scraped.

Dermatoses—Skin conditions or skin eruptions.

Developmental delay—Condition in which child's development is slower than normal.

Diagnostic test—Test done to determine if a problem is present. It is often done after a screening test indicates a problem *may* be present. See *screening test.*

Diastasis recti—Separation of abdominal muscles.

Diethylstilbestrol (DES)—Nonsteroidal synthetic estrogen; used in the past to try to prevent miscarriage.

Dilatation—Amount, in centimeters, cervix has opened before birth. When woman is fully dilated, she is at 10cm.

Dizygotic twins—Twins born from two different eggs. Also called *fraternal twins.*

Dominant gene—Trait will be evident even if only one gene is present (from one parent); an example is dimples.

Doppler—Device that amplifies a fetal heartbeat so the doctor and others can hear it.

Down syndrome—Chromosomal disorder in which a baby has three copies of chromosome 21 (instead of two); results in mental retardation, distinct physical traits and various other problems.

Due date—Date baby is expected to be born. Most babies are born near this date, but only 1 of 20 are born on the actual date.

Dynamic cervix—Describes dilatation of the cervix seen during ultrasound. It is often associated with a history of an incompetent cervix or preterm labor and preterm delivery.

Dysuria—Difficulty or pain when urinating.

Early labor—Woman experiences regular contractions (one every 20 minutes down to one every 5 minutes) for longer than 2 hours. Cervix usually dilates to 3 or 4cm.

Eclampsia—Convulsions and coma in a woman with pre-eclampsia. Not related to epilepsy. See *pre-eclampsia.*

Ectodermal germ layer—Layer in developing baby that produces skin, teeth and glands of the mouth, nervous system and pituitary gland.

Ectopic pregnancy—Pregnancy that occurs outside the uterus, most often in the Fallopian tube. Also called *tubal pregnancy.*

ECV (external cephalic version)—Procedure done late in pregnancy in which doctor manually attempts to move a baby in the breech presentation into a normal head-down birth presentation.

EDC (estimated date of confinement)—Estimated due date for delivery of a baby.

Effacement—Thinning of the cervix; occurs in latter part of pregnancy and during labor.

Electroencephalogram—Recording of the electrical activity of brain.

Embryo—Organism in early stages of development; from conception to 10 weeks.

Embryonic period—First 10 weeks of gestation.

Endodermal germ layer—Area of tissue that produces digestive tract, respiratory organs, vagina, bladder and urethra in a baby. Also called *endoderm* or *entoderm.*

Endometrial cycle—Regular development of mucous membranes that line inside of uterus. Begins with preparation for acceptance of pregnancy and ends with shedding of the lining during menstrual period.

Endometrium—Mucous membrane that lines inside of uterine wall.

Enema—Fluid injected into the rectum for the purpose of clearing out the bowel.

Engorgement—Filled with fluid; usually refers to breast filled with milk in a breastfeeding mother.

Enzyme—Protein made by cells; improves or causes chemical changes in other substances.

Epidural block—Type of anesthesia; medication is injected around the spinal cord during labor or other types of surgery.

Episiotomy—Surgical incision in the area behind vagina, above rectum; used during delivery to avoid tearing the vaginal opening and rectum.

Essential nutrient—Nutrient that can't be made by the body; must be provided in the diet.
Estimated date of confinement—See *EDC.*
Exotoxin—Poison or toxin from a source outside the body.
Expressing breast milk—Manually forcing milk out of the breast.

Face presentation—Baby comes into the birth canal face first.
Fallopian tube—Tube that leads from the uterine cavity to the area of the ovary. Also called *uterine tube.*
False labor—Tightening of uterus without dilatation of the cervix.
Fasting blood sugar—Blood test to evaluate the amount of sugar in blood following a period of fasting.
Fertilization—Joining of the sperm and egg.
Fertilization age—Dating a pregnancy from the time of fertilization; 2 weeks shorter than gestational age. Also see *gestational age.*
Fetal anomaly—Birth defect.
Fetal arrhythmia—See *arrhythmia.*
Fetal fibronectin (fFN)—Test done to evaluate premature labor. A sample of cervical-vaginal secretions is taken; if fFN is present after 22 weeks, indicates increased risk for premature delivery.
Fetal goiter—Enlargement of baby's thyroid gland.
Fetal monitor—Device used before or during labor to listen to and to record fetal heartbeat. Monitoring baby inside the uterus can be external (through maternal abdomen) or internal (through maternal vagina).
Fetal period—Time period from after the first 10 weeks of gestation until birth.
Fetal stress—Problems with a baby that occur before birth or during labor; often requires immediate delivery.
Fetoscopy—Test that enables a doctor to look through a fiberoptic scope to detect subtle problems in a fetus.
Fetus—Refers to an unborn baby after 10 weeks of gestation until birth.
Fibrin—Elastic protein important in blood coagulation.
Fistula—Abnormal opening from one part of the body to another, such as from the vagina to the rectum.
Forceps—Instrument sometimes used to deliver a baby. It is placed around a baby's head, inside the birth canal, to help guide baby out of the birth canal.
Fortification—Addition of one or more essential nutrients to a food.
Frank breech—Baby presenting buttocks first. Legs and knees are straight.
Fraternal twins—See *dizygotic twins.*
Fundus—Top part of the uterus; often measured during pregnancy.

Genes—Basic units of heredity. Each gene carries specific information and is passed from parent to child. Child receives half of its genes from its mother and half from its father. Every human has about 100,000 genes. Codes determine specific characteristics, such as hair color.

Genetic counseling—Consultation between a couple and specialists about the possibility of genetic problems in a pregnancy.
Genetic screening—Performing one or more genetic tests.
Genetic tests—Various screening and diagnostic tests done to determine whether a couple may have a child with a genetic defect. Usually part of genetic counseling.
Genital herpes simplex—Herpes simplex infection involving the genital area. Can be significant during pregnancy because of danger of newborn becoming infected with herpes simplex.
Genitourinary problems—Problems involving genital organs and bladder or kidneys.
Germ layers—Layers or areas of tissue important in fetal development.
Gestational age—Dating pregnancy from the first day of the last menstrual period; 2 weeks longer than fertilization age. Also see *fertilization age.*
Gestational diabetes—Occurrence of diabetes only during pregnancy.
Gestational trophoblastic disease (GTN)—Abnormal pregnancy in which embryo does not develop. Also called *molar pregnancy* or *hydatidiform mole.*
Globulin—Family of proteins from plasma or serum of blood.
Glucose-tolerance test (GTT)—Blood test done to evaluate body's response to sugar. Blood is drawn from mother-to-be once or at intervals following consumption of a sugary substance.
Glucosuria—Glucose (sugar) in urine.
Gonorrhea—Contagious venereal infection, transmitted primarily by intercourse.
Grand mal seizure—Loss of body control and functions during major seizure.
Group-B streptococcal (GBS) infection—Serious infection occurring in mother's vagina, throat or rectum.
Group-B streptococcus (GBS) test—Near the end of pregnancy, samples may be taken from woman's vagina, perineum and rectum to check for GBS. Urine tests may also be done. If test is positive, treatment may be started or given during labor.

Habitual miscarriage—Occurrence of three or more miscarriages.
Health Information Portability and Accountability Act (HIPAA)—Enacted in 1996, legislation includes privacy rule creating national standards protecting personal health information. Also addresses transfer and continuity of health-insurance coverage.
Heartburn—Discomfort or pain that occurs in the chest, often after eating.
Height of fundus—Top of the uterus is the fundus. Doctor looks for this point, and measures from here to bottom of uterus, around pubic bone, to see if growth of baby is normal.
Hematocrit—Determines proportion of blood cells to plasma; important in diagnosing anemia.
Hemoglobin—Pigment in red blood cells that carries oxygen to body tissues.
Hemolytic disease—Destruction of red blood cells. See *anemia.*
Hemopoietic system—System that controls the formation of blood cells.

Hemorrhoids—Dilated blood vessels, most often found in rectum or rectal canal.

Heparin—Medication used to prevent blood clotting and to treat or to prevent thrombosis.

Hepatitis-B antibodies test—Test to determine if a pregnant woman has hepatitis B.

High-risk pregnancy—Pregnancy with complications that require special medical attention, often from a specialist. Also see *perinatologist.*

HIPAA—See *Health Information Portability and Accountability Act.*

HIV/AIDS test—Test to determine if a person has HIV or AIDS; test cannot be done without person's knowledge and permission.

Homan's sign—Pain caused by flexing toes toward knees when a person has a blood clot in the lower leg.

Home uterine monitoring—Pregnant woman's contractions are recorded at home, then transmitted by telephone to the doctor. Used to monitor women at risk of premature labor.

Human chorionic gonadotropin (HCG)—Hormone produced in early pregnancy; measured in a pregnancy test.

Human placental lactogen—Hormone of pregnancy produced by the placenta and found in the bloodstream.

Hyaline membrane disease—Respiratory disease of a newborn.

Hydatidiform mole—See *gestational trophoblastic disease.*

Hydramnios—Increased amount of amniotic fluid.

Hydrocephalus—Excessive accumulation of fluid around baby's brain. Sometimes called *water on the brain.*

Hyperbilirubinemia—Extremely high level of bilirubin in the blood.

Hyperemesis gravidarum—Severe nausea, dehydration and vomiting during pregnancy. Occurs most frequently during the first trimester but can continue throughout pregnancy.

Hyperglycemia—Increased blood sugar.

Hypertension, pregnancy-induced (PIH)—High blood pressure that occurs during pregnancy.

Hyperthyroidism—Higher-than-normal levels of thyroid hormone in the bloodstream.

Hypoplasia—Defective or incomplete development or formation of tissue.

Hypotension—Low blood pressure.

Hypothyroidism—Low or inadequate levels of thyroid hormone in the bloodstream.

Identical twins—See *monozygotic twins.*

Imaging tests—Tests that look inside body; includes X-rays, CT scans (or CAT scans) and magnetic resonance imaging (MRI).

Ileoanal pouch—Pouch or sac connecting the ileum (small intestine or small bowel) to the anus (the lower opening of the digestive tract).

Immune globulin preparation—Substance used to protect against infection with certain diseases, such as hepatitis or measles.

In utero—Within the uterus.

Incompetent cervix—Cervix dilates painlessly, without contractions.

Incomplete miscarriage—Miscarriage in which part, but not all, of uterine contents are expelled.

Inducing labor—Medication is used to start labor. See *oxytocin*.

Inevitable miscarriage—Pregnancy complicated with bleeding and cramping. Usually results in miscarriage.

Infertility—Inability or decreased ability to get pregnant.

Insulin—Hormone made by the pancreas; promotes use of sugar and glucose.

Intrauterine-growth restriction (IUGR)—Inadequate fetal growth during pregnancy.

In-vitro fertilization—Process in which eggs are placed in a medium outside the body to which sperm are added for fertilization. Fertilized egg is then placed inside the uterus in attempt to result in pregnancy.

Iodides—Medications made up of negative ions of iodine.

Iron-deficiency anemia—Anemia produced by a lack of iron in the diet; often seen in pregnancy.

Isoimmunization—Development of a specific antibody directed at the red blood cells of another individual, such as baby inside the uterus. Often occurs when an Rh-negative woman carries an Rh-positive baby or is given Rh-positive blood.

Jaundice—Yellow staining of skin, eyes and body tissues. Caused by excessive amounts of bilirubin. Treated with phototherapy.

Ketones—Breakdown product of metabolism found in blood, particularly from starvation or uncontrolled diabetes.

Kick count—Record of how often a pregnant woman feels her baby move; used to evaluate fetal well-being.

Kidney stone—Small mass or lesion found in the kidney or urinary tract. Can block urine flow.

Labor—Process of expelling fetus from the uterus.

Laparoscopy—Less-invasive surgical procedure performed for tubal ligation, diagnosis of pelvic pain or diagnosis of ectopic pregnancy.

Leukorrhea—Vaginal discharge characterized by white or yellowish color. Primarily composed of mucus.

Lightening—Change in the shape of a pregnant uterus a few weeks before labor. Often described as the baby "dropping."

Linea nigra—Darker-than-normal line that often develops during pregnancy; line runs down the abdomen from bellybutton to pubic area.

Lochia—Vaginal discharge that occurs after delivery of the baby and placenta.

Macrosomia—Abnormally large-sized fetus.

Malignant GTN—Cancerous change of gestational trophoblastic disease. See *gestational trophoblastic disease.*

Mammogram—X-ray study of breasts to identify normal and abnormal breast tissue.

Mask of pregnancy—Increased pigment over the area of face under each eye. Commonly looks like a butterfly.

Maternal serum screen—Blood test done between 15 and 20 weeks of pregnancy on mother-to-be to screen for Down syndrome, trisomy 18 and neural-tube defects.

McDonald cerclage—Surgical procedure performed on an incompetent cervix; drawstring-type suture holds cervical opening closed during pregnancy. Also see *incompetent cervix.*

Meconium—First intestinal discharge of a newborn; green or yellow in color. Consists of epithelial or surface cells, mucus and bile. Discharge may occur before or during labor or soon after birth.

Melanoma—Cancerous pigmented mole or tumor.

Meningomyelocele—Birth defect of baby's central nervous system. Membranes and spinal cord protrude through an opening in the vertebral column.

Menstrual age—See *gestational age.*

Menstruation—Regular or periodic discharge of endometrial lining and blood from the uterus.

Mesodermal germ layer—Embryonic tissue that forms connective tissue, muscles, kidneys, ureters and other organs.

Metaplasia—Change in structure of tissue into another type that is not normal for that tissue.

Microcephaly—Abnormally small development of head in a developing fetus.

Microphthalmia—Abnormally small eyeballs.

Miscarriage—Premature end of pregnancy; giving birth to an embryo or fetus before it can live outside the womb, usually defined as before 20 weeks of pregnancy.

Missed miscarriage—Failed pregnancy without bleeding or cramping. Often diagnosed by ultrasound weeks or months after a pregnancy fails.

Mittelschmerz—Pain that coincides with release of an egg from the ovary.

Molar pregnancy—See *gestational trophoblastic disease.*

Monilial vulvovaginitis—Infection caused by yeast or monilia; usually affects the vagina and vulva.

Monozygotic twins—Twins conceived from one egg. Often called *identical twins.*

Morning sickness—Nausea and vomiting usually occurring during the first trimester of pregnancy. Also see *hyperemesis gravidarum.*

Morula—Cells resulting from early division of a fertilized egg at the beginning of pregnancy.

Mucus plug—Secretions in the cervix often released just before labor.

Multiple-markers test—See *quad-screen test* and *triple-screen test.*

Mutations—Change in the character of a gene. Passed from one cell division to another.

Natural childbirth—Labor and delivery in which a woman has as few interventions as possible. May include no medication or monitoring. Woman usually has taken classes to prepare her for labor and delivery.

Neural-tube defects—Abnormalities in the development of the spinal cord and brain in a fetus. Also see *anencephaly; hydrocephalus; spina bifida.*

Nonstress test (NST)—Test that records fetal movement felt by a woman or observed by a healthcare provider, along with changes in fetal heart rate. Used to evaluate fetal well-being.

NSAIDs—Nonsteroidal anti-inflammatory drugs, such as ibuprofen, Motrin, Alleve and Advil.

Nuchal translucency screening—Detailed ultrasound that allows doctor to measure the space behind a baby's neck. When combined with blood-test results, it can help measure a woman's probability of having a baby with Down syndrome.

Nurse-midwife—Registered nurse who has received extra training in the care of pregnant women and delivery of babies.

Obstetrician—Medical doctor or osteopathic physician who specializes in the care of pregnant women and delivery of babies.

Oligohydramnios—Lack or deficiency of amniotic fluid.

Omphalocele—Birth defect resulting in outpouching of the bellybutton containing internal organs in a fetus or newborn infant.

Opioids—Synthetic compounds with effects similar to those of opium.

Organogenesis—Development of organ systems in an embryo.

Ossification—Bone formation.

Ovarian cycle—Regular production of hormones from the ovary in response to hormonal messages from the brain. Ovarian cycle governs endometrial cycle.

Ovarian hyperstimulation syndrome—Complication of infertility treatment involving ovarian enlargement and abdominal swelling, with changes in blood-fluid volumes. Can be life-threatening. May occur when infertility drugs, such as Clomid, are used to stimulate ovulation.

Ovarian torsion—Twisting or rotation of the ovary.

Ovulation—Cyclic release of the egg from the ovary.

Ovulatory age—See *fertilization age.*

Oxytocin—Medicine that causes uterine contractions; used to induce or to help along labor. May be called by brand name *Pitocin*. Also hormone produced by pituitary glands.

Palmar erythema—Redness of palms of the hands.

Pap smear—Routine screening test to evaluate the presence of premalignant or cancerous conditions of the cervix.

Paracervical block—Local anesthesia to relieve pain of dilating cervix.

Pediatrician—Medical doctor or osteopathic physician who specializes in the care of babies and children.

Pelvic exam—Inside of pelvic area is felt to assess various uterine conditions. At the beginning of pregnancy, it is done to assess uterine size. At the end of pregnancy, it can help determine if the cervix is dilating and thinning.

Percutaneous umbilical cord blood sampling (PUBS; cordocentesis)—Test done on a fetus to diagnose Rh-incompatibility, blood disorders and infections.

Perinatologist—Physician who specializes in the care of high-risk pregnancies.

Perineum—Area between the rectum and vagina.

Petit mal seizure—Brief seizure, with possible short loss of consciousness. Often associated with blinking or flickering of eyelids and mild twitching of the mouth.

Phosphatidyl glycerol (PG)—Lipoprotein present when fetal lungs are mature.

Phospholipids—Fat-containing phosphorous; most important are lecithins and sphingomyelin, which are important in maturation of fetal lungs before birth.

Phototherapy—Treatment for jaundice in a newborn infant. Also see *jaundice.*

Physician assistant (PA)—Qualified healthcare professional who may take care of you during pregnancy. He or she is licensed to practice medicine in association with a licensed doctor. Also called *physician associate.*

Physiologic anemia of pregnancy—Anemia during pregnancy caused by increase in the amount of fluid in blood compared to the number of cells in blood. Also see *anemia.*

Placenta—Organ inside the uterus attached to baby by the umbilical cord. Essential during pregnancy for growth and development of an embryo and fetus. Also called *afterbirth.*

Placenta previa—Attachment of the placenta very close to, or covering, the cervix.

Placental abruption—Premature separation of the placenta from the uterus.

Pneumonitis—Inflammation of lungs.

Polyhydramnios—See *hydramnios.*

Postmature baby—Baby born 2 weeks or more past its due date.

Postnatal—After baby's birth.

Postpartum—6-week period following baby's birth. Refers to mother, not baby.

Postpartum blues—Mild depression after delivery.

Postpartum distress syndrome (PPDS)—Range of symptoms including baby blues, postpartum depression and postpartum psychosis.

Postpartum hemorrhage—Bleeding greater than 17 ounces (450ml) at the time of delivery.

Postterm pregnancy—Pregnancy of 42+ weeks gestation.

Pre-eclampsia—Group of important symptoms unique to pregnancy, including high blood pressure, edema, swelling and changes in reflexes.

Pregnancy diabetes—See *gestational diabetes.*

Premature birth—Birth before 37 weeks of pregnancy.

Premature delivery—Delivery before 37 weeks gestation.

Premature rupture of membranes (PROM)—Rupture of fetal membranes (bag of waters) before onset of labor.

Prenatal care—Program of care for a pregnant woman before birth of her baby.

Prepared childbirth—Woman has taken classes so she knows what will happen during labor and delivery. She may request pain medication if she needs it.
Presentation—Describes which part of the baby comes into the birth canal first.
Preterm premature rupture of membranes (PPROM)—Rupture of fetal membranes before 37 weeks of pregnancy.
Proteinuria—Protein in urine.
Pruritus gravidarum—Itching during pregnancy.
Pubic symphysis—Bony prominence in pelvic bone found in the middle of a woman's lower abdomen. Landmark from which doctor often measures the growing uterus during pregnancy.
Pudendal block—Local anesthesia during labor.
Pulmonary embolism—Blood clot from another part of body that travels to the lungs. Can be very serious.
Pyelonephritis—Serious kidney infection.

Quad-screen test—Measurement of four blood components to help identify problems—alpha-fetoprotein, human chorionic gonadotropin, unconjugated estriol and inhibin-A.
Quickening—Feeling baby move inside uterus.

Radiation therapy—Method of treating various cancers.
Radioactive scan—Diagnostic test in which radioactive material is injected into a particular part of the body then scanned to find the problem there.
Recessive gene—Both parents must have the same gene for a trait to be present, such as the occurrence of cystic fibrosis.
Rh-factor—Blood test to determine if a woman is Rh-negative.
Rh-negative—Absence of rhesus antigen in the blood.
Rh-sensitivity—See *isoimmunization.*
RhoGAM—Medication given to Rh-negative women during pregnancy and following delivery to prevent isoimmunization. Also see *isoimmunization.*
Ripening the cervix—Medicine is used to help the cervix soften, thin and dilate.
Round-ligament pain—Pain caused by stretching ligaments on the sides of the uterus during pregnancy.
Rubella titers—Blood test to check for immunity against rubella (German measles).
Rupture of membranes—Loss of fluid from the amniotic sac. Also called *breaking of waters* or *water breaking.*

Screening test—Test to determine if a problem may be present. If a problem may be present, a *diagnostic* test may be done to determine if the problem actually *is* present. See *diagnostic test.*
Seizure—Sudden onset of a convulsion.
Septate uterus—Uterus is divided into two cavities by a membrane (septum).
Sexually transmitted disease (STD)—Infection transmitted through sexual contact or sexual intercourse.

Sickle-cell disease—Anemia caused by abnormal red blood cells shaped like a sickle or cylinder.
Sickle-cell trait—Presence of the trait for sickle-cell anemia. Not sickle-cell disease.
Sickle crisis—Painful episode caused by sickle-cell disease.
Silent labor—Painless dilatation of the cervix.
Skin tag—Flap or extra buildup of skin.
Sodium—Element found in many foods, particularly salt. Consumption of too much sodium may cause fluid retention and lead to swelling.
Sonogram or sonography—See *ultrasound.*
Sperm motility—Spontaneous movement of sperm; ability of sperm to swim or move.
Spina bifida—Birth defect in which membranes of the spinal cord and the spinal cord itself protrude outside the body. Can cause paralysis and other problems.
Spinal anesthesia—Anesthesia given in the spinal canal.
Spontaneous miscarriage—Loss of pregnancy during first 20 weeks of gestation.
Stasis—Decreased flow.
Station—Estimation of baby's descent into birth canal in preparation for birth.
Stillbirth—Death of a fetus before birth, usually defined as after 20 weeks of gestation.
Stress test—Test in which mild uterine contractions are induced; fetal heart rate in response to contractions is noted.
Stretch marks—Stretched areas of skin; often found on abdomen, breasts, buttocks and legs.
Superovulation—Ovulation of a larger than normal number of eggs, usually from administration of fertility drugs.
Supplementation—Nutrients that are added to a normal diet.

Tay-Sachs disease—Inherited disease of the central nervous system. Most common form affects babies, who appear healthy at birth and seem to develop normally for the first few months of life. Then development slows, and symptoms begin to appear.
Teratology—Study of abnormal fetal development.
Term—Baby is considered "term" when born after 38 weeks. Also called *full term.*
Thrombophilia—Disorder that causes blood to clot when and where it shouldn't.
Torsion—Twisting or rotation.
Trait—Refers to a characteristic of a person, such as blue eyes.
Transition—Phase after active labor during which the cervix fully dilates. Contractions are strongest during this stage.
Trimester—Division of pregnancy into three equal periods of about 13 weeks each.
Triple-screen test—Measurement of three blood components—alpha-fetoprotein, human chorionic gonadotropin and unconjugated estriol—to help identify problems.

Ultrasound—Noninvasive test that shows picture of a fetus inside womb. Sound waves bounce off fetus to create picture.

Umbilical cord—Cord that connects placenta to the developing baby. Brings oxygenated blood and nutrients from mother through placenta to baby, and removes waste products and carbon dioxide from baby.

Unicornuate uterus—Only one side of the uterus is developed; the other side is undeveloped or absent.

Urinalysis and urine cultures—Tests for infections and to determine levels of sugar and protein in urine.

Uterine didelphys—Uterine abnormality in which a woman has a double uterus with a double cervix and double vagina.

Uterine rupture—Splitting open of the uterus during labor or delivery. Occurs most often in the area of a surgical scar, such as previous Cesarean delivery or uterine surgery.

Uterus—Organ the embryo/fetus grows in. Also called a *womb.*

Vacuum extractor—Device sometimes used to provide traction on the fetal head during delivery; used to help deliver a baby.

Vagina—Birth canal.

Varicose veins—Dilated or enlarged blood vessels (veins).

Vasa previa—Condition in which blood vessels of the umbilical cord cross the interior opening of the cervix. When the cervix dilates or membranes rupture, unprotected vessels can tear and baby bleeds to death. Or vessels can become compressed, which shuts off blood and oxygen to the baby.

Vena cava—Major vein in the body that empties into the right atrium of the heart. Returns unoxygenated blood to the heart for transport to the lungs.

Venereal warts—See *condyloma acuminatum.*

Vernix—Fatty substance that covers fetal skin inside the uterus.

Vertex—Head first.

Villi—Projection from mucous membrane. Important in exchange of nutrients from maternal blood to placenta and fetus.

Weight check—Weight is checked at every prenatal visit; gaining too much weight or not gaining enough weight can indicate problems.

Womb—See *uterus.*

Yeast infection—See *monilial vulvovaginitis*

Zygote—Cell that results from union of sperm and egg at fertilization.

Following is an excerpt from Your Baby's First Year Week by Week. *The excerpt deals with the first week of your baby's life.*

If you want information about preparing for baby's birth and the first 48 hours after baby is born, the book contains detailed discussions of each.

Week 1

Baby Care and Equipment

Baby's First Visit to the Doctor

In the past, a baby didn't go to the doctor's office for her first visit until she was between 1 and 2 weeks old. Today, baby's first well-baby checkup usually occurs within 4 to 6 days after birth to help make the evaluation and treatment of jaundice more reliable.

When you go to this appointment, be sure to bring your insurance card and be ready to fill out various forms. Your baby is a "new patient."

You will be asked for all sorts of information, such as date, time, place and the name of the doctor for your delivery. You will need to supply the doctor's office with information on problems during pregnancy or delivery, and baby's weight and length at birth. If you have other children, leave them at home for this visit. You have a lot to discuss.

Your doctor will give baby a pretty thorough checkup. He or she will weigh baby, measure her length and the circumference of her head, check for jaundice, be sure her arms and legs move properly, listen to her heart and lungs, and check for abdominal obstructions. It's a good time for you to ask any questions you have.

Umbilical-Cord Care

In the hospital, triple dye, an antibacterial substance, may be applied to the stump of the umbilical cord to prevent infection and to help it dry out more quickly. If it is used, the area is blue-purple.

At home, if the area becomes dirty, use soap and water to cleanse the area gently. Don't clean your baby's bellybutton area with rubbing alcohol. Studies show it may actually delay how long it takes for the cord to fall off. Air drying—also called *dry care*—seems to work the best. It takes from 7 to 10 days for the stump of the cord to heal and fall off.

If the area appears irritated, you may want to buy newborn diapers with a half circle cut out at the waist. Or fold down baby's diaper so it doesn't rub against the cord. If the umbilical cord oozes pus or leaves more than a couple of drops of blood on baby's diaper, call the doctor. If skin at the base of the cord is red or if baby acts as if it is painful when you touch it, let your doctor know.

Penis Care for Circumcised and Uncircumcised Boys

For Circumcised Boys. After the circumcision, you may notice your son's penis is a little red, and there may be a yellow secretion. Both are signs the incision is healing.

During this first year, your baby will probably grow about 10 inches and triple her birthweight.

The penis should be healed within a week; however, if you notice any swelling or sores, call your doctor. He or she may suggest using mild antibiotic gels or advise you to clean the area more often. Sometimes ice or a cold pack is used, but do this *only* when directed to do so by your doctor.

For Uncircumcised Boys. If your son is not circumcised, care for his penis will be different from care of a circumcised baby. The penis is made up of a shaft with a bulb at the end, called the *glans.* The glans is covered by the *foreskin,* which is a layer of skin. The foreskin is not removed or cut on an uncircumcised baby boy.

Do not force the foreskin back. This can cause bleeding and can lead to skin adhesions. *Skin adhesions* are folds of skin along the penis shaft that become stuck to the head of the penis. They are fairly common, so do not become worried if they develop. They aren't painful, so you don't need to do anything to deal with the situation; they will naturally resolve by themselves.

The foreskin will eventually retract on its own, so avoid cleaning the penis vigorously. Gently wash the area with soap and water, just as you do any other parts of the baby's body.

Feeding Your Baby

Feeding your baby is one of the most important things you do for him. You'll know when he's hungry; he'll exhibit definite signs of hunger,

In the first 2 weeks of your baby's life, he should be feeding every 2 or 3 hours during the day. At night, he should be feeding every 3 to 5 hours.

including fussing, putting his hands in his mouth and turning his head and opening his mouth when his cheek is touched.

A newborn infant's stomach can hold only 2 to 3 ounces of milk. His metabolism burns this amount of nourishment in 2 to 3 hours, then he'll be ready to eat again. A newborn spends over 3 hours of every day feeding and usually eats 8 to 12 times in a 24-hour period.

A newborn gains about an ounce of weight a day. You may feed at regular intervals to help your baby get on a schedule. Or you may decide to let your baby set his own schedule—some babies need to eat more often than others. There are times a baby needs to feed more often than usual, such as during periods of growth.

A baby is usually the best judge of how much he needs at each feeding. He'll usually turn away from the nipple (mother or bottle) when he's full.

It's a good idea to burp your baby after each feeding. Some babies need to be burped during a feeding.

You may want to ask your doctor about vitamin-D supplements for baby. Vitamin D is necessary to help children build strong, healthy bones. A child needs at least 200IU a day of vitamin D. If you feed your baby formula, he'll get the vitamin because formula is fortified. However, if you breastfeed, beginning at 2 months, baby should receive liquid supplements of vitamin D. Be sure you discuss this with your pediatrician.

Babies frequently spit up some breast milk or formula after a feeding. It's common in the early months because the muscle at the top of the stomach is not fully developed. When a baby spits up enough to propel the stomach contents several inches, it is called *vomiting*. If your baby vomits after a feeding, don't feed him again immediately. His tummy may be upset; wait until the next feeding.

Picking Up and Handling Baby

If you're like most first-time parents, the thought of handling baby fills you with trepidation. She's such a tiny, delicate being. You want to be sure you pick her up correctly, and you don't want to drop her. Rest easy—she's not as fragile as you think.

There are ways to handle her so you'll both feel confident. *Always* support her head with your hand or arm, and keep an arm or hand under her back. You may hold her close or a little more loosely. Use smooth motions when moving her, and always protect her head with your arm or hand.

Never shake your baby—shaking can result in "shaken baby syndrome." This causes bleeding and bruising of the brain, injury to the eyes and damage to the spinal cord. See the discussion of *Shaken-Baby Syndrome* in Week 17.

Diapering Baby

Changing your baby's diapers is a necessary task; once you get the hang of it, you'll be able to do it quickly and efficiently. Many dads soon become experts! See the illustration on the opposite page.

Change baby's diapers whenever she's wet or soiled to prevent irritation and diaper rash. A newborn wets between 6 and 10 times a day. Bowel movements are more variable; some babies poop two or three times a day, others only every few days. Whether your baby is breastfed or bottlefed may also make a difference in her bowel movements.

You don't need to clean baby with baby wipes if she has only a wet diaper. Urine is germ free; using a baby wipe every time you change her

A Quick Method to Change Baby

Try this method for changing baby; it's quick and easy. Lay baby on the changing table; strap her in or keep your hand on her tummy. Undo pins or diaper tabs, and gently lift her ankles. (You can do this with one hand.) With your other hand, wipe any feces into the dirty diaper and put it to the side. Using baby wipes or wet cotton balls, clean the genitals; with a girl, wipe from front to back to avoid contaminating the vaginal area, which could cause a urinary-tract infection. Let her air dry for a bit, or dry her with a soft washcloth. Slide a clean diaper under her as you again lift her ankles. Fasten diaper with pins or tabs, and adjust leg openings so there are no gaps.

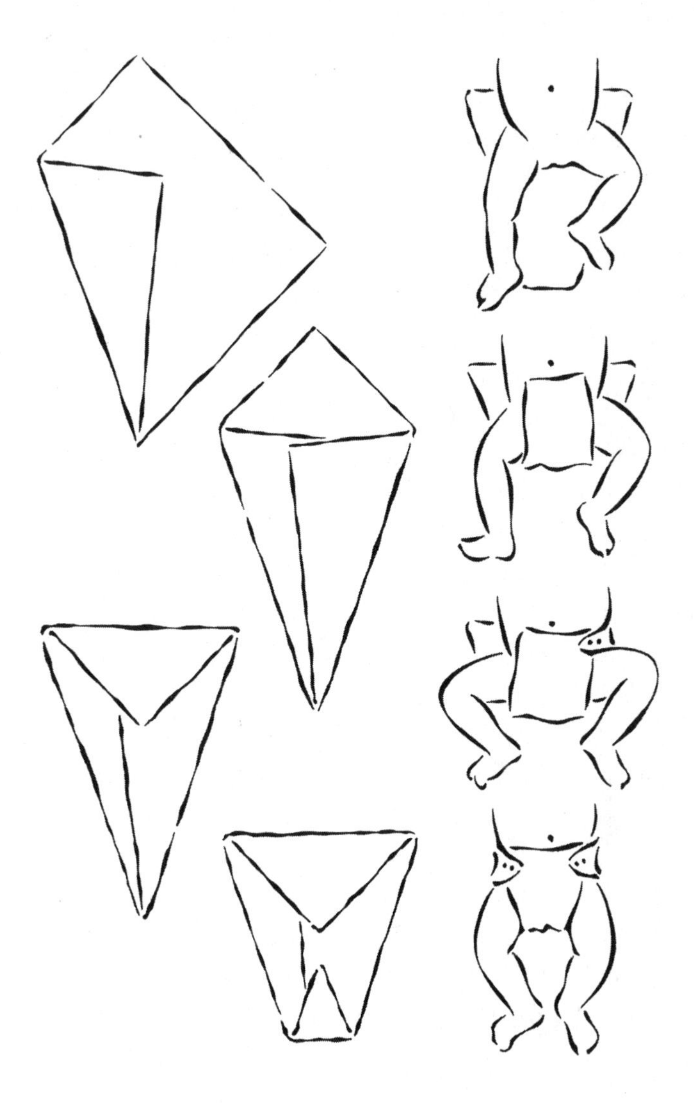

Folding a diaper then positioning
it under baby's bottom.

could be irritating. If possible, let her "air out" (go without a diaper for a while) between diaper changes. It helps reduce the risk of diaper rash.

Dressing Your Baby

One of the most challenging tasks for a new parent is dressing baby. It's not like dressing a baby doll—baby dolls don't wiggle and squirm! But there are a few tricks we can pass along to help make your first attempts a little easier. Our best advice is to take it slow, and don't get frustrated. With practice, you'll soon be an expert!

Some tips we've learned over the years deal with the types of clothing you choose for baby. If you use T-shirts with a snap bottom, it'll be a snap to get them on! In addition, you won't find baby nearly engulfed in his T-shirt because it won't ride up his chest when he squirms or rolls around. A snap-bottom shirt helps keep his diaper in place. A onesie with feet is the easiest outfit to put on and take off. It may be the perfect outfit for Dad to start with.

After you've diapered baby, put on his undershirt. Hold the shirt neck open with your fingers, and slip it over his head. Reach into the end of one sleeve, grasp his hand and gently pull it through. Adjust the body of the shirt once you've got both arms in. When you put his pants on, first reach through the bottom leg opening and grasp one foot. Slide it through the opening, then do the same for his other foot. Once both feet are through the leg openings, pull pants up to his waist.

If you're putting on overalls, we've found sliding them on from the bottom works best. Adjust them, snap the legs, then hook the straps. With a sleeper or one-piece outfit that opens down the front, lay it down on the changing table, then lay baby on top of it. Slide baby's arms, one at a time, through the sleeves, adjust, then slip baby's feet through the openings. When everything's in place, snap the snaps or zip up.

A word of advice: When changing your newborn, keep the room warm. A small baby can get cold quite quickly when undressed.

Swaddling Your Infant

Before her birth, your baby was in a pretty tight environment, with little room to move. When she's born, the lack of confinement may make her feel a little insecure. *Swaddling*, wrapping her snugly in a soft blanket, can help if she seems discontented. It can help make her feel secure and comfort her. In fact, research shows that swaddled babies (under 3 months of age) are less restless and don't startle as easily as babies who are not swaddled. Swaddling also helps a baby sleep well on her back. She may wake up less often and sleep longer when she is swaddled.

Lay a blanket (a square receiving blanket works well) on a flat surface in a diamond shape. You can fold the top down inside or leave it up, if it's cold and you want to protect baby's head. You may want to use a "swaddling blanket," a special blanket designed to swaddle baby. Many different types are available. Check local stores or the Internet if you are interested.

Place baby on the blanket, with her head at the top of the diamond, and place her arms by her face or her side. Some babies are comforted when their hands are left by their faces—this is often the case with a premature baby.

Fold the top-left edge of the blanket across her body, pulling it taut. Tuck excess material under her back. Bring the bottom corner of the blanket up over her body. Some babies like their legs tucked into a fetal position; others don't. Fold the top-right edge of the blanket across her body, and tuck excess material under her back. She can be laid in her crib in this manner, or you can hold her. Be sure you don't swaddle her so tightly that it affects her breathing.

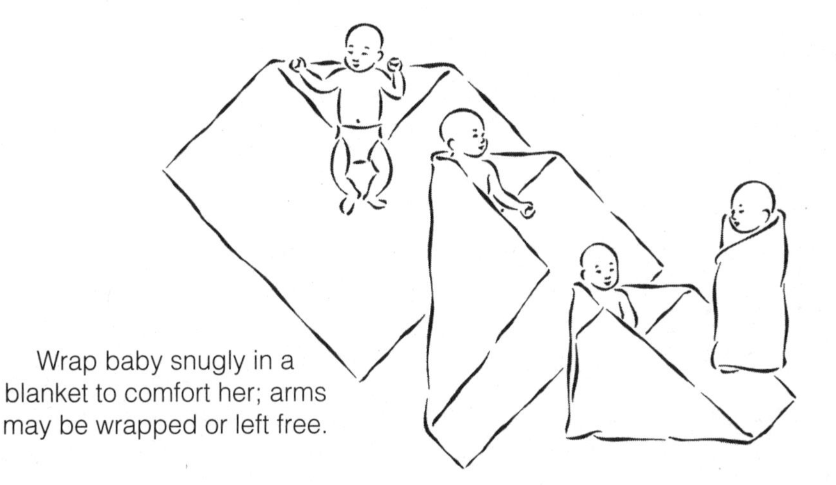

Wrap baby snugly in a blanket to comfort her; arms may be wrapped or left free.

Changes You May See This First Week

During the first year of life, your baby grows and changes according to stages of development. The four most important developmental categories include the following.

- **Motor Development**—Your baby's large and small muscle groups develop dramatically this first year. At this time he moves very little, yet by the end of 12 months, he will be walking or ready to walk!
- **Language Development**—Development of language includes his speech and his attempts to listen to and to understand language around him.
- **Intellectual Development**—As your baby's brain grows, his thinking skills develop.
- **Social Development**—Social skills he learns help your baby relate to the world around him.

As the weeks and months pass, your baby will move from one learning task to another, and his focus will shift when this happens. Developmental milestones can be very different among children. There is a wide range of what is considered normal. So don't worry if he seems to be slow in one area for a while; it's his overall development you are concerned with.

At birth, your baby's brain is not fully developed, and a great deal of growth must still occur. A baby's brain grows most rapidly from the last trimester of pregnancy through the first 3 months of life. Even when your baby seems to be lying still, with nothing happening, his brain is expanding as he adjusts to his new world.

Baby's Sight

From the moment your newborn opens her eyes after birth, she can see her world, although it is a bit fuzzy. She is nearsighted; her best field of vision is about 8 to 12 inches away from her. She will stare at objects placed in this range of her vision. She can also tell the difference between a human face and other objects—she prefers faces. (If the baby is smiling at you at this point, it's probably gas.)

A Newborn's Hearing

When born, your baby's middle ear is still a bit immature. The sound-processing center of his brain is also not fully developed.

Your baby hears most noises in the first few weeks as echoes, not distinct sounds. However, he hears voices; he recognizes his mother's voice at or shortly after birth and will soon recognize the voices of other people around him. Speak to him often, about everything, to help develop his hearing and help him begin to relate to language. A baby can't learn to talk or begin to understand the subtle nuances of language if he doesn't hear a lot of conversation.

Other Newborn Development

Many babies are quiet and alert for a few days after birth, then they start crying. This is normal—crying is the only way baby can communicate with you!

Soothing a crying or fussy baby takes experimentation on your part. After all, you don't know each other very well yet, so you may need to try different tactics to help her settle. You may find your baby calms when she is swaddled. (See the discussion on page 643.) Rocking and patting her or offering her a pacifier are other options. Some babies calm down when they listen to monotonous "white" sounds. Try different things when baby needs to be comforted.

When you snuggle and/or feed your baby, your skin-to-skin contact makes her feel secure and safe. It also provides gentle stimulation. Offer her this contact as much as possible.

A newborn's hands and lips have the largest number of touch receptors. This may be the reason your newborn enjoys sucking on her fingers.

When your baby is sleeping or drowsy, you may notice her smiling. She's in a dream state—her eyes may be moving at the same time. Enjoy watching her. It's a beautiful sight.

Note: See also the box *Milestones This First Week.*

What's Happening 1st First Week?

Some Changes You May See in Baby

Incredible as it may seem, infants often go through a growth spurt very soon after birth. At 7 to 10 days after birth, your baby may grow in length; when you take him to the pediatrician for his next checkup, he may have grown more than you realized.

Your baby's heart rate is faster than yours; his heart beats between 100 and 150 beats a minute. When he yawns, hiccups or has a bowel movement, his heart rate may decrease. He also breathes quite rapidly—up to 50 breaths a minute. This is normal.

Some babies don't like to cuddle; it's normal. If he stiffens and arches his back when you hold him close, hold him with his back against your chest. This may be better for him.

When he cries, you may not see tears. His tear ducts are not yet mature enough to produce tears. Tears normally flow out of tiny openings—tear ducts—located on the inner part of the lower lid. Occasionally, a tear duct is blocked by a thin membrane, which usually opens after birth. Sometimes it doesn't, so tears don't drain. They back up in the eye. This causes mucus to form on the eyes, lashes and lids.

Most tear ducts open by the time baby is 9 months old. Until this happens, gently massage the ducts with a clean index finger. Move in a circular motion toward the nose; do this throughout the day. The gentle pressure will help open the duct.

In this book, we've included information in each weekly discussion about a baby's mental, physical and social development. However, *when* these developmental changes occur (the weeks we put them in) are merely *estimates* of where your baby may be at any given time. Each developmental step represents an average; a baby could be anywhere from 6 to 10 weeks on *either side of the week* in which the discussion occurs and still be perfectly normal! Don't be worried if your baby doesn't do something exactly at the time it's discussed in the book. Every baby develops in her own way, at her own pace.

Before your baby was born, he was exposed to various flavors when he swallowed amniotic fluid. He prefers sweet tastes at this point—breast milk and formula are sweet.

Baby and Sleep

Newborns sleep between 17 and 20 hours a day; however, they don't usually sleep longer than 5 hours at one stretch. You'll notice your baby sleeps a lot in these first weeks. Sleep gives your baby energy. She'll slip between waking and sleeping with little regard for day or night and will eat every 2 to 4 hours.

In another 6 to 8 weeks, she'll sleep longer at night and will be awake more during the day. Exposing her to daylight during the day and putting her in a dark room at night to sleep help establish this pattern. Because a newborn's nervous system is immature, she won't sleep as deeply as she will when she gets a bit older.

Your baby may hold her breath for a short time when she sleeps. This is called *periodic breathing*. It's OK if she does this occasionally and for less than 10 seconds, then resumes breathing on her own. It happens because the part of the brain that controls her breathing is not yet fully developed. Research shows that periodic breathing is *not* linked in any way with SIDS.

You may be given the advice by a relative, friend or someone else to put baby on her tummy so she'll sleep better. Don't—we know that ***"back is better."*** Put your baby to sleep on her back *every* time you put her down. Why? Research has shown that with a healthy, full-term baby, sleeping on her back lowers the chance she will have problems, especially with SIDS.

Studies also show that a normal baby doesn't usually have problems choking or aspirating vomit if she spits up while lying on her back because she has a well-developed gag reflex. Don't be tempted to put your baby to bed on her tummy.

Exceptions to the rule may be premature babies who have breathing problems, babies with certain upper-airway problems, babies with birth defects of the nose, throat or mouth, and babies with swallowing or vomiting problems. If your baby experiences any of these, discuss the situation with her doctor.

Milestones This First Week

Changes You May See This Week as Baby Develops Physically

- responds to sudden changes with entire body
- when startled, arches her back, kicks her legs and flails her arms
- can lift head
- moves head from side to side
- controls arm, leg and hand movements by reflex
- when palms are pressed, baby will open her mouth and lift her head up slightly
- sleeps and wakes on a continuum
- head flops forward or backward when in sitting position
- controls swallowing and rooting by reflex
- stroking bottom of baby's foot from heel to toes causes toes to flare up and out
- sleeps between 17 and 20 hours/day
- moves bowels often and sporadically
- feeds 7 to 8 times or more each day

Changes You May See This Week in Baby's Developing Senses and Reflexes

- blinks at bright lights
- focuses between 8 and 12 inches away
- eyes tend to turn outward
- is sensitive to direction of sound
- hands remain fisted much of time
- distinguishes volume and pitch of sounds; prefers high-toned voices
- lifts head when on stomach or at someone's shoulder
- moves head from side to side
- distinguishes tastes—likes sweet already
- will grasp and grip something if hand accidentally strikes it

Changes You May See This Week as Baby's Mind Develops

- quiets when picked up or in response to any firm, steady pressure
- stops sucking to look at something
- shuts out disturbing stimuli by going to sleep
- makes animallike sounds
- learns to expect food at certain times
- looks at person briefly

(continues)

Changes You May See This Week in Baby's Social Development

- shows excitement and distress
- seems to respond positively to soft human voice
- becomes alert to and tries to focus on human face or voice

Every baby is an individual, and your baby may do some of these things more quickly or more slowly than another baby. If you are concerned about your baby's progress, discuss it with your healthcare provider.

What Baby's Crying Can Mean

Crying is one of the ways your baby communicates with you. It's his way of telling you he's uncomfortable, hungry or needs some attention. As you get to know your baby better, you'll be able to understand what his crying means. However, it's important to understand that not every newborn cries a great deal—some don't cry much at all.

Don't worry about picking him up when he cries—you won't spoil him. You'll actually be building a stronger bond with him. You are teaching him that you will take care of him, and he will feel secure with you.

As you get to know your baby, you'll understand his crying and what it means. Crying usually falls into basic categories:

- boredom—may sound like a fake cry and stops as soon as you pick him up
- discomfort—sounds whiny, similar to boredom but doesn't stop when you pick him up
- fatigue—soft, rhythmical cry as baby attempts to soothe himself
- hunger—a short, low-pitched cry that rises and falls, and doesn't stop when you pick him up but does if you feed him
- pain—a sharp scream, followed by no breathing, then another sharp scream

As you become more experienced as a parent, you'll find ways to soothe your crying baby. You might want to try some of the techniques below to help you discover what works best with your baby. Ways to calm a crying baby include the following:

- swaddle him in a blanket
- put him in a front carrier
- put him in his stroller and walk him around the house
- sing to him
- play white noise
- go outside
- take a drive in the car
- give him a bath

It may seem like baby cries a lot, but on average, he cries only about 4 hours out of every day this first week. And that is usually only 5 minutes here and 10 minutes there. By the second week, he'll be crying only about 2½ hours a day.

If baby cries nonstop for more than 30 minutes, call his doctor. Be sure to call if his crying is accompanied by fever, vomiting, a lack of appetite or a change in his bowel movements. It could mean he is having a problem that needs to be taken care of by his doctor.

Cradle Cap

Your baby may have chunks of yellow or brown waxy material on her head—this could be *cradle cap*. Also called *seborrheic dermatitis of the scalp*, it is common in newborns and infants. It usually occurs from 1 week to 12 weeks following birth and is usually gone between 8 and 12 months. It's very common—50% of all infants get it. If your baby has cradle cap, you'll notice patches of thick scaly skin on the scalp; these may also appear in other areas of the face or at the hairline. It's not painful or itchy, but it looks cruddy.

What You Can Do at Home. You can treat the symptoms at home with mineral oil or olive oil. Dampen your baby's scalp with water before applying the mineral oil. Apply the oil to your baby's scalp to loosen the material enough so you can shampoo it off the scalp. Or rub a small amount of diluted adult dandruff shampoo into baby's scalp. Be sure to keep it out of her eyes! Rub into a lather, rinse, then brush out the flakes.

It's OK to use a soft brush to remove skin patches after rubbing with lotion. Keep the area clean and dry. Don't pick at the patches because you might irritate them or infect them.

TROUBLE SIGNS

Until baby reaches 12 weeks old, anything out of the ordinary can qualify as a possible emergency, even if you might consider them minor in an older child. That's because baby's immune system has not matured yet and cannot fight infection.

As a new parent, you may be unsure what is normal and what is not with your baby; you may not know when to call the doctor. Be alert to the following signs and symptoms, and call your baby's doctor if he:

- has difficulty feeding
- has a bruise or bump on the head
- has difficulty breathing—if he sucks his ribs in when he breathes or if his lips look blue
- vomits after most feedings, especially if vomit is brown or green, or is ejected with force (projectile vomiting)
- if you see mucus or blood in his stools or if he has diarrhea after each feeding
- doesn't have a bowel movement during the first week
- has a fever of 100.6F or higher, measured rectally
- appears yellow; it could be jaundice
- looks and/or acts differently, such as extreme lethargy or sleepiness, is highly irritable or is very pale

Call your pediatrician if your baby sleeps longer than 6 hours, is hard to wake up or skips more than three feedings. Repetitive movements in your newborn that don't stop when you hold your baby are serious. Contact your doctor immediately.

Baby's soft spot may also alert you to illness in your baby. If it remains sunken for longer than a few minutes, it may be a sign of severe dehydration, especially if accompanied by fever, vomiting and/or diarrhea. Take your baby to the hospital immediately!

Don't worry about calling the doctor—your pediatrician and his or her staff are there to help you. Your questions won't sound silly. They've probably heard any question you can think to ask many times before!

When to Call the Doctor. There should be no signs of infection on the scalp; contact the doctor if the area seems to be infected. Call the doctor if the problem lasts longer than 8 weeks. Call if the area shows signs of oozing or pus, if the cradle cap fails to respond to the measures listed above, if the skin becomes red or scaly, or if the area becomes inflamed.

If there are signs of inflammation or redness on other parts of the body, it could indicate another problem, so be sure to call your pediatrician. This form of dermatitis may be treated by your physician with a cortisone lotion.

Jaundice

Studies show that more than 50% of all newborns develop jaundice, also called *hyperbilirubinemia*. It may be up to you to detect if your baby has jaundice. Most cases of jaundice develop between 2 and 5 days after birth—your baby may be home from the hospital by then! It is most obvious by day 4.

Jaundice occurs when levels of bilirubin get too high. This can occur more often if a baby is premature, ill or at risk. Left untreated, it can cause hearing loss and even brain damage.

Phototherapy is used to treat jaundice. Baby is exposed to ultraviolet light, which changes the bilirubin into a substance that can be disposed of more easily by the body.

In the hospital, determining the level of bilirubin in your baby's blood may involve a blood test or the *Colormate TLc BiliTest*, in which a handheld device is used to measure the yellow tinge of baby's skin. The test is 95% accurate, and results are available in minutes.

Symptoms of jaundice include yellow appearance of the skin (caused by excessive amounts of bilirubin), which is often first seen in the face. The whites of the eyes (the sclera) may also appear yellow. The yellowness of the skin spreads to the rest of the body. Even the nail beds may appear yellow; pinch the fingernail gently and release to check for yellow discoloration.

Most cases of jaundice resolve on their own in the first few days as the baby's liver develops. However, a small number of cases turn into *kernicterus*; see the discussion below.

What You Can Do at Home. You can test baby at home, if you believe she might have jaundice. With your finger, press on her forehead or nose. The imprint should be pale in color for *every* baby, no matter what ethnic background. If it's not, let your pediatrician know. He or she can do a blood test for definitive results.

When to Call the Doctor. Mild jaundice is not serious; follow your doctor's advice. Bili lights, also called *phototherapy*, may be used. These ultraviolet lights break down bilirubin, making it possible for it to pass from your baby's bloodstream. It also helps improve the condition if baby is feeding well because bilirubin is excreted in her bowel movements. Call your doctor if your baby appears to be getting more yellow, or if she is not feeding well. Your pediatrician wants to know if baby experiences any problems.

Kernicterus. Kernicterus is caused by severe newborn jaundice. It is a rare but serious disease that can affect a baby soon after birth. The level of bilirubin is monitored in newborns to determine whether treatment of jaundice is needed to prevent kernicterus.

Kernicterus is an abnormal accumulation of bilirubin in the brain and other nerve tissue. It causes yellow staining of the skin and sclera (whites of the eyes) and damage to the brain. Early diagnosis and treatment of jaundice are the keys to avoiding kernicterus.

Vaginal Discharge in Girls

After birth, your baby girl may have a vaginal discharge that is clear or white. This is caused by the excessive hormones in her body from her mother. It is rarely a problem. To take care of it, gently clean the vaginal area. The discharge should soon disappear. Call your baby's doctor if the discharge seems excessive or if the color is yellow or green.

Toys and Play This 1st Week

This first week of life is the beginning of a wonderful time of games and play you will share with your child for years to come. You'll find that as you get to know your baby better, games and fun will begin to present themselves. You'll make a game out of something very ordinary, and it will be a special time for you both.

Help Stimulate His Vision

To stimulate his vision, hold bold-patterned objects within 8 to 12 inches of him, and let him look at them. At this time, he prefers bold patterns and the contrast of black and white because he can't see the nuances of color yet.

Baby will also enjoy looking at pictures of people's faces. Cut some large pictures out of a magazine to hold in front of him. Let him gaze at them as long as he is interested. When he begins to squirm or look away, it's time to end the game.

Talk and Sing to Him!

Begin your journey of play and interaction with words and music. Talk to baby as often as you can; hearing your voice is what matters. Sing to him—even if you can't carry a tune! Tell him what you're doing and what's going on. Play soothing music for him when he's fussy; it may help settle him.

Talk to your baby throughout the day and when you interact with him. One study showed that a baby needs to hear 30 *million* words by the time he is 3 years old to be prepared for maximum learning when he goes to school. So talk to him!

Index

When we use (B) following a page number, it denotes the information can be found in a box on the designated page.